PYRAMID
TRUTH
GATEWAY
UNIVERSE

THE PURPOSE, INTENT, AND OVERVIEW OF EXTRATERRESTRIAL VISITATIONS

YAHWEH'S
SCIENTIFIC EXPLANATION OF
PYRAMID POWER, EARTH TRANSITIONS,
TRADERS, TRAVELERS, AND PERSONAL GROWTH

Reg T. Miller

Pyramid Truth Gateway Universe

Copyright 1997 by Pyra Publishing

Artwork and photos by Reg T. Miller
(Exception = 10.2, page 166. Thanks Puma)
Graphic arts assistant, Fiona King
Cover assistant, Eugene Epstein

ISBN# 0-9651546-4-5

Library of Congress CCN# 97-076420

First Printing May 1998

Printed in the United States of America
Medicine Bear Publishing
P.O. 1075 Blue Hill, ME 04614

Special Acknowledgments

Yahweh
the Love Energy and Consciousness channeled by
Chuck Little

Gloria Eblacus
special support and encouragement

Steve Hays
copy editing

Jeri Little
and the helpful Yahweh students: Magdalena Antilla, Allen Barnes, Bix Blankenship, Carolyn Capps, Carol Dodge, Margorie Fox, Joe Hall, Larry Hawes, Gwen Jorgensen, MJ Lachowicz, Boni Light, Chuck McCall, Bob Richards, Lisa Smith, and Jay Wilder.

The Travelers
Semjase for her time and effort that brought us clear UFO photographs, teachings, patience, and news of humans on other worlds. And to all of the others who have come in peace to teach, heal, and study the evolving Earth humans.

The Traders
Thank you for helping life flourish here and on other planets. The aerial maneuver was greatly appreciated.

Disclaimer

This book is being published to provide information on the topics covered, and is sold with the understanding that the author is not engaged in offering professional services directly related to the subject of this book.

It is not the purpose of this manual to reprint all the information that is otherwise available to the author, but to compliment, amplify and supplement other texts. You are urged to read all of the available material, learn as much as possible about pyramidology and metaphysics, and tailor the information to your individual needs. For more information, see the reference list.

Every effort has been made to make this book as complete and as accurate as possible, however, there may still be mistakes. The road to enlightenment is always under construction. Therefore, this text should be used only as a general guide and not as the ultimate source of pyramidology or metaphysical information. In addition, this work is a dynamic one and the story continues to evolve and unfold.

The purpose of this manual is to educate, entertain and provide a tool whereby the reader can help himself. The author and the publisher shall have neither liability nor responsibility to any person or entity with respect to any loss or damage caused, or alleged to be caused, directly or indirectly by the information contained in this book.

Belief Systems

The information contained herein may contradict what you were taught in the various schools you attended, or the life experience that has formed your belief structure. Although the author presents this material as factual, there is no reason to allow your own belief system to be shaken to the point of discomfort. If that begins to happen, set the book down and wait. You may never pick it up again and that is just as valid as starting to read it again later.

Table of Contents

THE PAST

THE PRESENT

THE FUTURE

INTRODUCTION

Even though it is one of the most studied and analyzed structures in the world, the Great Pyramid remains the world's greatest unsolved mystery. Who really built the Great Pyramid, when, for what purpose, and of course, how?

Where is the evidence that proves the most-accepted theory — the standard theory? How can such an ancient structure reflect the knowledge of advanced mathematics and astronomy, when the culture that surrounds it has not demonstrated an understanding of those principles until recent times?

Here the author answers questions that have never been definitively explained. He answers questions others seldom consider, such as, how the Great Pyramid dramatically affected the daily life of those living nearby. He refutes the accepted theories by which we currently define the Great Pyramid, and even ourselves.

While admired as a marvel of the ancient past, this unduplicated monument is so much more than generally believed. It is a history of not only the beginning of man's story on Earth, it is the key to understanding his future as well.

The story of the great civilization that built it and used it as a power source, and that civilization's rapid decline, very possibly mirror our fate. Understanding how that happened and the nature of that civilization reveal our common roots.

The author has worked in applied science for the Department of Defense, Aerospace, and many other private enterprises. In 1987 he visited the Great Pyramid and experienced its residual energy vibrate the very core of his being. Since then he has devoted his knowledge to unraveling the secret of the Great Pyramid. To understand the phenomena he draws on the information of the channel Yahweh, also known as The Storyteller, to present the history of our planet. The Earth chronicles begin on other planets and involve other beings, The Traders, who have the ability to move quickly among the stars.

A misunderstood group, these Traders and their companions, the Travelers, have played no small role in our history. What was that role? Why were they involved? What are their present intentions? What is the link between us, the Traders, the Book of Revelations, and the asteroid Nemesis, the still-orbiting destroyer?

Arguably, the most important part of this work is how the energy that powered the Great Pyramid is still available to us today. Some understand that and use it now. The nature of this energy and how to draw it out in a balanced manner is told here. Ultimately, it is available to each of us as we learn to recognize it within ourselves.

Not only will understanding this energy reveal our own individual path to a fulfilling life, whether or not we develop it will determine our individual and collective futures. How well we do, in fact, will influence how long humans will live on Earth, whether or not he will ever be able to leave the planet and join the Traders and other Travelers, and in time, even determine the future of the planet Earth itself.

Those stories, our true history and legacy, won't fit everyone's religious history, but it doesn't necessarily contradict them either. This work is both profoundly spiritual as well as scientific. Some may be disturbed at our turbulent history and what lies ahead. All avatars, however, have taught the same essential truth. The seed for properly writing the upcoming final chapter (how it all turns out) lies within these pages.

For some, this book will contain too much supporting data, but the book was written for skeptics, and much care was taken to ease them from what is commonly known into the region of the unknown. For the most part, the reader will find this the greatest adventure story of them all — it's our story. It would be difficult to read this book and not view human beings and the universe from a new perspective afterwards. I found myself thinking, "that's why," and "of course!" It simply fits. It feels like it's familiar, like returning home, but gives a brand new appreciation and understanding of the rich heritage of our Earth home, our universe, and the challenges ahead of us.

Steve J. Hays
publisher of The Light Connection
June 1997, Vista, California

AN EARTH CHRONICLE

Based on information from Yahweh, The Storyteller

In the distant past, farther back than most dare to imagine, long before the supposed "Stone Age" humans of 20,000 years ago, and more precisely at the time of the Neanderthal, the total population of *Homo erectus* types was 600 million worldwide. These types were the true Earthmen, but they shared the planet with a more advanced version of themselves. The Earthmen, for the most part, ate roots and hunted for meat. Today they would appear to be primitive and truly of the Stone Age, but they had rational minds, lived in societies, and shared stories around the campfire. Some of what they observed during their hunting expeditions shaped their belief systems and their religious practices.

Occasionally it went like this: The buzzing of insects, the cry of the birds, and the other natural sounds of the forest were disturbed by an unearthly vibration. The whirring and swishing sounds were so unusual that they demanded investigation. With a sense of apprehension, the expert hunters, in stealth mode, slowly and cautiously crept closer to the unusual sound. Finally, the last leafy branch was swung aside just enough to provide the view of a lifetime.

There, in the clearing, not more than 150 feet from them, they saw first-hand what had only been rumors. A large green-platinum pedestal glowing brightly, hummed softly, and actually hovered above the ground. Suddenly, a doorway formed itself and in a moment, a being appeared silhouetted in the blazing light of the interior. The being was much like them only strangely clothed, oddly long-legged, tall, and too thin to be very strong. Frozen in awe, they watched the beings emerge, one after another. The beings went about their business with an amazing lack of concern about the close presence of the dangerous hunting group. They moved about in magical ways, hovered in mid-air, and effortlessly raised themselves to the top of the pedestal and down again. Over time, many such sightings revealed that they could make food appear for themselves without the long hunt, and they could even wink out and appear in the blink of an eye a vast distance away, requiring the hunters to walk many hours to catch up.

The hunters now knew that the stories and myths told to them as children were true. They had witnessed the great ones first-hand and excitedly they made their way back to their village. Enthusiastically, the legends would be reinforced again that night. The story telling from father to son continued and formed the basis of their mysticism in language and words that were understandable to those of the Neanderthal hunting culture. The *Homo erectus's* rational minds could only conclude that what was observed was a first-hand witnessing of the gods. Examples of these god beings is evident from the art of the hunting cultures.

The Neanderthals were unaware that ten-thousand advanced humans arrived to share the planet in the year 50,000 B.C. Through a soul connection — not his present physical body — the author was one of them. The journey to this planet would not have been possible without the benevolent efforts of a group of aliens known as the Traders, who supplied not only the means to get here, but also the technology and energy to build a new civilization. These small humanoids with large head, large eyes, and hands with only four fingers are still around, and are continually monitoring our progress. Because they keep to themselves and do the whole process with such extreme stealth, most of us know nothing about them.

One of the first items we needed was a power source, so the Great Pyramid at the Giza Plateau near Cairo, Egypt was constructed. The top third was surfaced with a gold alloy that sparkled in the sunlight. The apex blazed with a perpetual plasma ball by night because the Great Pyramid was a microwave power source that powered the entire civilization, including the floating discs that moved us everywhere we wanted to go. This sustainable life style went on for 3,000 years until a global cataclysm brought it all to an end.

The complete history of the Great Pyramid Society was chiseled into the limestone casing-blocks just beneath the gold cap. It began with our names, the builders of the monument and fathers of a new civilization upon this, our new planet. The historical events of importance that followed continued to be recorded in this cuneiform fashion, so the complete work could be read as one spiraled from the top towards the bottom. Unfortunately, this history was completely destroyed when the limestone blocks were removed 13-hundred years ago to rebuild Cairo after a devastating earthquake. Consequently, the Great Pyramid, who built it, how, when, and why, has become an enigma.

Through the millennium, we the originators, have lived many incarnations in and around the Great Pyramid. Because of the special transition that the planet is now going through, many of us have returned to help disseminate the teaching originally given to the Earth-human for harmonious behavior. This particular transition is an extreme one that will largely determine the fate of Earth-humanity. These teachings can be taught in a great variety of ways, and the challenge here is to show that the monument was many things to the Great Pyramid Civilization: Not only a power generator, but a library of knowledge and a healing center. Above all, it was and still is the "Sermon in Stone." Simply put, the purpose of this book is to show how to live from moment to moment in **balance**.

It is a teaching of self-imposed responsibility, a doctrine of absolutely no absolutes. Living each event in balance is essential to being able to ride out the extreme events of the Transition that are rushing into the present. These are the techniques to live a life of joy and excitement.

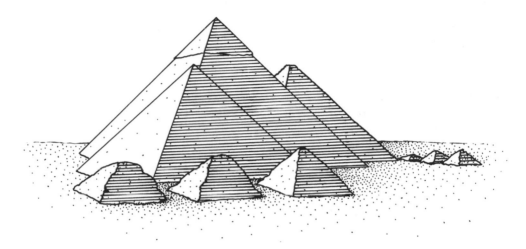

Figure Int.1 Which pyramid is considered the Great Pyramid? From this vantage point of the pyramids at Giza, the tallest might well be considered to be Greatest, but that is an error of perspective. The pyramid furthest from the artist is the most voluminous and is the Great Pyramid. There are many reasons, besides sheer volume, that earns this monument the title **Great**. This can only be understood by a careful study and comparison of the outer and internal features of all the pyramids. This book will guide you in that pursuit.

PREFACE

Existing metaphysical works lack the detailed subatomic foundation to convince a scientifically trained student that a connection to the spiritual realm actually exists. As a result the polarity between the religious and the scientific communities increases. This work attempts to bridge that gap. New information is given that shows that both sides are partly right. The arguments cease here.

BOOK OUTLINE

The Master Sections

The story of the Great Pyramid has been divided into **THE PAST, THE PRESENT,** and **THE FUTURE**.

THE PAST

Chapters One through Twelve detail events of the past, and are divided into the standard theory and the new theory. The currently accepted history credits the Egyptian civilization of approximately 5,000 years ago as being the builders of the pyramids. The revolutionary idea presented here argues that the original pyramid the Great Pyramid, was built by an even more ancient civilization, called the Great Pyramid Society. Other civilizations in between it and the Pharaonic Egyptian civilizations have erroneously been accepted as the first.

The Chapters

Chapter 1 through 5

These chapters show in detail that the units of weights, measures, and time as used on this planet are globally accepted. In stark contrast, no language, religion, or song is. These units and the Great Pyramid are Earth commensurate, that is, related to the size and rotation of the earth. This is true of one pyramid alone, the Great Pyramid, and that was part of the clue encoded in its shape so that descendants could discover who built it, when, and where they came from. The great interrelated nature of these units suggest that a computer or some advanced method beyond the papyrus and reed pen technique of Pharaonic Egypt were used to establish them.

Chapter 6 and 7

With the realization that the builders of the Great Pyramid knew the exact size of the Earth, the standard theory attempts to credit this knowledge as having originated with the Egyptians. By examining the techniques that were available to them, however, it becomes apparent that the precision needed to determine the measurements could not be achieved by anything less than an orbiting, artificial satellite, something that our modern civilization has achieved only recently. The standard theory leaves much unexplained and provides many contradictions about the design and shape of the Great Pyramid. These are discussed in fine detail. The open minded will strongly question many long accepted theories about the Great Pyramid, especially that its sole function was to be a tomb for a Pharaoh.

1

Chapter 8 and 9

These chapters examine the specific technology of the solid-state power converter, the Great Pyramid. It becomes obvious why the truth has escaped researchers for so long: Too many pieces are missing. Consider this analogy. Imagine that an engine block is abandoned because it has an unrepairable crack in it, and that all the pieces attached to the block are removed to be used on another engine. Then the technical society that produced the engine suddenly disappears because of a combination of active volcanoes, bad weather, and famine. Few would survive.

In time a new society would begin to explore that region and find the metal block with holes in it. They couldn't fathom what it was, because heat engines were not part of their civilization. They relied on horses and wind-driven ships. The weight and size of the object, however, were sufficient as an anchor for a fairly large vessel. The line was easily attached because of the existing piston cylinders. That there were more holes than were needed didn't matter, they had a new anchor. In a similar manner, the burial of Khufu in the Great Pyramid has obscured the correct understanding of the many overly-precise features of an object that originally was a power source.

Chapters 10 through 12

History buffs will appreciate learning how aliens interacted with our species from the very beginning of our evolution, and still do. These chapters describe how, left on our own, we often resort to war, and become our own worst enemy. The root of this human problem and how to correct it are also contained in these chapters. Explained are the days of Pharaonic Egypt, the use of the Great Pyramid with its many chambers, and how one of them was used as Khufu's tomb, a secondary use similar to converting an engine block to an anchor. The propensity of later Egyptian civilizations to copy the grand style of the more advanced earlier society has left it nearly impossible to define the civilizations that came before. Imagine you were the researcher who discovered the engine block tied with an anchor line to a sunken vessel of Norse origin. You would conclude on the face of it, that the ones who built the boat, had also built the anchor. Time has buried the mystery of the Great Pyramid for too long. The answers are there if you know where to look. By uncovering the truth of this ancient civilization, we discover our connection to them.

THE PRESENT

Chapter 13

The thirteenth chapter represents the most recent events, including the present transition that we are experiencing every day. Rapid changes will intensify, and good health is the best insurance to joyfully experience the coming roller coaster ride. Unlike the Great Pyramid society, which used clean energy and sustainable technological practices, our society has often taken short cuts at the expense of the environment. The toxic by-products and residue of our technology means that a large portion of the population has acquired maladies, some related to immune deficiencies. Don't be passive and leave your state of health up to doctors to "fix." Take responsible steps to insure your optimum health. If you are desiring positive changes to your health, you may want to start here.

THE FUTURE

Chapter 14

Chapter Fourteen summarizes coming events, including the passing of a huge comet that might tear off part of the Earth's atmosphere, or at least trigger massive earthquakes and volcanoes. It could cause such chaos that the benevolent aliens might finally appear in mass to observe or even to intercede. In worst case scenarios, they often save part of the species so that extinction does not occur. Divulged are interesting facts with regard to the so-called abduction experiences and why they occur repeatedly to a minority of the population. Also covered is how to travel with the aliens. If you have fears of the aliens, the coming comet, or the unknown in general, this chapter will be of great help.

THE PAST

Chapter One

Synopsis

Long ago, someone decided the basis for the unit of time to be one rotation of the planet. This, of course, is one day. Despite the fact that we have ten fingers, ten toes, ten dimes to a dollar, and ten pennies to a dime, the smaller units of the day — the hour, minute, and second — are related to the day by the factor 12. Why there are 12 hours in the day, 12 hours to the night, 12 x 5 minutes to the hour, and 12 x 5 seconds to the minute, is a puzzle. Isn't it curious that the different cultures around the globe developed different alphabets, languages, and measurements, but when it came to time, all cultures agreed? Why? The key to unraveling this mystery is the Great Pyramid.

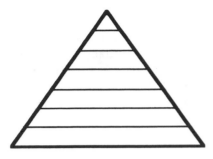

Chapter One

TIME

The Origin of the Units of Time

The Egyptians did use copper tools, papyrus rope, and other primitive techniques to build pyramids, but they built just about everything except the Great Pyramid. To realize the truth of this, one must look at the subtle details most often overlooked. With a little effort and study, the gateway to the universe will be opened.

Time flies or time drags depending upon what we are doing, but we know intellectually there is a mechanical time that is not concerned with our emotional swings, and it beats a steady rhythm in tune with the celestial orbs. The Earth revolves quite regularly about its own axis and makes about 365 such revolutions in one complete orbit of the Sun. This periodic motion is the basis of our mechanical time.

Day and night periods have always been subdivided into twelve hours each, yielding a total of twenty-four hours for one complete revolution of the planet. Since the dawn of the Industrial Revolution and the need to show up at a factory to work for a prescribed amount of hours, the use of mechanical clocks has pervaded society. We now take them, and the units of time, very much for granted. It's as if they have always been with us, and one of the first things we learn are those units of time: 24 hours in a day, 60 minutes in an hour, and 60 seconds in a minute. This, however, yields a strange number: 24 x 60 x 60 = 86,400 seconds in one complete day.

This system of measuring time is completely arbitrary. There are an infinite number of ways to divide the day, so why not use 50,000 seconds per day, 80,000 seconds per day, or better yet, 100,000 seconds per day? The value 100,000 is the base ten multiplied by itself five times. It is quite common in our society to use the base ten: ten pennies make a dime, ten dimes make a dollar, and 100,000 pennies makes a thousand dollar bill. In step with this system, wouldn't it be better to adopt a time scheme with ten hours in a day, 100 minutes in each hour, 100 seconds in each minute, and thus: 10 x 100 x 100 = 100,000 seconds per day?

Sporting events in which contestants win by 1/100 of a second, prove that the second, as it is currently defined, is too large a unit, so perhaps 1,000,000 seconds per day would be the ideal. Industrial and scientific uses would benefit with a newly defined second. The 1,000,000 second-per-day system would also be neat and tidy — 100 hours per day, 100 minutes per hour, and 100 seconds per minute — and easy to remember.

Another thing to puzzle over is the entirely arbitrary method of dividing the hour into two subdivisions: minutes and seconds. Why aren't there three subdivisions? Besides minutes and seconds one could also have "subhours." In this scheme, hours would have three subdivisions and twelve subhours to the hour, 30 minutes to the sub-hour, and only ten seconds to the newly defined "minute." In this new scheme with three subdivisions there would still be 24 x 12 x 30 x 10 = 86,400 seconds in a day. So even if our research reveals that 86,400 seconds is required in each day, this in itself does not preclude there being three subdivisions to the hour. In other words, why are there three subdivisions to a day: hours, minutes, and seconds? Why not four, as in the above example, or even five, or six?

It is interesting to ponder why, with an infinite number of possibilities to measure time, there is one scheme that is accepted worldwide. Isn't it a wonder that everyone on earth accepts this unusual division, and yet there is no worldwide agreement about which language to speak? There is no universally accepted alphabet to write the written word. There is no song that everyone agrees is most melodious. There is no one color that is considered the ideal hue.

On the contrary, there is diversity in everything, except with time. The contrived division of the day is our only common scheme — it seems to defy the odds. The things that everyone agrees upon are only commonly observed things given to us by nature. For example: the sun will rise in the east and set in the west. There are 365 days in one year. Summers are hot and winters are cold. Fish live in the water. Creatures with wings can fly in the air. Lions eat meat and cows eat grass.

The importance of this is that it must have been invented by someone at some point in history. Who is the genius of that time who invented this division that we all have come to accept: 86,400 seconds per day?

A public television presentation on the evolution of clocks showed that before the industrial revolution, some industrious monks wanted to chant a favorite prayer at a certain time each day and so they invented a workable clock. It had wooden wheels with wooden pegs for gears. Water poured into a bucket for weight unwinding the wooden shaft connecting wheels with protruding spokes that were the gears for the device. This wooden clock, employing the properties of a pendulum into the design, unwound at a consistent rate. The device was reportedly the earliest recorded example of a mechanical clock. Certainly these monks have to be given credit for the mechanical invention, but did they invent time? A device that existed centuries earlier, the sun dial, already had twelve divisions for the day. One wonders where they got the idea.

In researching this book, many knowledgeable people, including college students engineers, mathematicians, and professors, were questioned about the divisions of time.

Amazingly not one had ever thought about these distinctions. What may appear to be trivia, however, turns out to be an important clue in uncovering the truth of the Great Pyramid. Who, when, and why were the units of time invented? Why was it so perfect that it was accepted worldwide?

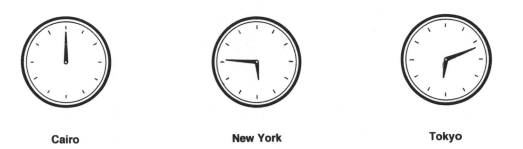

Cairo   **New York**   **Tokyo**

Figure 1.1 Why is time calculated in the same manner worldwide? Who invented it? When?

Chapter Two

Synopsis

The basis for the standard angle was long ago decided to be the division of a circle. Despite the obvious method — using the base ten — the base twelve was used. There are 12 x 30 degrees in one complete circle. The smaller units — minutes and seconds — are the same as the units of time. There are 12 x 5 minutes in one degree, and 12 x 5 seconds in one minute. The key to unraveling this mystery is the Great Pyramid.

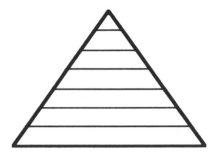

Chapter Two

ANGLES

The Origin of the Standard Angle

The units used to measure common angles are accepted without question, and their universal acceptance is similar to that of time. This is apparent after considering several common angles. The most familiar is the "right angle," which is defined as radii intersecting to form a quarter of a circle, and thus the lines are mutually perpendicular.

Carpenters use this right angle to position two pieces on a perpendicular line or to mark a line on a board to make a "square" cut. The carpenter's tool looks like a large "L" which has a right angle designed into it, and since a circle is defined as having 360 degrees, the right angle has one quarter of 360 degress, or 90 degrees. (See Figure 2.1.)

The next most familiar angle is the 45 degree angle, and two such angles are found in the 45 degree triangle used by draftsmen. The 45 degree angles are found in opposite corners as shown in the diagram below and each 45 degree angle is exactly one-half of a right angle. Note that the 45 degree triangle has equal legs. It typically is used to mark the miter lines used in picture frames or in door frames. (See Figure 2.2.)

Other common angles are found in another standard draftsman triangle known as the 30-60-90 degree triangle, which has a 30 degree angle in one corner, a 60 degree angle in another corner, and a 90 degree angle in the remaining corner. The 30 degree angle is exactly 1/3 of the right angle, and the 60 degree angle is exactly twice the 30 degree angle, or 2/3 of the 90 degree angle. The 30-60-90 triangle is noteworthy in that the hypotenuse, which is the side opposite the 90 degree angle, is always twice the shortest leg, the side opposite the 30 degree angle. (See Figure 2.3.)

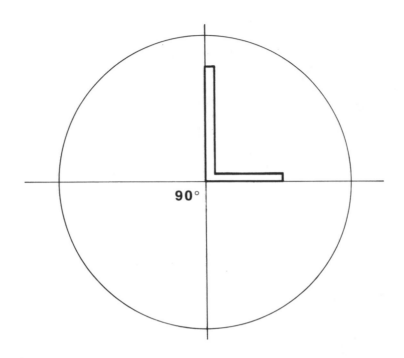

Figure 2.1 The carpenter's right triangle, square, or L-angle, is defined by the quarter of a circle formed by the intersection of two perpendicular radii.

A basic geometry tool that is introduced to children is the "protractor." This device enables one to draw any angle from 1 to 180 degrees, and even half degrees if care is taken. This is possible because of its shape as a half circle and the small graduations printed on it. The protractor is the basic tool for drawing and is based on the universally accepted fact that there are 360 degrees in a complete circle, or one revolution. We learn as children to become familiar with the degrees, the basic angles, the common drafting triangles, and for most of us it becomes part of our general knowledge. We use it, it works, and we never think twice about it.

It is interesting to look at the basic assumption of the system. Is the right triangle really right, that is, why is it accepted that there are 90 degrees in one quarter of a circle, or 360 degrees in one complete revolution? Just as there are many possible divisions of the day, the division of one revolution of angular measurement can be defined in an infinite number of ways. For example, a system based on multiples of 10 would result in one revolution having 100 degrees, or 1,000 degrees — even 1,000,000 degrees. Thus the quarter revolution or right triangle would contain 25 degrees, or 250 degrees, on up to 250,000 degrees. This would be an entirely logical scheme and match our money system since 1/4 of a dollar is a "quarter" and equal to 25 pennies.

Another useful system might be 400 degrees in one revolution so that a quarter revolution, a right triangle, would contain an even 100 degrees. Since carpenters are usually dealing with right angles this 100 degrees-per-quarter version might prove easy to divide when in the field.

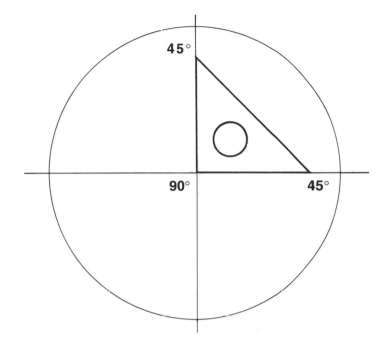

Figure 2.2 The 45-degree triangle is typically used as the common miter angle for frames. It is one half of a right angle and has equal legs.

Contrasting this with theoretical systems no longer in use, there was an alternate system used by the navigators of sailing vessels hundreds of years ago with 256 divisions in one revolution. The reason it was adopted over the standard 360 degree version was because of the use of the divider tool which divided an angle on navigation maps in two equal parts. The new line that divided the original angle was called the bisector. Note how it worked. With the divider, which usually has a metal point on one leg and a pencil point on the other, place the point on the apex of the angle and sweep a quarter circle. Then lift the tool and place the point where that circle crosses the legs of the right angle. Draw two arcs and where they intersect, that point and the original apex of the right angle defines the bisector. In this case each angle will be 45 degrees. (See Figure 2.5.)

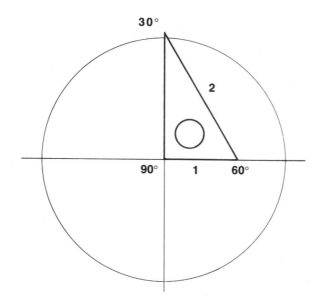

Figure 2.3 The 30-60-90 degree triangle has a small 30 degree angle which is exactly 1/3 of the right angle, a 60 degree angle which is 2/3 of the right-angle, and a hypotenuse leg which is always twice as long as the short leg.

The 45 degree angle can be divided by the same process, yielding 22 1/2 degrees on each side of the bisector. The method is continued and the next angles obtained by this practical graphical technique are: 11.25 degrees, 5.625 degrees, 2.8125 degrees, 1.40625 degrees. At this point the divisions are increasingly difficult to obtain by graphics, but with dead reckoning and angles of 1.40625 degrees, there is sufficient plotting definition on navigation maps to get anywhere in the world. As a result, the compass rose that gained popularity with navigators that is divided into at least 32 segments, called points. A point is defined as one 11.25 degree division. Sometimes more divisions are shown and in some cases up to 256 segments are represented.

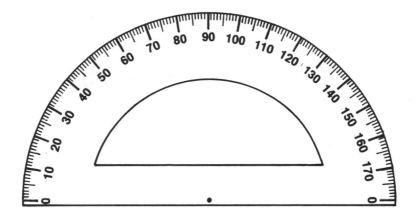

Figure 2.4 The protractor is a graduated arc that defines 180 degrees to a semicircle. It is a basic instrument for laying down and measuring odd angles that are needed for drawing and plotting.

Another unique system that differs from the standard division, and in use in one branch of physics, is known as the radian system. This alternate system takes the radius of a circle and measures that radial length along the arc of the same circle. The angle subtended by the arc is defined as the radian. Mathematically, this yields the fact that in one revolution there are exactly 2π radians whose numeric value is 6.263185307... (an endless number). Although this appears to be unwieldy, the reason this system is preferred is that the mathematical equations that describe that branch of physics would be very cumbersome to solve otherwise. That is because the value π in these equations appear in the numerator and the denominator and most often cancel out. However, one could spend a lifetime in the applied sciences and never once have to use this system, which remains a useful tool for those involved with theoretical studies.

Obviously it is easy to invent alternate schemes, and a few actually are in use, but the standard is that one revolution contains 360 degrees. This system is used on a world-wide basis in the applied science of manufacturing, all household appliances, cars, boats, airplanes, and even our space vehicles.

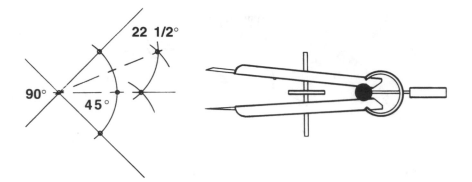

Figure 2.5 The divider tool, used extensively in navigation, can graphically locate the bisector of any angle, thus dividing the angle in two equal parts. The process can continue, eventually dividing a whole circle into as many as 256 divisions.

Another unquestioned standard is why the degree is always divided by 60 minutes, and why those minutes are divided by 60 seconds. In the radian system just discussed there is only a decimal subdivision for the radian: 1/4 of one radian is 0.25 radians and 1/3600 of a radian is 0.000277777 radians and so on. By contrast, in the standard degree system: 1/4 of a degree is 15 minutes and 1/3600 of a degree is 1 second. Once again we note that there are two subdivisions for the degree, minutes and seconds. It is surprising that there are only two subsets and not 1, 3, 4, or 5. Of all the names that could be given to these subsets, of all the divisions that could be designed into the subsets, it is the same minutes and seconds normally associated with time. (See Chapter 1.) The radian method, designed for theoretical physics, is not in any way connected to time. Why would the designer of degrees choose 360 for one revolution and then use the same number of subsets, two, and assign to them the same identity, the same name as for the subdivisions of the time scheme? Is there an implied relation between the two? Are angles in some way related to time? Who was the inventor of these universally accepted units of geometry?

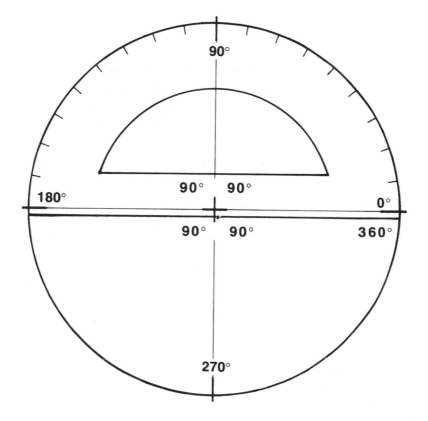

Figure 2.6 Who determined that a circle (one revolution) contains 360 degrees; one degree, 60 minutes; and one minute, 60 seconds? When did this system begin? Why?

Chapter Three

Synopsis

The basis for the unit of length was long ago decided to be the foot. The obvious question is whose foot? Also, why are there twelve inches per foot, and not ten? The answer to this mystery is revealed in a study of the Great Pyramid

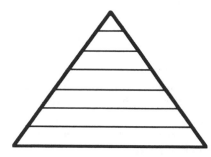

Chapter Three

HEIGHT, WIDTH, DEPTH

The Origin of the Standard Foot

At some moment in history humans had to invent how to measure the height, width, and depth of his environment. Perhaps not long after man first began to use language, the concept of distance was agreed upon by necessity. It would be very useful, for example, to point in a particular direction and communicate how many steps it was to the water source. What primitive man understood about these concepts is speculation, however, the evidence suggests that by the time of ancient Egypt, at least, very definite units had been established. The cubit, the foot, the palm, and the finger were all well established. Understandably, for this agrarian society, all units were conveniently based upon the human anatomy. Thus from a practical point of view they could never get lost.

Obviously for bipedal humans, it was a "basic step" to create the most basic unit of distance in relation to the human gait. The finer definition of the step would naturally follow and be the short step, made by placing the heel of the lead foot adjacent to and touching the toe of the trailing foot. This unit, of course, is the foot and there are normally three feet to one long step.

For measuring things at table height or waist height, the basic unit is the arm or the "cubit." This unit of length is basically the distance from the elbow to the tip of the middle finger. Although in ancient Egypt there came to be a "royal" cubit used for special purposes and of a different length than the "common" cubit, it is this common cubit that is equal to one and one-half feet. Thus, two cubits equals three feet, which also equals one step.

The cubit and the foot are further divided by the palm and by the finger. There are two types of palms. There is the foot composed of four palms and the foot composed of three palms. Probably it is the latter definition that is the common palm, measured at the widest part of the hand where the fingers are almost exactly one inch thick. The British system apparently has inherited from this system, as there are twelve inches or "fingers" to the foot.

Of all of these units the foot is obviously the basic unit, and even though everyone easily understands his own foot, a "standard" foot would eventually need to be defined. Given human differences there are far ranging opinions over the ideal standard foot. Somewhere in history there must have been some powerful leader who stepped in to define the standard, and quite possibly it was the length of his own foot. So in each country there must have been a definite historical event in which the length of the "official" foot was scribed onto a stone stele or recorded in some other way.

Such decisions would have been basic even in an agrarian society, since otherwise accurate trading would have been impossible. That is because volume and weight are related to an official foot. Units of volume are obtained by cubing units of length. Units of weight are obtained by filling the units of volume with rainwater at ordinary temperature. Thus the weight of gold or silver can be related to a unit of volume of water, thereby establishing an international measure for fair and accurate trade.

In modern times units of space and time are related to radioactive decay and to properties of the atom. Units of time are defined by a specific number of decay particles emitted by a unit volume of a cesium isotope, and length is defined by a specific number of wavelengths of krypton 86 in a vacuum. Assuming that these atomic relationships remain unchanged in the various gravity fields of the universe, this modern definition, based on atomic physics, may very well prove to be globally and even intergalactically stable as well.

This atomic physics definition was predated by many interesting macro definitions of the foot. For example, the development of the official British foot, which historically was the length of 36 grains of barley placed end to end. The 36 grains were taken from the middle ear for better accuracy, but undoubtedly during drought conditions such a practice would yield a slightly shorter foot. The officials of course always understood the wisdom of having an official standard somewhere that could be referred to as needed, so one yard was defined as a three-foot length. This unit is scribed onto a material with a low coefficient of expansion and is kept at Whitehall in England.

After the French Revolution great changes were the norm and the official unit of length in France became the meter, defined to be earth commensurate and specifically the 1/10,000,000 distance from the equator to the pole, as measured along the surface of the earth. The French have had this new scientific standard of measure scribed onto a metal bar that is placed in a vault at constant temperature, humidity, and barometric pressure, and kept by the French version of the bureau of standards in France. The true earth commensurate meter, as we now know it as measured by satellite technology, would be slightly longer. The relation of the French meter to the English foot of twleve inches yields 39.37007874 inches to one meter. This may seem cumbersome, but reduces handily to 2.540 centimeters = one inch (one hundred centimeters = one meter). This relationship is the memorized conversion factor known by engineers of the modern world. Although it would be possible to invent new units of height, width and depth, these two systems, in use for centuries, are here for good. The cost of converting tons of blue prints to any new system would be astronomical and in all probability will never be done, so practically speaking, both systems belong to our modern society.

A survey of the ancient world reveals that in ancient Egypt, ancient Greece, and ancient Rome, different foot standards existed that varied from the official British foot of today. In the ancient world the official foot was not only scribed upon a stone, but was also enshrined in either a temple or a coliseum. The length and width of a courtyard was designed to be a precise, even number of feet, for example 100 feet wide and 300 feet long. Thus anyone visiting these public courtyards could step them off and thereby determine his own correction factor for the purpose of doing accurate trade.

Has the foot always been a variable or was there ever one ideal standard foot in use by some long-vanished proto society, perhaps from the precursor to the ancient worlds of Rome, Greece and Egypt? Or was Egypt the cradle of the original foot standard? With this in mind and with the knowledge that the foot may be enshrined in a temple, coliseum, or pyramid, consider what table of measure secrets are found in Egypt.

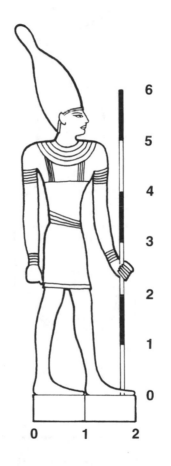

Figure 3.1 Was there a standard foot defined in prehistoric times? Was it the precursor to the standard foot used by later civilizations?

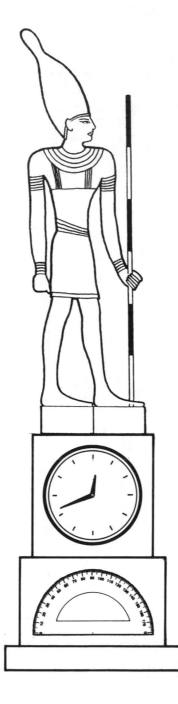

Figure 3.2 Is there a coliseum or monument that embodies all the units of measure —
time, angles, and the standard foot?

Chapter Four

Synopsis

If the base perimeter of the Great Pyramid is defined as three thousand feet, this is nearly three thousand British feet. One Great Pyramid foot (G.P. ft) = 1.00756 British feet, an error of less than one percent. The value pi (π) is defined as twice the height divided into the base perimeter. The value phi is 1/2 the base divided by the apothem (slope length at the major section). If the base perimeter of the Great Pyramid is set along the equator, it equals the exact angular rotation of the Earth every two seconds. It is also one-half minute of meridian-arc length. There are many more of these relationships. Obviously the size and shape of the Great Pyramid define important mathematical relationships and they relate to the exact size of the Earth!

Chapter Four

DIMENSIONS OF THE GREAT PYRAMID

The Earth Commensurate Monument

The psychological impression of being next to the Great Pyramid is difficult to convey. With one hand on a five-foot tall and twelve-foot wide corner block, one can view these huge stones, one after another, until they fade into mere specks due to the extreme length of the base and the law of perspective. Likewise, by looking upward, the definition between courses blurs near the top, and on some days the apex itself is at sufficient altitude to part the clouds. The awe-inspiring experience boggles the mind because unlike a skyscraper, which is mostly hollow, the Great Pyramid is nearly 100% solid masonry made up of massive, individually quarried blocks. It is hard to imagine a gang of men cutting, transporting, and sliding even one block into such precise positions, yet the Great Pyramid is constructed of almost three million of these colossal pieces.

To get a grasp of the size of the Great Pyramid, it is natural for a researcher to walk around it and to step it off. If one were to count the steps of just one side, the number would depend on the individual, and be between 240 to 260 steps. Since the monument has four such sides, that yields about 960 to 1040 steps to the complete perimeter. These values are very close to 1000 steps, which leads to the speculation, could the designers have intended exactly 1000 steps for the base perimeter? Since one step is three feet, it would yield 3000 feet to the entire base length.

Greek and Roman temples were often designed with court yards of even multiples of the official foot, thus enshrining the value for merchants desiring accurate trade. Suppose the designers purposefully created a perimeter to be exactly 3000 official feet. Then, just like Roman and Greek temples, it would serve many functions, one of which being a sort of bureau of standards.

If the Great Pyramid geometry did serve as a standardization of measurement, then what would the height represent? Unfortunately, the peak, many of the upper courses, and most of the fine limestone outer casing blocks were dismantled to rebuild Cairo after the devastating Earthquake around 840 A.D. With the apex missing, the height of the Great Pyramid must be calculated by trigonometric means using remaining clues about the slope angle. Besides the slope outline of the core masonry and several casing stones at the base, there are many chips and pieces of damaged casing stones that have been saved in museums. The slope of the Great Pyramid has been estimated from these various sources by several investigators (Reference 5). The reported values range from 51 degrees 49 minutes to 51 degrees 52 minutes 15.5 seconds. Smyth used an "averaging" technique and came up with 51 degrees 51 minutes 14.3 seconds, as his best average.

Using Smyth's value, the height and the apothem length can be calculated. The height is 477.4648 Great Pyramid feet. (See Figure 4.2.) The apothem length is the length from the mid-point of the base to the apex, known to designers as the main section line of the Great Pyramid, and it calculates to be 607.1218... (indicates an endless irrational number) in units of Great Pyramid feet.

These values are not the even numbers that one would expect, and in fact these strange, irrational numbers confused researchers for some time. Eventually, however, John Taylor, a 19th century amateur astronomer and mathematician, concluded that the designers intended the height and perimeter (P) of the base to relate exactly as the radius and circumference of a circle: P/2H (of the Great Pyramid) = π = C/2R (of a similar circle).

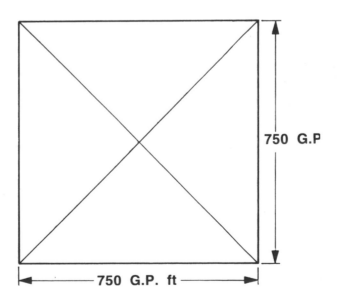

Figure 4.1 Base length = 750 Great Pyramid feet. Perimeter length = 4 x 750 = 3000 Great Pyramid feet.

The value of π is one of the unique or "magic" numbers in the universe, and is the value defined by the circumference of any circle divided by its diameter (or twice its radius), and it always equals 3.141592654.... It has been hypothesized that this number could be the basic "hello" for mathematicians anywhere in the universe, because it is a fact of the geometry of nature, of three-dimensional reality, and would be universally recognized by anyone who lives in three-dimensional reality and considers its mathematical relationships. It has been suggested by scientists that with a few equations and unique universal numbers, the value of π among them, the language barrier that would exist between races of distant worlds could be deciphered. For that reason this value has been included on a gold plate attached to the Voyager space craft, which is expected to leave our solar system and perhaps be found by an alien intelligence in the future. Thus, our society actually has left a little message about ourselves to be deciphered by some future discoverer even though the prospects of anyone ever finding and decoding it are extremely remote. Could a message of similar intent already exist on this planet, could it be encoded into the geometry of the Great Pyramid, and can it now be deciphered?

Discovering the value π within the geometry of the Great Pyramid is a significant discovery. There is no question that the value of π was deliberate. Of the more than 75 large and small pyramids in Egypt, no other pyramid has a slope of 51 degrees 51 minutes 14.3 seconds. A few are close to 52 degrees, but the major angle, the apothem angle, of most pyramids ranges from 43 degrees to 75 degrees. (See Reference 1.)

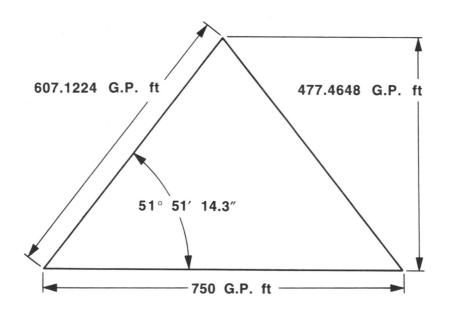

Figure 4.2 Section view of the Great Pyramid relating the base, height, apothem length, and major angle.

A logical extrapolation of the clue that π has been intentionally designed into the Great Pyramid could be drawn if the following were considered. Since π is derived from the diameter and circumference of a circle, and since a circle is derived by slicing the Earth at the equator, the resulting hemisphere has a specific mathematical π-link to the Great Pyramid. To see this clearly, expand the pyramids of Egypt until they have a base perimeter equal to the circumference of the Earth. Only the Great Pyramid has its apex touching the North Pole. That link suggests that perhaps the Great Pyramid is intended to be Earth commensurate.

Do the units that are defined by the monument also apply to known facts about the size of the Earth itself? There is a clue to this effect given to us from the period 500 to 400 B.C. by several of the Greek scholars and historians (Pythagoras, Siculus, Strabo, and Agathurchides. These scholars had written that the apothem length of the Great Pyramid is 1/600 of one degree arc length, and that the base length of the Great Pyramid is 1/8 of one minute arc length. (See Reference 5.)

It would seem improbable that an agrarian society like the Egyptians would know much about the exact dimensions of the planet, but for us, with facts from satellites compiled neatly in almanacs, it is easy to test this idea. If the standard division for one revolution, 360 degrees, is used and if the standard subdivision, 60 minutes in one degree, is used, then a simple calculation should yield the circumference of the planet.

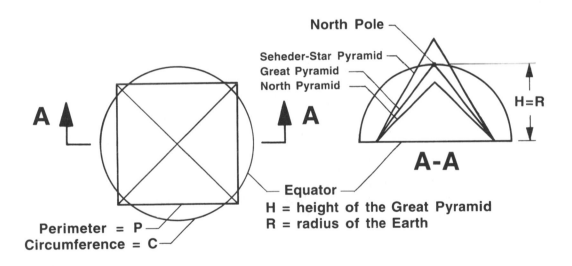

Figure 4.3 Depicted is the hemisphere of the Earth and three Egyptian pyramids expanded until the base of each pyramid equals the Earth circumference at the equator — Circumference = Perimeter. Which pyramid is the closest to hemisphere geometry? The one where its height equals the radius of the Earth: H = R. This is the Great Pyramid. It has by virtue of the slope angle, selected by its designers, the value π encoded into its geometry. The hemisphere and the circle have the value π encoded into their geometry. Thus: Earth circumference = 2 x radius x π, and Great Pyramid perimeter = 2 x height x π. This is the clue that the Great Pyramid is Earth commensurate. Mathematicians naturally look for other relationships.

Since the Great Pyramid base = 750 Great Pyramid feet (G.P. ft), and if this is equal to 1/8 minute arc length along the surface of the Earth, this yields 129,600,000 G.P. ft per revolution. (See Note 4.1.) By checking several sources and the almanac we will see how close this is. *Secrets of The Great Pyramid* by Peter Tompkins, a companion reference, lists four "modern" values which were perhaps part of an earlier survey and valid at the time of his book. The value is 130,188,084.1 in units of G.P. ft. (See Note 4.2.)

The ratio of the two yields the error:

130,188,084.1 / 129,600,000.0 = 1.004537686

This is the same value with a less than one-half per-cent error, or precisely: 0.45% error. The 1989 Almanac lists a slightly different value for the size of the Earth based on the International Union of Geodesy and Geophysics adopted in 1967, which used orbiting satellite technology. This Almanac value is 7,926.41 miles for the diameter at the Equator. The Equator bulges slightly and the poles are slightly flat. The length of an average meridian is 24,859.82 miles (British). The meridian would actually be the best estimate of a perfectly spherical Earth. By using the same simple formulas the conversion of 24,859.82 miles (British) into units of Great Pyramid feet yields: 130,275,015.9 feet. Comparing this to the ancient prediction gives:

130,275,015.9 / 129,600,000 = 1.005208456

This, again, is about a one half percent error, or precisely, 0.52% of the value predicted by the perimeter of the Great Pyramid. This is truly astounding and the implications are far reaching. The designers obviously intended the base to be an exact fraction of a degree, specifically 1/8 of one minute. The perimeter is 1/2 of one minute exactly, and the monument is truly Earth commensurate. But why would the designers choose 1/2 of one minute for the perimeter? Why not one minute for the perimeter, or 1/4 of one minute for the perimeter? Obviously the "one minute" monument would be extremely expensive compared to the "1/4 minute" monument, so was the "1/2 minute" monument simply an economic compromise?

Consider the problem from another perspective, the perimeter as expressed in units of time, and the answer becomes apparent. There are 24 hr x 60 min x 60 sec = 86,400 sec per day. There are 129,600,000 G.P. ft. in one revolution so 129,600,000 G.P. ft. divided by 86,400 sec per day = 1500 G.P. ft. as the angular velocity, at the equator, of the rotating Earth. In other words, the planet rotates a certain distance each second. Every *two* seconds, the distance traveled at the equator is exactly equal to the perimeter of the Great Pyramid. Of all the possibilities, why is the perimeter of the base of the Great Pyramid designed to equal the rotation time or angular velocity of the Earth precisely every *two* seconds, not every *three* seconds or *one* second, but exactly *two* seconds? The symbolic meanings are dealt with later. Unquestionably the two-second interval chosen is still accurate to within 0.5%, and experts know that the size of the Earth is a variable. It is entirely conceivable that when the value was calculated, it was even more precise!

No other pyramid in Egypt has this double Earth commensurate relationship. The fact that the Great Pyramid was related to the size of the Earth was known by classical writers of Greece 2500 years ago. It was part of the secret knowledge of the high priests of Egypt. Even though that clue was recorded by classical writers, it is very intriguing that today those Earth commensurate facts can be verified with great accuracy. Except for the reference to time, this exciting story is well documented and presented by Peter Tompkins in *Secrets of the Great Pyramid*. (See Reference 5.)

Also to be considered is the almost perfect north-south, east-west orientation of the faces of the Great Pyramid. In 1918, Cole cleared all four corners of the Great Pyramid and did an exacting survey (See Reference 5). Although the corner blocks were missing when Cole did the survey, he accomplished the task by scientific estimation. First there is a chiseled depression or socket in the bed rock into which the now-missing foundation block was originally positioned. Upon that the corner stone was fixed. Since there are two casing blocks still remaining on the north face, it is possible to estimate where the base and corner of the Great Pyramid actually existed in relation to the corner of the socket. Assuming that each corner casing block was located this same distance from the corner of the socket, the measurements were made with modern surveying equipment and the results are still considered the most accurate to date. The results verify that each corner is within six inches of the theoretical perfectly square location and no other pyramid can compare with this perfection.

The precision of this can only be appreciated by comparing it to a modern skyscraper, which looks perfectly aligned to the naked eye. Under the close scrutiny of modern surveying equipment, however, it does not come close to the accuracy of the ancient Great Pyramid. The obvious positioning of the Great Pyramid accurately to the meridians is in agreement with the nature of the Great Pyramid being an Earth commensurate monument. One can only wonder what other numbers lie hidden within the geometry of the Great Pyramid.

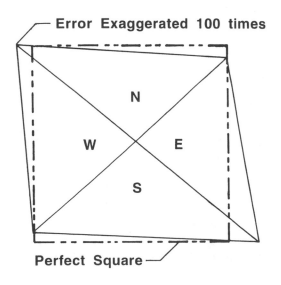

Figure 4.4 The corner precision of the Great Pyramid has to be exaggerated 100 times to be visible. No modern structure compares to this accuracy. (See Reference 50.)

NOTES

1. Calculation for the size of the Earth (assuming the planet is a perfect sphere.)

750 G.P. ft = 1/8 minute arc length

Transposing the 8 in the denominator yields:

8 x 750 G.P. ft = 1 minute arc length

Multiplying terms yields:

6,000 G.P. ft = 1 minute arc length

But since there are 60 minutes per degree, this yields:

60 x 6,000 G.P. ft = 360,000 G.P. ft = 1 degree arc length

And since there are 360 degrees per revolution, this translates into:

360 x 360,000 G.P. ft = 129,600,000 G.P. ft per revolution.

2. The circumference of the Earth according to Peter Tompkins in Secrets of the Great Pyramid. (See Reference 5.)

P. 46	3,955.80 mile radius
P. 202	3,956.59 mile radius
P. 207	3,955.77 mile radius
P. 209	3,947.54 mile radius

The average of these values is 3,953.925 miles. (English Units). This value for the radius, converted to the circumference of the Earth, is calculated by the simple formula:

$C = 2\pi R$

Substituting the value for the radius yields:

$C = 2 \times \pi \times 3,953.925 = 24,843.24347$ miles (British Units)

This, however, is stated in units that need to be converted. Convert miles to feet by substituting 5,280 feet/mile (British):

$24,843.24347 \times 5,280 = 131,172,325.5$ feet (British Units)

British units, though, are slightly less than Great Pyramid units. The base of the Great Pyramid would measure 755.67 feet with a British tape measure. The correction factor is easily obtained since the base, in Great Pyramid units, is 750 feet by definition, thus:

755.67 / 750 = 1.00756015 (See Note 3.)

Dividing the circumference of the planet expressed in British feet by the correction ratio yields the "known" true circumference of Earth expressed in units of the ancient world, Great Pyramid feet:

131,172,325.5 / 1.00756015 = 130,188,084.1

3. The values of Cole have been averaged to obtain the average length of the base of the Great Pyramid. (See Reference 5, page 202.) The values were originally published in Deter-mination of the Exact Size and Orientation of the Great Pyramid of Giza (Survey of Egypt, paper 58). Cole gives 230.215 meters (+/- 6 millimeters) for the south side; 230.454 meters (+/- 10 millimeters at the west end and +/- 30 millimeters) at the east end) for the north side; 230.391 for the east side; and 230.253 for the west side. These values were simply divided by 750 G.P. ft per side, listed, then averaged:

G.P. ft	=	Base in meters / 750 G.P. ft (Meters / G.P. ft)
1		.30695333 (S)
1		.307004 (W)
1		.307272 (N)
1		.307188 (E)
1.000		.307104333 (Avg)

One G.P. ft equals 1.007560146 British feet. This is determined by ratio: One inch (British) is defined as 2.54 cm, one foot (British) is thus: 12 x 2.54 = 30.48 centimeter (cm), or .3048 meter (m). The ratio of G.P. ft to British ft is: .307104333 / .3048 = 1.007560146 as shown.

Chapter Five

Synopsis

The orientation, size, and slope angle of the Great Pyramid was designed so that units of length, time, and degrees would be based on 12 or its harmonic 360 (12 x 30), and simultaneously be sub-multiples of some physical aspect of the planet. Thus the Great Pyramid is Earth commensurate. This concept unfolds in many bizarre ways. Spiral down from the apex dropping two G.P. feet every revolution and upon reaching the base, 360,000 G.P.ft (12 x 30,000) have been traversed — exactly one degree of average meridian-arc. The volume of every casing block equals 360 G.P. ft (12 x 30). The standard G.P. volume is 12 G.P. inches per side. Fill it with rainwater and it yields the G.P. standard weight. Sub-units of this weight based on 12 as the divisor equals the common units of dry and liquid volumes — the gallon, the quart, and the pint. Even units of pressure and temperature are based on the G.P. system. The original bureau of weights and measures for planet Earth is the Great Pyramid.

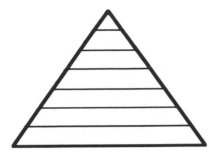

Chapter Five

SONG OF THE GREAT PYRAMID

The Harmony of Encoded Numbers

The beauty of the Great Pyramid can begin to be appreciated when it's realized that its dimensions are Earth commensurate not only once, but twice. It corresponds not only to the size of the Earth, but also to the angular velocity of the Earth. The dimensions of the Great Pyramid, shown by a special table (Figure 5.1), reflect everything discussed so far. At the top is a comparison of a hemisphere and an equivalent π pyramid. The height (H) of the pyramid is drawn equal to the radius (R) of the hemisphere so that H = R. The apothem angle is adjusted until the perimeter (P) at the base of the pyramid is equal to the circumference (C) of the circle which is the base of the hemisphere. The angles that could have been chosen were almost infinite, yet this unique pyramid contains the slope angle of 51 degrees 51 minutes and 14.3 seconds. This is the sole π pyramid, and mathematically it relates to the circle by a simple equation:

$$C/2R = \pi = P / 2H$$

Where:

C = Circumference of circle
P = Pyramid perimeter = 4 x Base
B = Base of the pyramid
R = Radius of the circle
H = Height of the pyramid
π = Universal Constant: 3.14159...

As examined earlier, the π pyramid infers a similarity to a hemisphere, especially to the hemisphere of the Earth, and was intended to be a bureau of standards for the planet. Part of this knowledge is summarized in Figure 5.1. Here the units of time, angles, height, width, and depth are clearly Earth commensurate. (See Note 1.)

The basic unit of time is recognized as one orbit of the planet about the sun, one year. During that time there are about 360 revolutions of the planet about its axis and each spin is one day. The actual number of days in one year, of course, is closer to 365.24 days, but 360 is correct to within 1.4%. Smaller divisions of the day are hours; one day has 24 hours. The hour is further divided by minutes; one hour = 60 minutes. The minutes are further divided by seconds; one minute = 60 seconds, and this means there are 3,600 seconds per hour. For angles, a complete circle, or one complete revolution, is equal to 360 subdivisions known as degrees. Degrees are further divided by minutes, one degree = 60 minutes. Minutes are further divided by seconds, one minute = 60 seconds and this means there are 3,600 seconds per degree. Space — or height, width and depth is measured by a unit of length, herein defined as the Great Pyramid foot (G.P. ft). There are 3,000 G.P. ft in one Great Pyramid base perimeter, which is one "revolution" at the base. There are 3,000 G.P. ft in every *two* seconds of Earth rotation at the equator so the perimeter accurately defines the angular velocity of Earth. There are 6,000 G.P. ft in every minute of arc length along a meridian, and there are 360,000 G.P. ft in one degree of arc length along a meridian. This fact is more accurate when the Earth, which really bulges slightly at the equator, is considered a perfect sphere of the same volume. This layout of Figure 5.1, depicted as a pyramid, was chosen to display the uncanny repetition of certain values, especially 60 and 360, and all values shown are divisible by twelve. This is more than coincidental and this fact is summarized in Table 5.1. It is obvious that all the units were deliberately designed around the value twelve or multiples of twelve, especially the harmonic 360.

There are two more mystifying facts related to this. Spiral down from the apex of the Great Pyramid to the base, dropping exactly *two* Great Pyramid feet per revolution, and the length of this spiral on the surface of the Great Pyramid is 360,000 G.P. ft — the same as in one degree of arc. In addition, when each casing block was designed, its height, width, and depth were selected so that the volume would be equal to 360 cubic Great Pyramid feet.

These very precise and intentional mathematical relationships are reminiscent of the harmony that is found in uplifting music. Think of these relationships as being written in the key of "12" with the harmonic "360" sounded at appropriate times, a sort of mathematical poetry or "Song of the Pyramid."

This inspired description comes after attempting to develop a better version of weights and measures for this planet, after all, 360 and 12 are but two numbers out of an infinite selection. The reader should arm himself with a scientific calculator, a far more powerful tool than anything the Egyptians could have had for calculating numbers, and then try the obvious. If the actual days in a year, 365.24 days, is the inspiration, and from that fact, the value 365 is used for the basis of one revolution, one cycle, and so on, then the number of degrees in a circle would be 365. The problem with this course lies in the fact that a "right" triangle would have 91 1/4 degrees in it, and a "45 degree" triangle would have 45.625 degrees in it, and this would complicate layout work for designers, craftsmen, and carpenters.

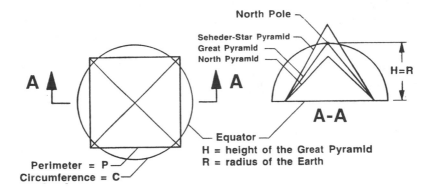

North Pole

Seheder-Star Pyramid
Great Pyramid
North Pyramid

H=R

A

A A

A-A

Equator
H = height of the Great Pyramid
R = radius of the Earth

Perimeter = P
Circumference = C

The diagram above depicts a top view of the Great Pyramid enlarged until the base perimeter equals the circumference of the Earth — the equator. The side view shows the apex of the pyramid just touching the North Pole. Amazingly, the Earth hemisphere and the Great Pyramid are related by the universal constant π. Thus, $C/2\pi = R = H = P/2\pi$.

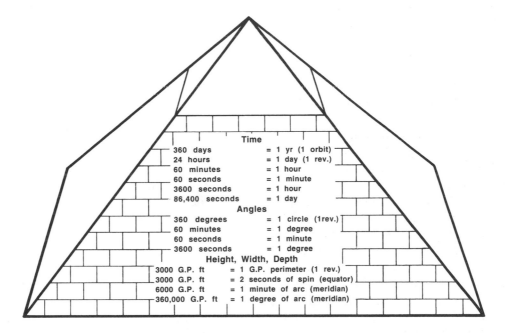

Time

360 days	= 1 yr (1 orbit)
24 hours	= 1 day (1 rev.)
60 minutes	= 1 hour
60 seconds	= 1 minute
3600 seconds	= 1 hour
86,400 seconds	= 1 day

Angles

360 degrees	= 1 circle (1rev.)
60 minutes	= 1 degree
60 seconds	= 1 minute
3600 seconds	= 1 degree

Height, Width, Depth

3000 G.P. ft	= 1 G.P. perimeter (1 rev.)
3000 G.P. ft	= 2 seconds of spin (equator)
6000 G.P. ft	= 1 minute of arc (meridian)
360,000 G.P. ft	= 1 degree of arc (meridian)

5.1 The bureau of weights and measures for the planet is the Great Pyramid. It defines the necessary units of space and time. Notice that each value is a multiple of twelve. (See Note 1.)

To match the rhythm as set forth in Table 5.1 other problems would unfold. The calculation for a 365 degree/revolution scheme implies 365,000 feet/degree which results in:

365 degrees/revolution x 365,000 feet/degree = 133,225,000
feet/revolution or feet/circumference of the Earth

In itself, this is no great obstacle. This would simply redefine the length of the foot which is easy to calculate by using the ratio of the circumference in units of G.P. ft to the new foot:

129,600,000/133,225,000 = 0.9727904

Thus, the new foot is 97.27904% of the existing G.P. ft. The difficult occurs when correlating this new foot into units of time, since shrinking the foot doesn't slow the Earth down. In this new system the Earth would not travel 3,000 feet every two seconds as hoped for, but it would travel 3,084.606 feet as measured by the new foot. This is also because these *two* seconds were defined by the G.P. ft. Perhaps it would be wiser to invent a new second. The better second would be 97.27904% of the G.P. second so there would be more seconds per day, which is easy to calculate with our conversion factor:

86,400/.9727904 = 88,816.66666667

With 88,816.66666667 seconds per day, the Earth would rotate 3,000 new feet every two seconds. Opposing this nice rhythm would be the fact that each hour, assuming 24 hours per day is still used, would have 3,700.694444445 sec/hr and this of course implies by simple division that there would be 60.833333333 min/hr and 60.833333333 sec/min. The more this system is explored the clearer it becomes that a scheme with irrational numbers would be unworkable in everyday situations. Additionally, this system has no harmony, no basic divisor like the 12 in the "Song of the Pyramid". Now the beauty and interrelatedness of the Pyramid numbers can be more fully appreciated, as it becomes obvious that changing one value imbalances all the other numbers. This is shown in Table 5.2, which presents the lack of a harmonic divisor by a question mark.

This poor attempt at mathematical poetry has an analogy in music — discord. It is like random slamming on the keyboard of a piano with very little thought about which keys to use. The rhythm is not there and it appears to be a crude solution, but there are many directions to try. Some of them are cataloged in the note section of this chapter. Those handy with a calculator might try a few systems to get a feel for what is involved. In reality, this is a highly complex problem.

Consider the advantage one has with a modern scientific calculator that accurately multiplies, divides, and solves square roots in a matter of seconds, greatly speeding up the necessary trial and error involved in attempting such a project. It is hard to imagine that someone in ancient times used an ink pen on papyrus paper and calculated by long hand, similar figures out to ten decimal places.

The mathematical relationships of the Song of the Pyramid, however, even extend into other units of measure. Another interesting connection is found when looking at British Imperial liquid and dry measures. The tabulation under "measures" in

		HARMONIC OF "360"	KEY OF "12"
TIME			
365 days	= one orbit	360 x 1 (a)	12 x 30
24 hours	= one day	360 x 1/15	12 x 2
60 min	= one hour	360 x 1/6	12 x 5
60 sec	= one minute	360 x 1/6	12 x 5
3,600 sec	= one hour	360 x 10	12 x 300
86,400 sec	= one day	360 x 240	12 x 7200
ANGLES			
360 degrees	= one revolution	360 x 1	12 x 30
60 min	= one degree	360 x 1/6	12 x 5
60 sec	= one minute	360 x 1/6	12 x 5
3,600 sec	= one degree	360 x 10	12 x 30
LENGTH			
3,000 feet	= one rev (base)	360 x 25/3	12 x 250
3,000 feet	= 2 sec at equator	360 x 25/3	12 x 250
6,000 feet	= 1 min arc	360 x 50/3	12 x 500
360,000 feet	= one degree of arc (meridian)	360 x 1000	12 x 30,000
SPIRAL LENGTH (at two foot increments of elevation)			
360,000 feet	= one degree	360 x 1,000	12 x 30,000
VOLUME OF ONE CASING STONE			
360 ft^3	= one casing block	360 x 1	12 x 30

(a) error = 1.4%

Table 5.1 Shows Great Pyramid units of measure based on the key of twelve, the harmonic of 360 seconds as hoped for, but travels 3,084.606 feet as measured by the new foot. This is also because these *two* seconds were defined by the G.P. ft.

		HARMONIC OF "365"	KEY OF "12" ?
TIME			
365 days	= one orbit	365 x 1	?
24 hours	= one day	?	?
60.833 min	= one hour	?	?
60.833 sec	= one minute	?	?
3,700.6944 sec	= one hour	?	?
88,816.666 sec	= one day	?	?
ANGLES			
365 degrees	= one revolution	365 x 1	?
60.833 min	= one degree	?	?
60.833 sec	= one minute	?	?
3,700.694 sec	= one degree	?	?
LENGTH			
3,000 feet	= one rev. (base)	?	12 x 25
3,000 feet	= 2 sec at equator	?	12 x 25
6,000 feet	= 1 min arc	?	12 x 50
365,000 feet	= one degree of arc (meridian)	365 x 1,000	?
SPIRAL LENGTH (@ two foot increments)			
365,000 feet	= one degree	365 x 1,000	?
VOLUME OF ONE CASING STONE			
365 ft^3	= one casing block	365 x 1	?

Table 5.2 Inharmonic hypothetical system based on 365 degrees per revolution. Each "?" represents a point of disharmony; changing one value affects all other relationships in the mathematical "song."

Webster's dictionary is that one fluid dram = 60 minims. (See Reference 39.) What is the familiar number 60 doing in liquid and dry measures?

By working backwards through the logic of the subdivisions, it is obvious that the subdivisions are based on the key of 12:

British Imperial Liquid and Dry Measures

Unit	Equivalent in Other Units of the Same System
bushel	4 pecks (2219.36 cubic inches)
peck	2 gallons (554.84 cubic inches)
gallon	4 quarts (277.420 cubic inches)
quarts	2 pints (69.355 cubic inches)
pints	4 gills (34.6775 cubic inches)
gill	5 fluid ounces (8.669375 cubic inches)
fluid ounce	8 fluid drams (1.733875 cubic inches)
fluid drams	60 minims (0.216734375 cubic inches)
minim	1/60 fluid rams (0.003612239 cubic inches)

To see this relationship, first assume that the Great Pyramid foot was used to define a unit for liquid and dry measure called **The Standard Volume**, which was a box one foot high, one foot wide, and one foot deep. The standard volume would be used to define liquid and dry amounts and eventually define weights. This standard volume is easily converted to G.P. inches since there are twelve inches per foot:

12 inches x 3 sides = 12 x 12 x 12 = 1728 G.P. in^3 in one standard volume by definition.

Since the standard volume is quite large, subdivisions were needed. Assume the next subdivision was to be 1/6 of the standard volume. This would yield:

1728/6 = 288 cubic inches

And since the British foot is shorter than the G.P. ft (one G.P. ft x 1.007560146 = one British foot, see Chapter 4), the calculation needs to be corrected for direct comparison. There would be more British inches in the height, width, and depth, so there would be more British inches by the cube of the correction factor or:

1.007560146^3 = 1.02285234

Using this to correct volume calculations:

1.02285234 x 288 = 294.58 cubic inches

This is very close to the value for the gallon in the above tabulation. The ratio is:

$$294.58 / 277.42 = 1.062$$

The British Imperial gallon is within 6.2% of 1/6 of a G.P. ft³. When these subdivisions are examined, it is found that all of them are multiples of twelve.

British Imperial Liquid and Dry Measures

Unit	Equivalent Compared to G.P. FT³	
6 gallons	1.00 G.P. ft³	1/(1/12 x 12) G.P. ft³
peck	1/3 G.P. ft³	1/(1/4 x 12) G.P. ft³
gallon	1/6 G.P. ft³	1/(1/2 x 12) G.P. ft³
quarts	1/24 G.P. ft³	1/(2 x 12) G.P. ft³
pints	1/48 G.P. ft³	1/(4 x 12) G.P. ft³
gill	1/192 G.P. ft³	1/(16 x 12) G.P. ft³
fluid ounce	1/768 G.P. ft³	1/(64 x 12) G.P. ft³
fluid drams	1/6144 G.P. ft³	1/(512 x 12) G.P. ft³
minim	1/368640 G.P. ft³	1/(30720 x 12) G.P. ft³

Isn't it thought provoking that this system of measure has subdivisions based on the key of 12? Since the British foot is different from the G.P. ft, perhaps when the British foot was revised, the peck and the gallon were invented. One can speculate that the standard volume originally had six subdivisions. The first subdivision would have been something like a 1/2 gallon. If the next subdivision was 1/4 of the 1/2 gallon, the above tabulation would appear as in its original pure form:

Theorized Original Liquid and Dry Measures

Unit	Equivalents Compared to G.P. FT³	
12 (gal/2)	1.00 G.P. ft³	1/1 G.P. ft³
1/2 gallon	1/12 G.P. ft³	1/(1 x 12) G.P. ft³
pints	1/48 G.P. ft³	1/(4 x 12) G.P. ft³
gill	1/192 G.P. ft³	1/(16 x 12) G.P. ft³
fluid ounce	1/768 G.P. ft³	1/(64 x 12) G.P. ft³
fluid drams	1/6144 G.P. ft³	1/(512 x 12) G.P. ft³
minim	1/368640 G.P. ft³	1/(30720 x 12) G.P. ft³

In this hypothesized scheme, the subdivisions again show the harmony of the Song of the Great Pyramid. If this were the original scheme, then perhaps the peck, gallon and the quart were invented later, as corruptions of the original system. What is known for sure is that the currently used British Imperial Liquid and Dry Measures have subdivisions based on the key of 12. This key of 12 also appears in part of the units of two other common systems. Look at the troy system:

Units of the Troy System of Weights

Unit	Grains	Part of Pound
pound	5760	1/1
ounce	480	1/(1 x 12)
pennyweight	24	1/(20 x 12)
grain	1	1/(480 x 12)

In the apothecaries' system, the subdivisions are again part of a key of 12 divisor:

Units of the Apothecaries' System of Weights

Unit	Grains	Part of Pound
pound	5760	1/1
ounce	480	1/(1 x 12)
dram	60	1/(8 x 12)
scruple	20	1/(24 x 12)
grain	1	1/(480 x 12)

According to Reference 33, one British ft^3 filled with rain water at standard temperature and pressure weighs 62.37 pounds. Because it is slightly larger, one G.P. ft^3 would weigh more by the correction factor, 1.02285234, already discussed:

1.02285234 x 62.37 = 63.7953 pounds

One pound is very nearly 1/60 of one G.P. ft^3 of rain water. The exact calculation is:

63.7953/60 = 1.063255 pound

Which means 1/60 of one G.P. ft3 is within 6.3% of the commonly accepted weight of one pound.

The conditions of standard temperature and pressure are the pressure at sea level when the mercury barometer is at 29.92 British inches (29.70 G.P. inches) and 59 degrees Fahrenheit. These conditions reflect the average of all global weather pressures and temperatures. Somehow, this condition must have been considered in ancient times. If this standard temperature and pressure were originally defined as 60 degrees Fahrenheit and 30 inches of mercury, the error compared to the value used today would be:

$60/59 = 1.0169...$

and

$30/29.70 = 1.0101...$

Perhaps it was intended that the one volume in units of G.P. ft^3 defined units of volume, dry and liquid, units of weight, and even units of Fahrenheit temperature. Whether the temperature scale used today proves to have been a recent invention or not, what is sure is that it uses the ancient units of "degrees."

The same parallel can be observed when comparing U.S. and British gallons. The U.S. dry gallon, 231 cubic inches, and the U.S. liquid gallon, 268.8025 cubic inches, are different from each other and also different from the British Imperial gallon, 277.420 cubic inches. Despite this difference, their subdivisions follow the same formula already discussed. Since the French revolution brought about much change in that country, including new units of measure, it can be seen that political change in itself can cause a change in units of measure. When societies collapse due to catastrophic upheaval such as earthquakes, volcanic venting, or a combination of both, it is easy to imagine that the standard length used in a region could be lost. In such a case, the survivors would always remember the basis, but might not have access to it, and would invent a new standard based on what was remembered. This would likely induce a certain amount of error. What is summarized in this chapter points to exactly that.

It is sometimes thought that the British formulated all the units of measure used by today's civilized societies during the Industrial Revolution. The evidence seems to suggest that the British, like others, have borrowed from a more ancient system and the origin of it all may very well be the Earth commensurate Great Pyramid.

NOTES

1. To those who have suggested that these boring numbers be put away in a footnote or in the appendix, kindly consider that they are the proof of our ET heritage. William Flinders Petrie (whose book is all numbers!), Charles Piazzi Smyth, and other Pyramidology researchers, have examined the Great Pyramid numbers and geometry and either dispelled them as coincidence or marvelled at the wonder of it. Eventually one comes to the great revelation that the basis for weights and measures is all interrelated and coincides with the size and shape of the Great Pyramid which is an intoxicating thought.

Just think, the one-hundred-year-old argument between Smyth's camp and Petrie's camp can now be explained! Smyth and his followers believed that the British inch was defined by the Great Pyramid geometry and that one inch equalled one year in a Biblical prophecy as read by a linear progression down the Descending Passage and then up the Ascending Passage. Petrie, an astronomer and a staunch believer in hard facts, went to Egypt to examine the Great Pyramid in detail and measured it with special equipment to great precision. His value was slightly different than Smyth's value, and so dismissed the whole idea as hogwash. Petrie's scientific methods "would reach the ugly little fact which killed the beautiful theory." That and other quotes such as, "It is useless to state the real truth of the matter, as it has no effect on those who are subject to this type of hallucination. They can but be left with the flat Earth believers and other such people to whom a theory is dearer than a fact" fueled other academicians to critize Petrie. Professor F.A.P. Barnard's opinion was that the pyramids "originated before anything like intellectual culture existed; have been constructed without thought of scientific method, and have owed their earliest forms to accident and caprice."

I submit that Smyth was right in the fact that an inch is defined by the Great Pyramid. The inch defined in this work is different from the British inch. Each inch does equal one year of history, but the movement must be in a spiral down and then up the passages, since all movement in the universe is in spirals. The prophecy, however, is probably not Biblical. It is far older than the Bible, and is beyond the scope of this work. It does tell who built the Great Pyramid, when it was built, and where they came from. Petrie was right to insist on accurate measurements, but wrong to insist that the British inch is the only inch that exists.

2. Listed here are additional attempts to develop hypothetical schemes to rival the Song of the Pyramid. Although the effort to calculate a better system than the ancients was a failure, as indicated by the numerous question marks and comments at the bottom of each sheet, what was gained was a great appreciation for the harmonies of Table 5.1. Hopefully, the reader will be encouraged to obtain a scientific calculator and try to invent a scheme that can surpass the ancient scheme that humanity has inherited.

		HARMONIC OF "365"	KEY OF "5"
TIME			
365 days	= one orbit	365 x 1	5 x 73
20 hours	= one day	?	5 x 4
60.41523 min	= one hour	?	?
60.41523 sec	= one minute	?	?
3,650 sec	= one hour	365 x 10	5 x 730
73,000 sec	= one day	365 x 200	5 x 14,600
ANGLES			
365 degrees	= one revolution	365 x 1	5 x 73
60.41523 min	= one degree	?	?
60.41523 sec	= one minute	?	?
3,650 sec	= one degree	365 x 10	5 x 730
LENGTH			
3,650 feet	= one rev	365 x 10	5 x 730
3,650 feet	= 2 sec at equator	365 x 10	5 x 730
6,041.5229 ft	= 1 min arc	?	?
365,000 feet	= one degree of arc (meridian)	365 x 1,000	5 x 73,000

Comments: The "90-degree" angle has 91.25 degrees, the "45-degree" angle has 45.625 degrees, the "30-degree" triangle has 30.418888 degrees, and the "60-degree" triangle has 60.8333 degrees. Once again, each "?" does not compute and represents a point of disharmony.

		HARMONIC OF "364"	KEY OF "4"
TIME			
364 days	= one orbit	364 x 1	4 x 91
20 hours	= one day	?	4 x 5
60.3324 min	= one hour	?	?
60.3324 sec	= one minute	?	?
3,640 sec	= one hour	364 x 10	4 x 910
72,800 sec	= one day	364 x 200	4 x 18,200
ANGLES			
364 degrees	= one revolution	364 x 1	4 x 91
60.3324 min	= one degree	?	?
60.3324 sec	= one minute	?	?
3,640 sec	= one degree	364 x 10	4 x 910
LENGTH			
3,640 feet	= one rev (base)	364 x 10	4 x 910
3,640 feet	= 2 sec at equator	364 x 10	4 x 910
6,033.241 feet	= 1 min arc	?	?
364,000 feet	= one degree of arc (meridian)	364 x 1000	4 x 91,000

Comments: The "90-degree" angle has 91 degrees, which is convenient enough, however, the "45-degree" angle has 45.5 degrees, the "30-degree" triangle has 30.3333 degrees, and the "60-degree" triangle has 60.6666 degrees.

		HARMONIC OF "364"	KEY OF "4"
TIME			
364 days	= one orbit	364 x 1	4 x 91
24 hours	= one day	?	4 x 6
60.3324 min	= one hour	?	?
60.3324 sec	= one minute	?	?
3,640 sec	= one hour	364 x 10	4 x 910
87,360 sec	= one day	364 x 240	4 x 21,840
ANGLES			
364 degrees	= one revolution	364 x 1	4 x 91
60.3324 min	= one degree	?	?
60.3324 sec	= one minute	?	?
3,640 sec	= one degree	364 x 10	4 x 910
LENGTH			
3,033.3333 feet	= one rev (base)	?	?
3,033.3333 feet	= 2 sec at equator	?	?
6,033.241 feet	= 1 min arc	?	?
364,000 feet	= one degree of arc (meridian)	364 x 1,000	4 x 91,000

Comments: Once again the "90-degree" angle has 91 degrees and that is convenient enough. The "45-degree" angle has 45.5 degrees, the "30-degree" triangle has 30.3333 degrees, and the "60-degree" triangle has 60.6666 degrees. This is not convenient.

		HARMONIC OF "364	KEY OF "4"
TIME			
364 days	= one orbit	364 x 1	4 x 91
28 hours	= one day	?	4 x 7
60.3324 min	= one hour	?	?
60.3324 sec	= one minute	?	?
3,640 sec	= one hour	364 x 10	4 x 910
101,920 sec	= one day	364 x 280	4 x 25,480
ANGLES			
364 degrees	= one revolution	364 x 1	4 x 91
60.3324 min	= one degree	?	?
60.3324 sec	= one minute	?	?
3,640 sec	= one degree	364 x 10	4 x 910
LENGTH			
2,600 feet	= one rev (base)	?	4 x 640
2,600 feet	= 2 sec at equator	?	4 x 640
6,033.241 feet	= 1 min arc	?	?
364,000 feet	= one degree of arc (meridian)	364 x 1,000	4 x 91,000

Comments: The "90-degree" angle has 91 degrees, which is convenient. The "45-degree" angle, however, has 45.5 degrees, the "30-degree" triangle has 30.3333 degrees, and the "60-degree" triangle has 60.6666 degrees, and these are not workable.

		HARMONIC OF "362"	KEY OF "2"
TIME			
362 days	= one orbit	362 x 1	2 x 181
28 hours	= one day	?	2 x 14
60.1884 min	= one hour	?	?
60.1884 sec	= one minute	?	?
3,620 sec	= one hour	362 x 10	2 x 1,810
101,360 sec	= one day	362 x 280	2 x 50,680
ANGLES			
362 degrees	= one revolution	362 x 1	2 x 181
60.1884 min	= one degree	?	?
60.1884 sec	= one minute	?	?
3,620 sec	= one degree	362 x 10	2 x 1,810
LENGTH			
2,585.7142 feet	= one rev (base)	?	?
2,585.7142 feet	= 2 sec at equator	?	?
6,016.6435 feet	= 1 min arc	?	?
362,000 feet	= one degree of arc (meridian)	362 x 1,000	2 x 181,000

Comments: Unfortunately the "90-degree" angle has 90.5 degrees, the "45-degree" angle has 45.25 degrees, the "30-degree" triangle has 30.1666 degrees, and the "60-degree" triangle has 60.3333 degrees, all of which are inconvenient.

		HARMONIC OF "366"	KEY OF "2"
TIME			
366 days	= one orbit	366 x 1	2 x 183
26 hours	= one day	?	2 x 13
60.4979 min	= one hour	?	?
60.4979 sec	= one minute	?	?
3,660 sec	= one hour	366 x 10	2 x 1,830
95,160 sec	= one day	366 x 260	2 x 47,580
ANGLES			
366 degrees	= one revolution	366 x 1	2 x 183
60.4979 min	= one degree	?	?
60.4979 sec	= one minute	?	?
3,660 sec	= one degree	366 x 10	2 x 1,830
LENGTH			
2,815.3846 feet	= one rev (base)	?	?
2,815.3846 feet	= 2 sec at equator	?	?
6,049.7967 feet	= 1 min arc	?	?
366,000 feet	= one degree of arc (meridian)	366 x 1,000	2 x 181,000

Comments: The "90-degree" angle has 91.5 degrees, the "45-degree" angle has 45.75 degrees, the "30-degree" triangle has 30.5 degrees, and the "60-degree" triangle has 61 degrees, which are not workable.

		HARMONIC OF "368"	KEY OF "4"
TIME			
368 days	= one orbit	368 x 1	4 x 92
28 hours	= one day	?	4 x 7
60.663 min	= one hour	?	?
60.663 sec	= one minute	?	?
3,680 sec	= one hour	368 x 10	4 x 920
103,040 sec	= one day	368 x 280	4 x 25,760
ANGLES			
368 degrees	= one revolution	368 x 1	4 x 92
60.663 min	= one degree	?	?
60.6630 sec	= one minute	?	?
3,680 sec	= one degree	368 x 10	4 x 920
LENGTH			
2,628.5714 feet	= one rev (base)	?	?
2,628.5714 feet	= 2 sec at equator	?	?
6,066.3007 feet	= 1 min arc	?	?
368,000 feet	= one degree of arc (meridian)	368 x 1,000	4 x 92,000

Comments: The "90-degree" angle has 92 degrees and the "45-degree" angle has 46 degrees which are convenient. The "30-degree" triangle, however, has 30.6667 degrees, and the "60-degree" triangle has 61.3333 degrees, and these are difficult.

		HARMONIC OF "500"	KEY OF "5"
TIME			
500 days	= one orbit	500 x 1	5 x 100
50 hours	= one day	500 x 1/10	5 x 10
50 min	= one hour	500 x 1/10	5 x 10
50 sec	= one minute	500 x 1/10	5 x 10
2,500 sec	= one hour	500 x 5	5 x 500
125,000 sec	= one day	500 x 250	5 x 25,000
ANGLES			
500 degrees	= one revolution	500 x 1	5 x 100
50 min	= one degree	5 x 10	5 x 10
50 sec	= one minute	5 x 10	5 x 10
2,500 sec	= one degree	500 x 5	5 x 500
LENGTH			
4,000 feet	= one rev (base)	500 x 8	5 x 800
4,000 feet	= 2 sec at equator	500 x 8	5 x 800
10,000 feet	= 1 min arc	500 x 20	5 x 2,000
500,000 feet	= one degree of arc (meridian)	500 x 1,000	5 x 100,000

Comments: This is nearly a perfect song of a pyramid, harmony in every category. Unfortunately it's a song that doesn't fit our planet. The "90-degree" angle has 125 degrees, but the "45-degree" angle would have 62.5 degrees, the "30-degree" triangle has 41.6666 degrees, and the "60-degree" triangle has 83.3333 degrees.

		HARMONIC OF "100"	KEY OF "5"
TIME			
100 days	= one orbit	100 x 1	5 x 20
10 hours	= one day	100 x 1/10	5 x 2
100 min	= one hour	100 x 1	5 x 20
100 sec	= one minute	100 x 1	5 x 20
10,000 sec	= one hour	100 x 100	5 x 2,000
100,000 sec	= one day	100 x 1,000	5 x 20,000
ANGLES			
1,000 degrees	= one revolution	100 x 10	5 x 200
100 min	= one degree	5 x 20	5 x 20
100 sec	= one minute	5 x 20	5 x 20
10,000 sec	= one degree	100 x 100	5 x 2,000
LENGTH			
2,000 feet	= one rev. (base)	100 x 20	5 x 400
2,000 feet	= 2 sec at equator	100 x 20	5 x 400
1,000 feet	= 1 min. arc	100 x 10	5 x 200
100,000 feet	= one degree of arc (meridian)	100 x 1,000	5 x 20,000

Comments: Again almost a perfect song of the pyramid with harmony in every category shown, but unfortunately, this song is for the wrong planet. In addition, while the "90-degree" angle has 250 degrees, and the "45-degree" angle has 125 degrees, the "30-degree" triangle has 83.3333 degrees, and the "60-degree" triangle has 166.6666 degrees.

Chapter Six

Synopsis

There are many reasons to support the standard theory, the current explanation for the evolution of pyramid building in Egypt by the Pharaohs of five-thousand years ago. The burial buildings progressed from square mastabas, to one- or two-step mastabas, to four-step pyramids, to nine-step pyramids, to small smooth-sided pyramids, culminating with the large, smooth pyramids found at the Giza complex, which included the Great Pyramid. In all there are 80 pyramids. The religious-political structure supported the building of these monuments. No block was too small to move. There are not only 60-ton monoliths on sleds in the hieroglyphic record, but the mute testimony of four-thousand ton obelisks still standing, as well. The mathematics to calculate the circumference of the Earth was known by the Egyptians. They had the necessary tools, including hardened, bronze chisels to shape the millions of blocks used in the pyramids. The implication is that the bureau of weights and measures, the Great Pyramid, was conceived and built by the Pharaohs of Egypt, about three-thousand years B.C.

Chapter Six

DID THE EGYPTIANS BUILD
THE GREAT PYRAMID? YES!

The Technology of the Egyptians

The "standard theory" has evolved over hundreds of years and is based on logic that seems obvious and straightforward. It maintains that the ancient Egyptian builders, already creators of large, rectangular, solid burial buildings called mastabas, improved that basic design by stacking smaller mastabas on top to form step mastabas. As their mastery improved, more steps were added and this eventually led to what is known as step pyramids. The step pyramids evolved into the smooth-sided versions, the true pyramids, and this accounts for more than 80 pyramids, including several colossal ones at Dashur and Giza, and all of them are found on the west bank of the ancient Nile River. To an impressive degree, the detailed evidence supports this standard theory so convincingly that almost no one with an alternative theory has gained much support. To explain why this is so, some of the evidence must be examined in detail.

Deciphering the hieroglyphic writings of Egypt has helped to solidify the body of evidence into the accepted standard theory. That decoding of ancient written text was made possible when the Rosetta stone was discovered. Although the slab was damaged, it contained enough of an historical event (written not only in Egyptian hieroglyphics, but also in the Greek alphabet) that it allowed cross referencing and a quantum leap in understanding hieroglyphic analysis. One thing that evolved from this was a more precise understanding of the era's chronology of events since the lineage of the kings became understood. (See Reference 1 and 3.) The detailed King's List has a condensed form called a Dynasty List, which gives the time for each dynastic period of ancient Egypt. (See Table 6.1.)

A temple or other artifact found with a particular king's seal on it can be given an approximate date by using the King's List, so the probability of when each monument was built and which pharaoh constructed it can be determined. Many temples are literally covered with hieroglyphs and therefore an understanding of the religious and political concepts of the era became understood. What follows is a condensed version of the scientific interpretation, the standard theory, of how the religious belief system, the political structure, and the technology of ancient Egypt led to the building of colossal structures, including the Great Pyramid.

Dynasty	Period
I - II	Early Dynastic Period, 3100-2686 B.C.
III - VI	Old Kingdom, 2686-2181 B.C.
VII - X	First Intermediate Period, 2181-2133 B.C.
XI - XII	Middle Kingdom, 2133-1786 B.C.
XIII - XVII	Second Intermediate Period, 1786-1567 B.C.
XVIII - XX	New Kingdom, 1567-1080 B.C.
XXI - XXV	Late New Kingdom, 1080-664 B.C.
XXVI	Saite Period, 664-525 B.C.
XXVII - XXXI	Late Period, 525-332 B.C.

Table 6.1 Short version of the King's List

A religious belief of the Egyptians was that a human being was a physical body united with a spirit body, and that the spirit was immortal, but the body was not. Even after death the body played a vital part in this relationship and could not be discarded unceremoniously. Upon death the body had to be buried in such a way that it would be carefully preserved, so that the spirit could use it as the portal to reach the afterlife, the place of paradise. The more artifacts buried with the preserved body, the easier it would be for the spirit to survive in the afterlife. Many supplies, such as hunting implements, food, water, bangles, and beads, were considered "sacred articles" and buried with the body.

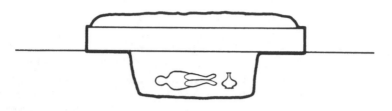

Figure 6.1 Depicts a common grave. The mound of sand is contained with a wooden frame. The pit, dug into sand, is lined with wood. The buried body is positioned in a fetal position, and close by are the sacred articles: food and drink, hunting equipment, jewelry, and so on.

Even before the dynastic period of the great pharaohs with great burial chambers, the bodies of nearly everyone were buried in shallow pits and placed on their sides with knees up to their chest. (See Figure 6.1.) The shallow grave meant that the body was surrounded by dry sand and the low moisture content discouraged microbial decomposition processes. Above the grave was a mound of sand held into position by a box-like structure of wood, locked at the ends. Under the mound and next to the body sacred gifts and articles were placed because it was thought the supplies would help the spirit in the next life. These simple burials would not last for too many years, because eventually the winds would blow the sand away, exposing the body to the sun and rain. Consequently, wealthy people made more elaborate burials.

Preparing for a proper Egyptian burial took on major importance in the lives of Egyptians and the devout spent most of their wealth on the tomb and other preparations for death. As a result, very little remains of the cities of the living, but much remains of the cities of the dead, the necropolises. Large and small burial tombs form many impressive necropolises scattered the length of Egypt which, fortunately for the investigators of antiquity, have become well-preserved time capsules.

Noblemen of great wealth constructed grand burial tombs called mastabas. The burial pit was usually dug into bedrock. Above the pit was the traditional mound of sand, and above that was a building composed of many cells. Each cell was first filled with sacred articles for the spirit, then filled with rubble. The final protective element was to cap the entire building with sun-baked mud bricks, a practice that evolved from the belief that the spirit could travel through walls and easily find the gifts. Surrounding the main building were two walls separated by a narrow pavement, again made of sun-baked mud brick. (See Figure 6.2.) Many of these mastabas remain today, proof of their effectiveness in preventing the elements from uncovering the buried body.

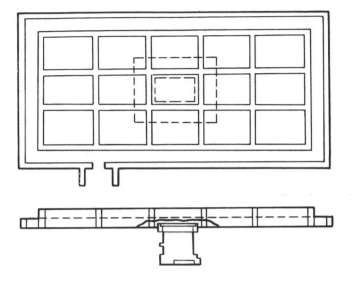

Figure 6.2 Ground plan and section view of a First Dynasty mastaba. Notice the mound of sand is still an essential feature and the numerous cells allow more room for the sacred articles.

As the burial practice evolved to the inclusion of precious jewelry and gold the wealth within the mastabas became targets for grave robbers who considered the sacred articles booty to be sold to the highest bidder. Determined grave robbers could burrow into the cells with relative ease, so the mastaba design was altered to prevent that. By the Second Dynasty, tombs were built by digging deeper into the bedrock and the body was placed in a room protected by a heavy portcullis door adjacent to the vertical shaft. This large, heavy slab of stone became a standard feature and was used for many centuries. The sacred gifts were no longer positioned in the cells of the mastabas, but were lowered and positioned into niches or small rooms at the bottom of the shaft to provide better protection. The final element of protection was that the entire shaft was filled with rubble and capped with sun-baked mud brick, over which the massive mastaba structure was built. (See Figure 6.3.)

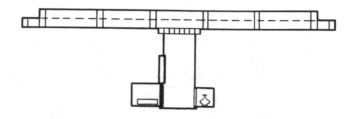

Figure 6.3 The Second Dynasty mastaba has a deep shaft filled with rubble and is capped with sun-dried brick. The body is protected with a massive stone portcullis door. The sacred articles are in a nearby niche.

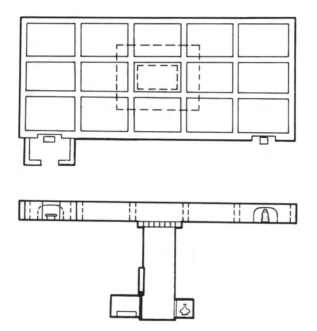

Figure 6.4 The Second Dynasty mastaba has niches on the east wall, the southernmost niche is an Offering room and the northern most niche contains a statue. The body is mummified and placed behind a protective portcullis. The sacred articles are in niches near the bottom.

Additional improvements at this time included small niches on the east side of the mastaba, which were used for offerings. The southernmost niche was sometimes surrounded by a small room, which evolved into the "offering room," a concept that was to continue even into the pyramid age, when an enlarged version of this special room was usually found attached to the east side of a pyramid.

One drawback to the deep burial technique was that the bodies quickly decayed because of the high moisture content at the lower depths. Recognition of the problem led to embalming or mummification, so with that improvement the mummified body and sacred articles could be buried at great depths, safe from both tomb robbers and moisture decay. (See Figure 6.4.)

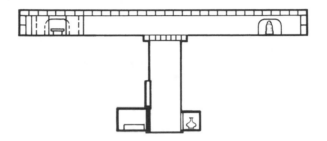

Figure 6.5 This diagram of a Third Dynasty mastaba shows the shaft cover and mastaba cover built of hard, durable stone.

A great technological improvement occurred in ancient Egypt at this time. The catalyst for the great renaissance was the arrival into Egypt of the famous intellectual, Imhotep, who introduced architectural improvements that resulted in the use of stone on a grand scale. Capping the monoliths with a layer of hard stone became the standard protective technique, and the use of sun-baked mud bricks was discarded. Limestone became popular because it was strong, hard and very durable. A high-quality version of the stone became known as Tura limestone, after the region in which it was mined. (See Figure 6.5.)

The king at that time, Zoser, employed Imhotep to design a grand mastaba using the new technology. This project was to be larger than anything of the time, 207 feet square and 26 feet high. It was built and surfaced with fine Tura limestone. This giant mastaba was a quantum accomplishment for that era, but this was not to be the final form for Zoser's monument. Apparently the success of the project inspired the builders to consider expanding the monument. First another fourteen feet were added all around, but at less than the original height, which gave it a step-like appearance. They must have considered the step architecture to be quite pleasing, because soon another step was added, this one 28 feet thick, to the east side. (See Figure 6.6.)

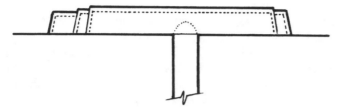

Figure 6.6 Zoser's huge mastaba was 207 feet square and 26 feet high. The mastaba was extended by a fourteen foot step all around. That project was followed by a 28-foot step to the east side.

Since each additional step was covered with the exquisite Tura limestone, it must have been considered the end of the project. The King and designer, however, must have been inspired by the appearance of the double step ascending into the sky. With a small leap of imagination a few more steps on top were added. In the process, the base was expanded, thus forming a truly huge step pyramid. Egypt became the home of the first step pyramid. It was a colossal structure by any standard, because when finished it was entirely capped in Tura limestone, and rose to a staggering 120 feet in four huge steps. (See Figure 6.7 and Note 1.)

The success of the four-step pyramid, however, was not the end of the project, as apparently the King and chief architect envisioned an even taller structure. A six-step pyramid that used the four-step pyramid as its core was designed and proved to be the last expansion of the pyramid. Even today it remains in this form in relatively good shape, proving that limestone surfacing is indeed an excellent protection against thousands of years of exposure.

In its final form the six-step pyramid, known as the Step Pyramid of Zoser, was 204 feet tall, a full ten times taller and 1,000 times more voluminous than any mastaba produced by previous dynasties. Add to that the fact that it was surrounded by a huge wall over 30 feet tall that formed an immense courtyard 912 feet by 1791 feet. Within the compound many ceremonial buildings were built.

The function of the complex, which contained offering chapels, is thought to have been the location for the "Heb-Sed," a jubilee ceremony. Kings enjoyed this ceremony after several years of fruitful rule. The ceremony was meant to be a reflection of and a reminder of the happiness to come in the afterlife. (See Reference 3.) Under the pyramid there exits not only a burial room with a coffer for the pharaoh, but eleven other shafts and burial chambers for members of the royal family. This maze of tunnels and niches is one of the most impressive Egyptian hypogea ever discovered. Scenes of King Zoser in religious ceremonies were carved on the walls of some rooms. Other niches were apparently for the sacred gifts and articles intended for the spirit.

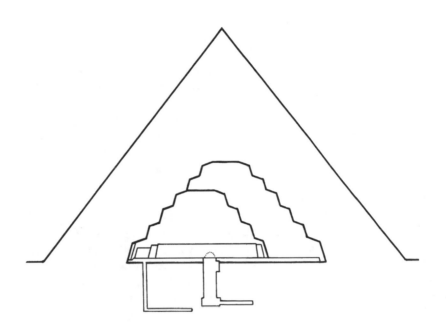

Figure 6.7 Depicted is Zoser's pyramid drawn at the same scale as the Great Pyramid, the largest pyramid in Egypt. The section view shows that the project evolved in distinct stages. The original mastaba was added to and completed with limestone to form a two-step mastaba. Next a third step was added, but to one side only. This success spurred the designers to expand the monument into a four-step pyramid. This, in turn, was enlarged to the final form, a six-step pyramid. Excavation below ground level formed a complex hypogeum that kept pace with the expansion project above. The section view gives a little hint of the interconnected shafts and passageways that were created on a level far below the surface. The tunnels, cut from the existing bedrock, were exquisitely finished with tile and decorations. Compared to mastaba monuments of that time, this mastaba-pyramid monument represented a work factor of over 1000, an impressive quantum leap for one pharaoh.

The building project, employing thousands of men, must have stimulated the economy, much like the road building projects of today. This is likely why each succeeding pharaoh attempted similar projects. The routine construction of pyramids resulted in almost 80 pyramids being started on the west side of the Nile River. The smallest of these pyramid monuments is 60 feet tall, which is ten times the volume of any mastaba ever built, and even more impressive when considering that the volume is not hollow, but solid masonry. The range of the size of the pyramid projects was quite dramatic. The Great Pyramid, which is almost 480 feet tall and rests on a base area of seven city blocks, is 2,000 times as voluminous as the 60 foot pyramid.

The Pyramid Comparison

To understand the standard theory, it is very important to look at some of the pyramids built in the period between Zoser's pyramid and the period of the great pyramids at the Giza complex. This study will show how the building technique and ceremonial complex design evolved, and on the face of it, supports the tenets of the standard theory.

The pyramids of Egypt generally look so old that many of them appear to be no more than mounds of sand. Because of their age, quite a physical and intellectual effort has been required to match each pyramid with its builder. The first 25 pyramids, including the small subsidiary pyramids, are attributed to builders of the Old Kingdom, the Second Dynasty through the Fourth Dynasty. (See Table 6.1.) During the end of this period the Great Pyramid was built. The standard theory states that the evolution of pyramid architecture followed a transition from mastabas to step pyramids, and finally to true pyramids, the pyramids with smooth sides. The facts seem to support this and, as stated, Zoser's complex at Saqqara documents many starts and changes proving that the original mastaba grew in width, then in height and evolved into the first step pyramid. As the stone masons mastered their skills, they apparently attempted larger and larger structures.

An early question that had to be resolved was how much masonry could the Earth support. Perhaps caution in this matter dictated the many starts and stops observed to Zoser's pyramid. Another question would have been how to deal with occasional earthquakes. The apparent solution used by the early builders was to build around a central core with a 75 degree slope. The core was faced with limestone before succeeding layers were built against it. Each layer was built with the inner stone, an inferior soft stone quarried locally, but finished with a protective covering of hard limestone. Most of the early pyramids employed this method, which evolved from the success at Saqqara. (See Figure 6.8.)

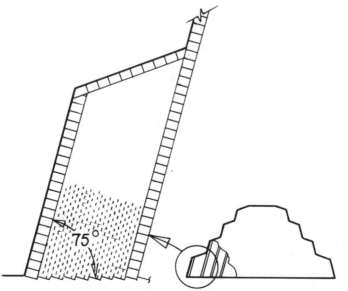

Figure 6.8 Ground settling and earthquake considerations may have been the reason why the builders of the first pyramids used the technique of building in layers around a sloping core.

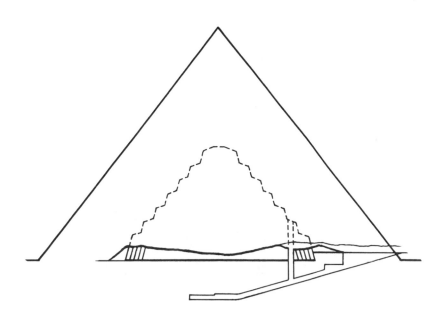

Figure 6.9 Depicted is the Buried Pyramid, the second pyramid of Egypt, drawn at the same scale as the great Pyramid. The dotted lines indicate that the pyramid, which was probably intended to have seven steps, was never completed. Solid lines indicate what remains of the layered core and part of the hypogeum beneath the aborted project.

The remains of the next pyramid, the second, were found just southwest and very close to Zoser's pyramid at Saqqara. Its foundation and shafts are buried in rubble and it has acquired the designation the Buried Pyramid. There is some evidence to suggest that the builder is Sekhemkhet. The pyramid was never finished because the king reigned for only six years. Based on what remains of the core, the Buried Pyramid was probably intended to be a seven-step pyramid. (See Figure 6.9.) In contrast to the rubble pile above, the hypogeum beneath was completed and a U-shaped long corridor had 132 compartments carved into it at staggered intervals.

The next pyramid, the third, is located at Zawiyet El-Aryan just north of Saqqara, but south of Giza. The rubble remains of the pyramid are very much like the second pyramid in style of construction and state of completion. Its core is visible and looks like layers from above, hence the name Layer Pyramid. It is thought that Khaba, a king of the Third Dynasty, started the pyramid, intending it to be a seven-step pyramid. Like the Buried Pyramid, it has a complex hypogeum beneath. It has 32 compartments arranged in very regular fashion. (See Figure 6.10.)

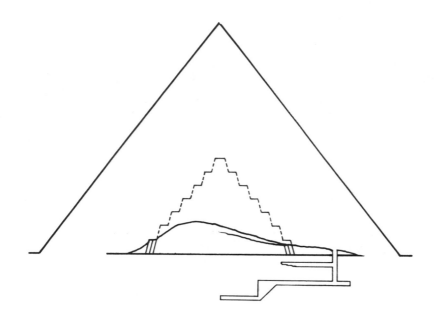

Figure 6.10 Depicted is the Layered Pyramid, the third pyramid of Egypt, drawn at the same scale as the Great Pyramid. The dotted lines indicate that the pyramid, which was probably intended to have seven steps, was never completed. Solid lines indicate what remains of the layered core and part of the hypogeum beneath the aborted project.

The fourth, fifth, sixth, and seventh pyramids are also step pyramids, but they are found away from the capital in outlying areas. There is some question as to whether they are royal pyramids at all. The fourth pyramid found at Seila and the fifth pyramid found at Zawiyet el-Mayitin are badly decomposed and probably had three steps. They are comparatively small, with square bases of about 84 and 59 feet respectively, and may have been finished economically in plaster and not limestone. No entrance has yet been found, but at the center of the base there may be a simple pit and tomb similar to another small pyramid with a square base of 62 feet, the sixth, which had four steps and was found at Nagada. Sir Flinders Petrie conducted excavations in 1896 and found, cut into the living rock, a simple pit at the baseline, positioned beneath the center of the pyramid. The pit was empty, yielding no clues as to the king or nobleman responsible for it. (See Figure 6.11.) The seventh pyramid found at El-Kula has a square base only 62 feet on a side, and the corners, not the faces, point to the cardinal points. It had only three steps, and being very distant from a source of good limestone, was finished with a plaster exterior. No entrance has been found and it, like the others, is assumed to have only a simple pit cut out of bedrock at the center of the base.

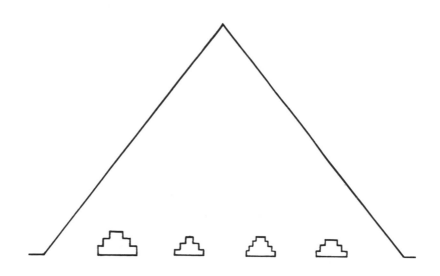

Figure 6.11 Four small step pyramids drawn to scale relative to the Great Pyramid

The eighth pyramid has had an interesting history and represents an important turning point in the design of pyramids. This pyramid was apparently designed and built in the established technique of building around a sloping core, and finished as a step pyramid, but later it was turned into a smooth-sided pyramid. This eighth pyramid is located at Maidum and is thought to have been started by King Huni, who completed it with seven steps. Later enlarged, it was turned into an eight-step pyramid. This pyramid, with a base of 482 feet square and a height of 307 feet, was the largest step pyramid ever finished after the time of Zoser.

The success of the step pyramid of Maidum inspired the next king, Snofru, to improve the megalith in an entirely new way. With great effort, his builders used limestone to fill in the steps and make the sides smooth. Snofru is accredited with being the first pharaoh to complete the first "true" pyramid. A small subsidiary pyramid, considered here as the ninth pyramid, is also found at the Maidum site and just to the south of his large pyramid. The precise size of the small subsidiary pyramid, as well as its function, is unknown as it remains in a state of almost total ruin, and whether it was a step or true pyramid remains unanswered. (See Figure 6.12.)

King Snofru not only created the first true pyramid, but also set a precedent for succeeding pharaohs with the level of perfection his multi-element complex reached. The walled complex contained not only the main true pyramid, but at least one smooth-sided subsidiary pyramid. In addition, the funeral would be conducted in complete privacy out of view of the laborers and, hopefully, the grave robbers. This was achieved by enclosing the grand "mortuary temple," usually built within the tall walls of the complex adjacent to and on the east face of the large pyramid. Additionally, the walls were extended along a long "causeway" to a "valley building" located either on the Nile River or a canal connected to the Nile.

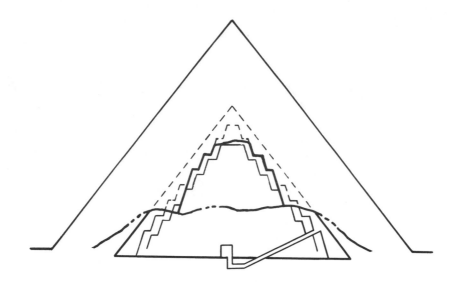

Figure 6.12 The First True Pyramid, the pyramid of Maidum, is drawn to the same scale as the Great Pyramid. The solid lines indicate what remains today. It appears that the sides collapsed exposing the sloping core. The hypogeum of the pyramid, if any, remains to be discovered.

The sequence of the funeral was this: the body of each pharaoh arrived by boat at the valley building, was moved via the causeway to the mortuary temple for embalming, and then finally carried through secret passageways to a coffer deep within, and usually beneath, the pyramid. After this, great effort was made to conceal the egress to the sarcophagus.

Snofru was a prolific builder. According to clues available, he also built the tenth pyramid, the "Bent" (named for its shape), the subsidiary pyramid or the eleventh pyramid, and the the North Pyramid or twelfth pyramid. This large pyramid is a short distance to the north of the Bent Pyramid complex. All of these pyramids are located at Dashur.

The Bent Pyramid is smooth sided except for the distinct change of angle about halfway up the sides, giving it two angles. The first is 54° 28" at the foundation level and then 43° 22" at the upper level. Like all pyramids up to that time, it is built of blocks sloping inward at 75 degrees. Within its protective layer of limestone, it survives amazingly well. The Bent Pyramid complex was planned with a large mortuary temple, one subsidiary pyramid, and a causeway leading to the valley building. (See Figure 6.13.)

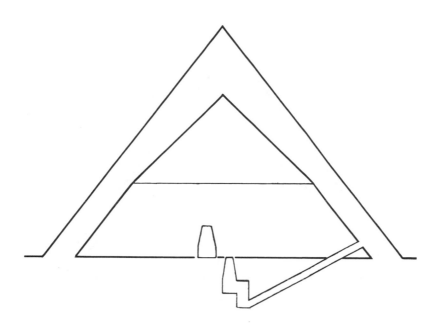

Figure 6.13 Depicted is the Bent Pyramid drawn to the same scale as the Great Pyramid. The name of the Bent Pyramid is obviously due to its bent appearance. The slope angle changes abruptly from about 54 degrees at the base to about 43 degrees at the upper half. Beneath the pyramid are two large chambers with corbeled ceilings. The pyramid also has two entrances to the interior, one from the north and a second from the west.

The North Pyramid, also called "Shining Pyramid" in some texts, represents an important architectural change, being the first pyramid built with rows of level, horizontally positioned blocks of soft limestone on the interior, and faced with hard, durable limestone on the outside. This technique was used in all succeeding major pyramids. The other unusual feature of the North Pyramid is the slope of its sides. Instead of nearly 52 degrees, as with many pyramids, it was only 43° 22". There is speculation that this angle, which is the same as the top half of the Bent Pyramid, was chosen for economy. The top half of the Bent also appears to have been a hasty effort.

Despite the lack of attention to building quality, Snofru appears to be the unsurpassed builder of pyramids. He experimented with Huni's step pyramid by turning it into the first True Pyramid. He then hastily finished the top of his own pyramid, the Bent Pyramid, so he could have time, or finances, to experiment with the first true pyramid built in horizontal rows, the North Pyramid. Besides these three large pyramids, just south of the Bent Pyramid, Snofru built the subsidiary pyramid, which is relatively large, measuring 107 feet at the base and 84 feet in height. In addition to the pyramids are the ceremonial buildings: the mortuary temples, the causeways, and the valley buildings, all of which are constructed of stone blocks. Even discounting these buildings, Snofru presided over the altering and building of four pyramids, the total volume of which far exceeds the volume of the Great Pyramid. That is quite an accomplishment.

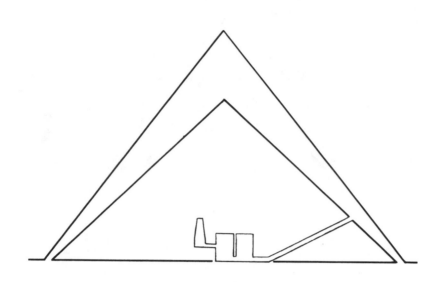

Figure 6. 14 Depicted is the North Pyramid drawn to the same scale as the Great Pyramid. There is one entrance on the north side and it leads to large corbeled chambers near the base and within the pyramid. This appears to be the first pyramid built in horizontal rows, a construction technique that was to be used on large pyramids thereafter.

Pharaoh Snofru had two sons who also became the rulers of Egypt. One of his sons, Khufu, or Cheops in Greek, is credited with building the Great Pyramid, which is located at Giza on a high plateau just west of the city of Cairo. This pyramid is not only the largest pyramid in terms of volume, it has the most complex internal features. Rising almost 480 feet to the apex, it is the tallest pyramid. (See Figure 6.15.)

A summary of the forced entry into the Great Pyramid in more recent times by Al Mamun is presented here, because it describes some of the unusual internal elements of this special pyramid. In 640 A.D. Al Mamun and his team of over 100 treasure-seeking men could not distinguish the door on the north side from the countless other blocks, so they gained entry into the Great Pyramid by brute force. They first built a huge fire on the north side to heat the smooth limestone red hot and then doused it with cold vinegar, thus cracking the limestone. They hammered and chiseled their way into the stone until the Descending Passage was found. A stone had fallen from the ceiling of this Descending Passage and it appeared that the stone was the cover for yet another passage, the Ascending Passage. Many granite plugs, however, were found to be blocking this passage. They were too heavy to move and so with great difficulty, Al Mamun's men chiseled their way upward and around the granite plugs.

The treasure seekers finally gained access to the Ascending Passageway that led to the two chambers within the body of the Great Pyramid. The lower chamber had a peaked ceiling, a typical feature found in burial chambers for queens of that time. It was thought to have been intended for the queen and so is usually referred to as the Queen's Chamber. The upper chamber had a flat ceiling, a typical feature found in the burial

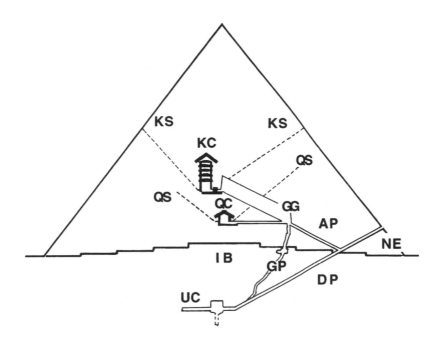

Figure 6.15 Depicted is the Great Pyramid, the largest pyramid in Egypt. The list of symbols that define some of the complex features of the pyramid are: NE = north side entrance to Descending Passage, DP = Descending Passage, UC = Unfinished Chamber, IB = irregular bedrock, AP = Ascending Passage, GG = Grand Gallery, QC = Queen's Chamber, QS = shaft from Queen's Chamber, KS = shaft from King's Chamber, GP = irregular Grotto Passage and Grotto Room, KC = King's Chamber.

chambers for the king. It was, therefore, thought to have been intended for the king, and is now called the King's Chamber.

This upper chamber contained one large sarcophagus without a lid. It was just such a coffer that had spurred Al Mamun on, believing it to be filled with gold and jewelry. Al Mamun was already a rich man, and was personally seeking maps of the planet reported to be hidden within the Great Pyramid.

Alas, to the disappointment of the workmen who were to share in the booty, the sarcophagus and the entire chamber were completely empty. Having found the sarcophagus empty, they concluded that other treasure seekers had somehow gotten there first. The fact that Al Mamun discovered torch marks on the ceiling of the pit at the bottom of the Descending Passageway convinced him that others had gained entry by another path in earlier times. Other investigators later discovered the "Grotto" and the irregular passage connecting it to the Descending Passage and to the upper passageways. It seemed obvious to them that this, in conjunction with some other passageway under the Great Pyramid or possibly the main entry door, was used by the original grave robbers. The rumor that the Sphinx and the Great Pyramid are connected via a tunnel or even a "maze of tunnels" is repeated in many writings, but at this time only the passageways and chambers shown in Figure 6.15 have been found.

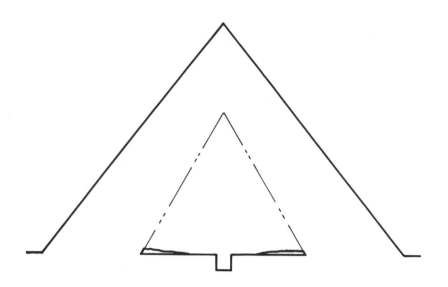

Figure 6.16 The Seheder-Star Pyramid of Djedefre drawn to the same scale as the Great Pyramid. The dotted lines indicate that the pyramid was never finished. What remains of the pyramid is indicated by solid lines.

Like the North Pyramid, the Great Pyramid was built with the new technique, horizontal rows capped with limestone casing blocks. Only two of these fine limestone casing blocks at the base are still in position for examination. After an earthquake destroyed Cairo in 840 A.D., the Great Pyramid became a convenient quarry for limestone to rebuild the buildings and the mosques of the damaged city.

There are three subsidiary pyramids on the east side and the remains of the offering temple, causeway, and valley building are evident. Khufu's name is found in the offering temple and the remains of his mother, Queen Hetepheres, reburied after her tomb at Dashur was plundered, has been found near the northeast corner of the Great Pyramid.

The sarcophagus of the Great Pyramid found by Al Mamun did not bear the name of Khufu. Tompkins, however, discovered a small access hole to the chamber above the ceiling of the King's Chamber and found what appears to be Khufu's name upside down on a block. The name on this inaccessible block is used to prove that the Great Pyramid was built during the reign of Khufu. Similar marks were found on the sixth course behind the now-missing casing blocks. Samuel Birch identified one as "belonging to Suphis, Shoto, or Khufu..." which is used as further evidence that Khufu was the true builder of the Great Pyramid.

After Khufu, a king by the name of Djedefre built the seventeenth pyramid at Abu Roash, five miles north of Giza. It was not faced with limestone, but with granite. It is quite obliterated, however, and whether it was ever finished seems questionable. The foundation outline of the causeway and offering temple have been found. The use of mud brick, and even the hasty finish of the offering temple implies that the king died before it was completed. (See Figure 6.16.)

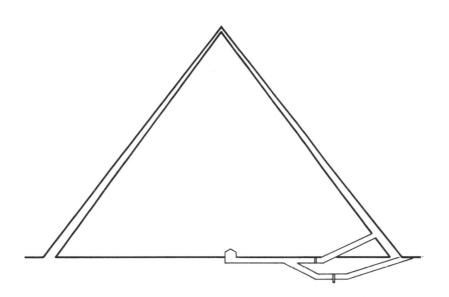

Figure 6.17 Khephren's Pyramid drawn to the same scale as the Great Pyramid. This pyramid still has limestone protecting its peak and is in relatively good condition. Entrance to the chamber is from the north side. An apparently abandoned passage is nearby and below the true entrance.

After the rule of Djedefre, another son of Snofru, Khephren, gained the throne and is credited with the building of the 19th and 20th pyramids. The 19th is known as the "second pyramid at Giza," and the 20th pyramid, a small subsidiary pyramid built just to the south, exists in a state of obliteration. Khephren's large pyramid is almost as large as the Great Pyramid in size. The square base of 707 feet is only 48 feet shorter than the Great Pyramid. Due to its steep slope, it rises to an impressive height of 471 feet, only ten feet shorter than the Great Pyramid. In photographs it actually appears to be taller than the Great Pyramid because it was built on ground of slightly higher elevation. (See Fig. 6.17.)

Khephren's Pyramid appears to have been as solidly built and of the same technology as the Great Pyramid. It is one of the best-preserved pyramids and still has its cap of limestone intact. Only the lower portions of the limestone outer casing blocks are missing. The Khephren complex had the traditional grand offering temple on the east side of the main pyramid connected by a causeway to the valley building. One unusual feature is the two entrances on the north side. It appears that the lowest was a remaining element of an aborted start. It is thought that because higher quality rock for the base was discovered nearby during the initial phase of construction the decision was to stop construction and restart 100 feet further to the south. This is another grand example of changes made after construction had commenced. Because of this change of plan, a second descending passage, the higher entrance, was built.

The 21st pyramid is located at Zawiyet el-Aryan. While it is unfinished and its builder unknown, its substructure is very similar to that of the 17th pyramid. With an open-trench design, it would have had a base of 686 square feet had it ever been completed. The unusual feature of the tomb of this pyramid is that the floor was paved in red

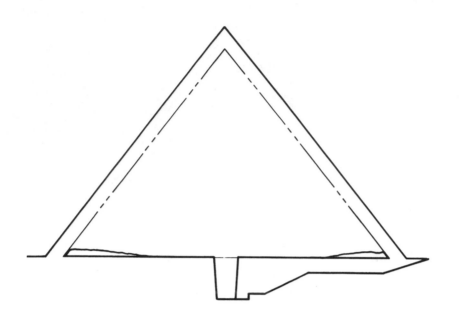

Figure 6.18 The Unfinished Pyramid drawn to the same scale as the Great Pyramid. The reference lines indicate that the pyramid was never finished. The lower solid lines indicate what remains of the project today.

granite. An oval granite coffer "without parallel in form," according to Edwards, was carved into the floor. (Figure 6.18.)

The 21st pyramid is the final main pyramid at the Giza complex, smaller than the other two main pyramids, but of similar construction. The 21st pyramid and its three subsidiary pyramids were built during the reign of Menkauré, or Mycerins in Greek. This pyramid, known as the Third Pyramid of Giza, has a 340-foot square base and a height of 212 feet. There is evidence that Menkauré died an untimely death. The valley building, the causeway, the offering temple, and two of the three subsidiary pyramids appear to have been finished hastily and with inferior materials. An interesting feature is that the double entrance leading to the burial chamber has three granite portcullises fitted in vertical slots and carved into the walls. They were similar to the ones found protecting the King's Chamber of the Great Pyramid according to Ricke, the investigator who claims the builders used rollers over the top of each slot and a system of ropes so that the heavy doors could be lowered into place. (See Figure 6.19.)

The three subsidiary pyramids at the Menkauré complex constitute the 22nd, 23rd, and 24th pyramids. While many more pyramids were built after this period, these first 24 pyramids truly reflect the old tradition, and demonstrate the evolution of the mortuary temple, subsidiary pyramids, the causeway, and the valley building. After these 24 pyramids and the surrounding temple buildings were built, the focus shifted away from pyramid building to statues, relief carvings, and hieroglyphic renderings on the walls of the valley building and within the mortuary temples.

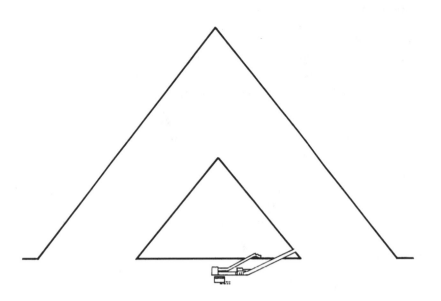

Figure 6.19 The pyramid of Mcnkurc´ at Giza drawn to the same scale as the Great Pyramid. This small pyramid is still in good condition. Solid lines indicate passage ways and chamber that were cut out of the bedrock.

In this post-pyramid era, if a pyramid was used as part of a complex, the materials for the interiors were either rubble or small, inferior stones. As a result, once the limestone covering was damaged or stolen, the interior quickly weathered. Today, piles of sand are the only evidence that these pyramids ever existed.

Following this 500-year Old Kingdom period was another period of over 500 years, during which the pyramid as an architectural element was discontinued altogether. What followed was another revivalist period of almost 1,000 years during which the pyramid structure was used more to add a decorative touch. For example, mortuary complexes favored columns as the main theme, but four or more columns were quite often used to support a small, elevated pyramid. Many of these architectural elements were used throughout the design. (See References 1 and 3.)

So it is the first 24 pyramids that constitute the real evolution of the pyramid in Egypt, from the simple burial pits to mud brick mastabas, from mud brick mastabas to stone mastabas, from stone mastabas to stone step mastabas or step pyramids, and finally from step pyramids to true pyramids. The grandest of these are found at the Giza complex where the Great Pyramid is located. The logic for the standard theory seems to leave little room for doubt. If the obvious evolution over time in the shape of these burial tombs is not enough evidence, there is more confirmation when considering the technology of the Egyptians and their use of canals to irrigate their crops along the Nile River. An explanation of this technology follows.

Technology of the Egyptians

Much has been written about the difficulty a low-technology agrarian society would have cutting, transporting, and lifting into place the two to three million blocks of the Great Pyramid. The average weight of the blocks is said to have been two tons, but each casing block weighed 36 tons. Could the Egyptians have accomplished this by hand labor? To investigate the possibility of moving heavy, dense objects by hand labor, the author performed an experiment to prove that on a small scale, the techniques are not only quite simple, but very effective. In one experiment a two-ton metal and fiberglass mold was easily moved about by first wedging it up enough to position two-inch-diameter steel pipes under the metal skids at the base. When all contact surfaces are dense and hard, friction is kept to a minimum. The floor was smooth, hard concrete so the steel pipes rolled easily. One man could easily move the object and as one roller exited at the rear, it was carried to the front to be reinserted and the process was repeated. (See Figure 6.20.)

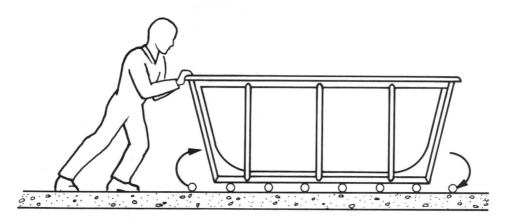

Figure 6.20 Heavy objects can easily be moved horizontally if the sled, rollers, and pavement are of hard materials. Note that the two-inch steel pipes are used repeatedly.

In the 1940s and 1950s, trains, homes and factories were still fueled with coal. Coal hoppers were regularly uncoupled and left on a side rail for unloading. A single workman could move 160-ton coal cars several car lengths to align with the conveyor belt at the unloading dock. Moving rail cars can be accomplished by wedging a long iron crowbar tool between the wheel and the track and then lifting upward. Although slow, a workman can move the heavy load because a hard metal wheel on a hard metal rail results in very low friction. Applying the same principle, the lubricated hard-axle bearings easily roll within the hard metal-bearing jacket, resulting in low friction for the axle.

These examples, however, demonstrate a single man moving massive weights along a horizontal plane. How could steep inclines be mastered? The answer is simply more man power. It has been calculated that gangs of men could move a heavy monolith mounted on a greased sled up a steep incline.

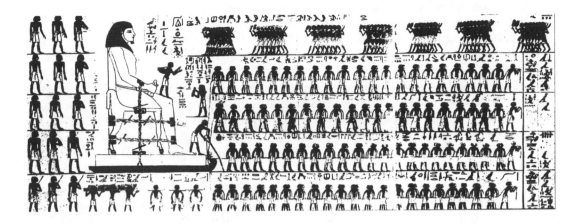

Figure 6.21 This Egyptian hieroglyph depicts details of moving a colossus. Notice especially the greaser lubricating the path for the sled, the cadence keeper, and 168 men in four rows.

There is hieroglyphic evidence that the Egyptians had mastered this, as shown in Figure 6.21, which is a scene from the tomb of Djehutihotpe at Deir-el-Bersha as copied by John Gardner Wilkinson before 1856. Commander F.M. Barber estimated that 900 men harnessed in double rank to four draft ropes could easily drag a 60-ton monolith mounted onto a greased sled up a ramp of 1:25 ratio. Such a gang would be 225 feet long and 16 feet wide. Men trained to heave on command "one, two, three, heave" produce a force more than the total weight of the men. Cattle or camels, by comparison, cannot be as well organized or drilled. (See Reference 5.)

The colossal temple complexes of Egypt occasionally contain obelisks, tall square columns topped with a pyramid shape. Some of these single stone structures weighing 4,000 tons are quarried hundreds of miles away. If moving a 60-ton monolith is comparatively easy with a properly greased sled and an organized and motivated work gang, how were the giant obelisks moved? The greased sled solution would require an extremely large army. Comparing the 60-ton monolith to the 4,000 ton obelisk, the calculation would yield:

$$4,000 \text{ tons} / 60 \text{ tons} \times 900 \text{ men} = 60,000 \text{ men}$$

Since a work gang of 6,000 men would have been impossible, there must have been a simpler solution. A clue is the many ten-foot diameter, cylindrical (untapered) columns found in many of the temples in Egypt. At Karnak, for example, 100-foot columns were made by stacking as many as ten of the sections that are ten feet in diameter and ten feet in length. Obviously it occurred to the builders that rolling a column section to its location was easier than dragging it on its square end, and that rolling it on a stone surface was much easier than rolling it through the sand. Similar stone "wheels" could have been positioned under an obelisk at the quarry and stone tracks could have been positioned to reduce the friction. (See Figure 6.22.)

In Figure 6.23, one solution for positioning the heavy obelisk upon the rollers is to carefully chisel the under portion of the obelisk as it is still in the quarry, then rolling many column sections into position and placing a wedge in the small gap as necessary. Once all rollers are in place and the last bit of living rock is carved away, the obelisk is ready to roll along the track. Within the first quarter rotation of the rollers, the wedges fall away and the obelisk settles directly upon the rollers. As rail and rollers exit at the rear they are rolled back to the front to be used repeatedly. The transit time to the site could even allow workers to smooth, polish and carve the top and sides while moving slowly on the long journey. Contrary to this speculation, however, there is at least one obelisk that was finished in place, and still remains in the quarry, with the bottom side unfinished.

If the workers could move an obelisk and average one thousand feet per day, the 400-mile journey would take six years, well within the time span of any ruler. Or, part of the trip may have been by large boat, as the Egyptians were skilled boat builders. Whatever method or combination of methods was used, Egyptian engineers moved 4,000 ton obelisks.

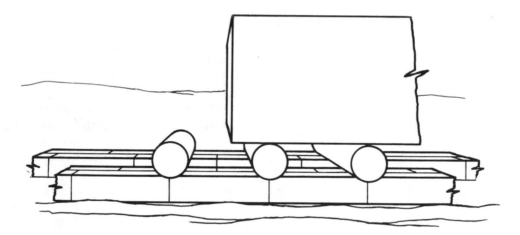

Figure 6.22 Depicted is a long obelisk riding on a stone track. The round rollers are similar to Egyptian column sections. The stone track is similar to Egyptian temple blocks. The hypothetical low-friction technique would eliminate the army size work force required to move the huge block by sled.

There is some evidence to suggest that hardened metal was used to shape granite and limestone rock into finished elements for the stone temples. Hardened copper tools dating as early as the First Dynasty have been uncovered at Saqqara. (See Reference 3.) This seems to lend some truth to the hypothesis that two-ton and larger stones were carved from distant quarries and moved by sled to the temple construction sites. This, however, brings up another question, could the Egyptians carve that many blocks in the reign of one pharaoh? Some brush this consideration aside saying that the Egyptians had thousands of years to patiently chip, carve, and move stone blocks. But what about the superhuman efforts of Snofru and his two sons? How, in the span of their 100-year rule, could the work force carve and move more blocks than the motivated pharaohs of the next 1500 years of Egyptian history? The answer is that the Egyptians often used concrete.

An excellent book that deals with this issue as well as the problem of stone density used in later Egyptian eras is *The Pyramids, an Enigma Solved* by Joseph Davidovits. (See Reference 7.) Davidovits is an expert in "agglomeration technique," which can form geopolymer stone possessesing the same properties of natural stone into any shape. Examples of this are very hard diorite granite and the most dense forms of limestone. Only a geopolymer expert can tell the difference between natural and man-made stone. Davidovits inspected the amazing Egyptian stonework: the tiny beads with hair-fine holes (very difficult to drill even today), the thousands of pots and vases beneath Zoser's Step Pyramid (there are no known tools that can fit down the thin necks of some of these vases), and the colossal blocks found in the temple buildings and the pyramids. He found evidence that they were actually made in molds and not carved from rock as previously believed.

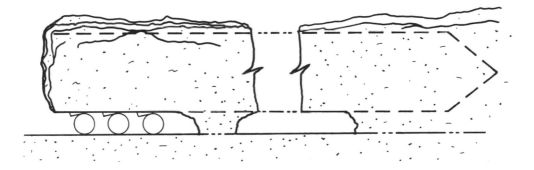

Figure 6.23 Hypothetical concept shows an obelisk partly carved from the quarry. The undersurface is finished first so that rollers could fit into place with wedges taking up the slack. The pavement is either quarry rock cut smooth, or block slabs, moved and used repeatedly like the rollers.

Concrete is an example of a common agglomeration formula that uses Portland cement as the binder and an endless variety of gravel and sand of various shapes, sizes, and compositions as the filler. When Portland cement, concrete, or any other formula of agglomeration mixture is poured into a mold and worked into position, several things can be noted with the naked eye. The resulting piece takes on the finish of the mold. A finely sanded mold, such as the long-necked vases and statues found in Egypt, will yield a stone piece with no tool marks. There will also be tiny air pockets visible on the surface, and some of the air pockets will be elongated, a sign of working the slurry into position.

When large blocks are made in a mold, it is sometimes necessary to stop the pour and let the exothermic reaction (heat given off during drying) take place to prevent cracking. Once cool, the pouring continues, but the delay causes a "weft" (usually a curving line) that is quite visible since small aggregates rise and are found near the top of a worked agglomeration. Any wavy line with large aggregates visible above smaller aggregates identifies the weft line. Examples are easily found in any modern concrete column where the mold has been removed and the surface left unpainted. Davidovits has photographed weft lines in many of the colossal stones of the Egyptian monuments.

Besides easily observed evidence, there is the evidence that can only be seen with a microscope. Naturally occurring nummulitic limestone is comprised of small calcium-carbonate skeletal remains called foraminifers. These accumulate over millions of years forming sedimentary layers of bedrock and as such, the fossil shells lie horizontally or flat in the natural bedrock that it forms. Upon close examination of the limestone in the Great Pyramid, however, one does not observe that pattern. Instead, the small fossil shells are in a randomly-oriented pattern as one would expect after a slurry has cured.

There are other details that support Davidovits' claim that the agglomeration technique was known and used by the Egyptians. The mining of huge blocks from quarries in the standard scenario implies the finishing of each side of these huge blocks and that type of construction is many times more difficult than pouring agglomeration into finished molds. These difficulties compound when extremely hard varieties of stone are considered. Also, had all the blocks of the Great Pyramid been quarried as in the standard theory, there would be huge mounds of chips rivaling the size of the pyramids themselves, but no such remains have been located. The reason is that all of the chips were crushed and turned into another agglomerated stone block. It is far easier to carry small sacks of gravel and binder to the top of a monolithic temple than one large finished block.

Davidovits shows that the agglomeration technique is a simple technology well within the grasp of the Egyptians and gives details of the formulas used by them. The formulas were easy to use since the slurries are formed and cure at room temperatures, and no kiln is needed. Several different binder formulations were used and each was of a higher quality than the Portland cement commonly used today. Part of the ingredients were readily available from the mud of the Nile River or the dried lake beds in various parts of Egypt, while the rare mineral part of the formula was obtained from mining.

An important text has been discovered by researchers that sheds light on Egyptian concrete technology. A cuneiform tablet, the Palermo Stone, holds records of Royal achievements. Among them are the efforts of Snofru, who sent expeditions to Lebanon for cedar wood, perhaps to make molds for the huge blocks for the many temples that he built, and also to retrieve the ingredients needed for the binder. Snofru's men obviously worked those mines with great activity and persistence as the mines were known as Snofru's mines 1,000 years after his rule. Snofru's name is also on a monument in the cliffs of the Sinai, which is what one would expect of the builder of so many temples and pyramids.

Although the Egyptians had the technology to build the Great Pyramid, what about the mathematics embodied by its geometry? How did they calculate the circumference of the Earth? The answer may be in the very obelisks that were built so smoothly and oriented so precisely. The shining sun at high noon on two 200-foot obelisks, separated north and south by a few miles, will produce different shadow lengths.

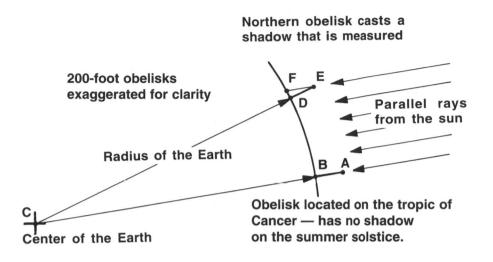

Northern obelisk casts a shadow that is measured

200-foot obelisks exaggerated for clarity

Parallel rays from the sun

Radius of the Earth

Obelisk located on the tropic of Cancer — has no shadow on the summer solstice.

Center of the Earth

Figure 6.24 Depicted is the center of the Earth, the curve of the Earth, and two oversize obelisks separated by about ten degrees, which was reasonable in Egypt. Sun rays, on the summer solstice, yield only the shadow FD on the northernmost obelisk.

Simple trigonometry can be used to calculate the radius of the Earth from which the circumference can easily be derived. (See Reference 5.) This is shown in Figure 6.24, in which similar triangles are formed by the shadow cast by obelisk ED and the alignment of the sun with obelisk AB on the summer solstice. Obelisk AB is located on the tropic of Cancer and casts no shadow. Obelisk ED is located many miles north and hence casts a shadow of length FD, which is carefully recorded. A mathematical ratio results:

ED/DC = FD/DB

The only unknown distance in the equation is the radius of the Earth, DC, and it is easily calculated by transposing terms:

DC = (ED x DB)/FD

Another way to calculate the Earth's circumference, called the rising star method, involves watching a rising star in the east. (See Reference 5.) In this case, two obelisks are separated east and west by about ten miles and observers are at the base of each. The observer to the east sees the rising star first. He instantly signals this event, perhaps by light signals, to the observer to the west. There are two observers to the west. The one at the top of the obelisk sees the candlelight and shouts for the start of the time count. Some 22 seconds later the ground observer sees the rising star and records the interval. Another variation of the same technique is to observe when the star crosses the meridian line above the peak of the obelisk. In either case the distance between the obelisk is known, as

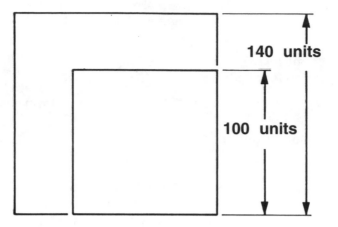

Figure 6.25 Depicted is a square in one corner of a larger square. The small square is 100 units on a side. The large square is 140 units on a side. The large square has twice the area compared to the small square.

is the number of seconds in one complete revolution of the planet, so the circumference of the Earth is calculated by simple trigonometry:

Circumference = 86,400/interval (in seconds) X distance between obelisks.

The slope of the Great Pyramid, as stated before, is such that the height of the Great Pyramid relates to the perimeter at the base in the exact proportion as the radius of a circle relates to the circumference of a circle. The evidence that the Egyptians knew of this ratio is quite clear. According to Stecchini, the Egyptians and other ancient civilizations used seven as a basis for counting linear distance and solving everyday problems of their agrarian society. (See Reference 5.) Hieroglyphic records show that problems involving distance, area, volume, and even a close approximation of the value for pi, were easily calculated and commonly used a handful of "magic ratios" involving seven and/or eleven. The following example illustrates how. If a farmer was a productive worker and was rewarded by giving him twice as much land as he had before, how would the new patch be calculated and measured? Assume he had a patch as in Figure 6.25.

If the existing patch was measured to be 350 feet long, how many feet would yield a patch double in area? First, divide the 350 in 100 equal units. This equals 3.5 feet. Make a rod 3.5 feet long and measure 140 rods in each direction. This new area is exactly twice the previous patch. Why? The "magic formula" used by the Egyptians is a sequence based on multiples of seven.

Base (any units)	Base^2 = Area	Error
70	4, 900 (about 1/2 x 10,000)	2%
100	10,000 (Set original to this size)	
140	19,600 (about 2 x 10,000)	2%

The modified form used for greater precision was:

Base (any units)	Base^2 = Area	Error
70	4,900 (about 1/2 x 9,801)	.01%
99	9,801 (set original to this size.)	
140	19,600 (about 2 x 9,801.)	.01%

Notice that compared to the 100-foot square, the 70-foot square has about one-half the area, and notice how the 140-foot square has about double the area (2% error). When the modified form was used, the 70:99:140 sequence, notice that when compared to the 99-foot square, the 70-foot square has very nearly one-half the area, and the 140-foot square has very nearly double the area. Yielding errors of less than one part in 10,000, the precision is quite remarkable.

Another "magic" method, based on seven, quickly accomplishes what the Pythagorean formula accomplished with great difficulty.

$$a^2 + b^2 = c^2$$

In the case of the Egyptian farmer, the diagonal of his square plot is:

$$Diagonal^2 = 350^2 + 350^2$$

The calculation by long hand is difficult, but fortunately for us this equation is easy to calculate with a $20 calculator and yields the value: 494.9747468. The Egyptian engineer with only a reed pen and papyrus paper could come very close by using the Egyptian formula based on multiples of seven:

Average the sum of 10/7 of one side and 14/10 of the other side:

350 x 10/7 = 3500/7 = 500
350 x 14/10 = 35 x 14 = 490
(500 + 490)/2 = 495

The error by this method is amazingly small:

495/494.9747468 = 1.000051 or .005%

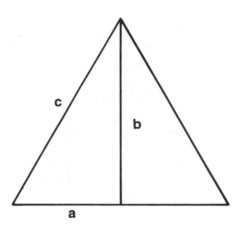

Figure 6.26 Depicted is an equilateral triangle with all sides equal to c, half sides equal to a, and a height equal to b.

Another Egyptian method quickly calculates the height of an equilateral triangle compared to one of its sides. We would use a calculator and the Pythagorean formula:

$$c^2 = a^2 + b^2$$

The problem is best solved by letting c = 1, so that a = 1/2. The value for b, the height, by using the calculator equals 0.866025403. The Egyptian method quickly solves the problem using a septenary ratio (multiples or divisions of seven) in which the height is 6/7 of one of the sides:

6/7 x c = 6/7 x 1 = 0.85714

The error in this case is about one percent, again quite good for a septenary "short hand" technique. An interesting solution to a practical volume problem was used by the Egyptian potter, using a "magic" ruler based on eleven. How can a square box be converted into a cylinder of equal volume? To solve this problem the potter divides the side of the square box into ten equal divisions. To calculate the cylindrical pot he takes eleven of those units in diameter and eleven units in height and puts a "brim line" mark just below the top on the inner edge.

What is the error? The volume of a box of ten units on a side is:

10 x 10 x 10 = 1000 cubic units of volume

A cylinder eleven units high and eleven units in diameter has a volume calculated by the formula: area of the base x the height of the cylinder. This is the radius squared x π x height. Again, fortunately for us, the calculator quickly yields the exact volume:

$(11/2)^2$ x π x 11 = 1045.364956 cubic units

If the potter puts a brim line equal to one-half of one unit, the volume would be less by:

$(11/2)^2$ x π x 1/2 = 47.51659 cubic units

Thus the difference between the two would be the true volume of the pot, if the user remembers to fill only to the brim line:

1045.364956 - 47.51659 = 997.848366 cubic units

The error is:

1000/997.848366 = 1.002156274

Or about 0.2%, again, quite remarkable.

The most incredible septenary ratio used by the Egyptians is the value to define π. We laboriously memorize π as "3.14 something", or pull it out of the memory of calculators for precise calculations: 3.141592654... (an endless number). The Egyptian engineers simply remembered the ratio: 22/7. The exact value of this ratio is 3.142857143. The ratio of π to 22/7 is:

3.141592654 /3.142857143 = 0.999597662

The comparison yields an error of .04%, that is, four parts out of 10,000, so the Egyptian engineer knew the magic number of the universe, π, to a very precise degree. The conclusion is that using these ratios, Egyptian engineers could circumvent the difficulties of longhand calculations, including difficult square root problems, and still maintain great accuracy without the use of calculators.

Some of the pyramids are oriented so precisely to the cardinal points (N, S, E, W) that it has to be questioned if such a feat were within the grasp of the Egyptians. Two devices, however, have been uncovered that indicate they were. Hieroglyphic evidence leads some to conclude that by using a "merchet" and a "bay", a true north-south meridian (spin axis of the planet) could have been determined anywhere in Egypt with great accuracy.

First a wall a few feet high was built with a water-filled mud canal on top of it. The canal walls were carefully leveled down to the height of the water and this provided the necessary artificial horizon needed in hilly terrain. Observations of rising and setting stars were accurately recorded on the level wall as shown in Figure 6.27. The bay was simply a rod, often wood or ivory, with a slot in it. This was placed in a hole drilled into the bedrock and rotated to line up with the sightings being taken. This bay could be one foot long or less, and the observer would signal his co-worker to move the merchet, which was a weight, a string, and a handle similar to a modern plumb line, to line up with any convenient rising or setting north star. The mark on the wall was carefully transferred to the bedrock, and the bisector, which was the true north-south meridian, was then determined. The east-west line could be determined from the meridian by the use of a large square or other geometric technique.

Apparently the technique works. The Great Pyramid is more precisely oriented to the cardinal points than any building built by modern society. (See Figure 6.28.) Close inspection of the Royal Observatory in England reveals a deviation of six seconds from true north, compared to the three second deviation of the Great Pyramid. (See Reference 51.)

Since the rising star method of measuring the circumference of the Earth requires the use of a timepiece to count seconds, it is only logical to assume the Egyptian engineers had an accurate means for counting seconds. Galileo in the 17th Century is usually credited as the discoverer of the isochronism of the pendulum. The length of the string determines the time period of the swing and the longer the string, the longer the time period. Pendulum clocks have evolved from this principle. One can safely assume that the Egyptians, with a merchet, essentially a pendulum, had realized the same principle and used a merchet with a string of the appropriate length to count seconds for their scientific work.

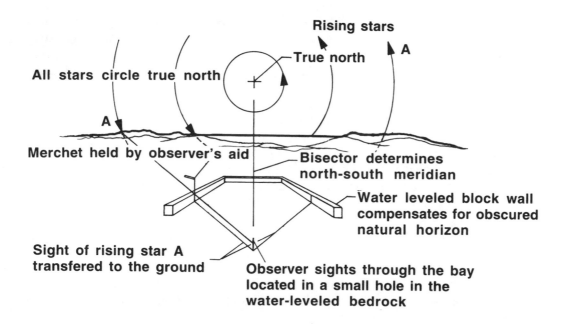

Figure 6.27 Depicted is a leveled artificial horizon, necessary because the true horizon is obscured by mountains. Rising and setting stars are marked on the wall with the aid of the merchet and the bay. The example shows that the bisector of the sight lines to star A is the true north-south spin axis of the Earth.

The base of the Great Pyramid has been found to be amazingly level. It is only one inch low at one corner, and that is thought to be due to settling. How could the Egyptians accomplish the leveling of such a large base area? These survivors of the wildly cyclic Nile knew how to cultivate using irrigation canals. Using mud banks to hold water was their forte. The bedrock was obviously chiseled down to a point where an equal depth of water was observed all around, while mud walls held the water in place.

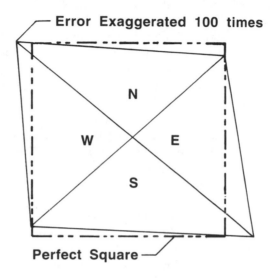

Figure 6.28 Depicted is a perfect square aligned to the cardinal points with the exaggeration of the distortion of the Great Pyramid corners, superimposed 100 times to make the error visible. No other man-made structure is so perfectly aligned.

North Face	2 minutes 28 seconds NE corner too far south
East Face	5 minutes 30 seconds SE corner too far east
South Face	1 minutes 57 seconds SW corner too far north
West Face	2 minutes 30 seconds NW corner too far west

By comparison, other carefully oriented pyramids are:

Name	Average Error	Location
Khephren	5 minutes, 26 seconds	Giza
Maidum	24 minutes, 25 seconds	Maidum
Bent	9 minutes, 12 seconds	Dashur
Mycerinus	14 minutes, 3 seconds	Giza

There is an interesting effect one can observe in every temple and pyramid found in Egypt. It occurs for the same reason there are erasers on one end of a pencil — human error. Some examples: the Step Pyramid of Zoser shows many obvious changes of plan with the many starts and stops of the underground maze of corridors and chambers; the original mastaba was finished and then extended twice; a four-step pyramid was finished over that; and finally, the six-step pyramid was finished over that. In other locations, monumental errors are obvious. Several pyramids were started and never completed. The pyramid at Maidum was finished as a seven-step pyramid, later turned into an eight-step pyramid, and finally filled in to form a smooth-sided pyramid. The Bent Pyramid upon close scrutiny shows comparatively inferior workmanship on the top portion, with the ten- degree change of slope angle, a late decision made, perhaps, for economic reasons. The huge pyramid of Khephren has two entrances on the north side, one above the other. The apparent explanation is that well after the project was started it was decided to relocate the base of the pyramid 100 feet to the south, rendering the lower passage obsolete and unfinished. The third pyramid of Giza by Menkaure´ has an unfinished entrance on its northern side, an apparent aborted effort. These are a few major examples of human error and changes made after work was in progress.

Did similar alterations take place when the Great Pyramid was under construction? It appears that the original burial chamber was planned for the "Unfinished Chamber," which is shown in Figure 6.15. This 12′ x 46′ x 27′ chamber was left in a very rough state. It has a trenched floor and rough walls, and it resembles the rough state of a quarry. That it was intended to be the burial chamber seems indisputable from its alignment with the apex of the pyramid, identical to all other pyramids. Another mistake seems to be the unfinished, roughly hewn corridor which leads south from the Unfinished Chamber and ends abruptly. Perhaps a second chamber was planned, but was not followed through on. It would not have been unusual to have a double chamber design; the North Pyramid had such an arrangement. The decision to abandon the lower chambers in favor of the rooms high in the body of the Pyramid came after several layers had already been completed. Sixty feet from the entrance of the Descending Passage, the Ascending Passage was cut through existing stones. Proof of this fact are the joints at the corners of these lower stones, which are irregular. From that point on the Ascending Passage was carefully constructed and the joints are executed with great accuracy. The Queen's Chamber seems to have been the original choice for the burial of the king, but a decision was made to abandon it and build the chamber even higher within the pyramid. This has been deduced by the fact that the floor was left unfinished. It is roughly cut and not faced with fine granite or limestone. Even after several hundred years of pyramid building, the Egyptian master builders, just like humans of today, were still changing their minds and correcting errors during the construction phase.

In summation, there is little room to doubt that the Egyptians were the builders of the Great Pyramid. It is located on the West Bank of the Nile in a cluster of other pyramids of similar shape and of similar construction. On that West Bank there are some 80 other pyramids up and down the Nile. The study of them leads to the conclusion that there was an obvious evolution from the mud brick mastaba, to stone mastaba, to step mastaba, to step pyramid, to true pyramid, and eventually to the Great Pyramid, the most voluminous and built at the height of power and wealth of Egypt. There is much evidence to believe that it was pharaoh Khufu who built the Great Pyramid because his name appears on the list of kings, several blocks of the Great Pyramid, and the mortuary temple built adjacent to the Great Pyramid. Just northeast of the Great Pyramid, a pit was found bearing the remains and some of the belongings of his mother, Queen Hetepheres. This sarcophagus was found empty, likely the result of grave robbers who carved a rough path through the Great Pyramid. King Khufu's sarcophagus, in contrast, was found within the Great Pyramid in the King's Chamber, still intact. So the Great Pyramid was obviously built as the protective tomb for the king. This sarcophagus is the typical Egyptian sarcophagus that bears the saw marks left by the craftsmen who quarried it.

That the Great Pyramid could have been built by Egyptian hand labor is entirely possible since the largest block weighs only 70 tons and most are only two tons. Since the Egyptians have demonstrated the ability to quarry and move 4,000-ton obelisks 400 miles, it is a relatively simple matter to move two-ton blocks with proper rollers and pavement. Tools of hardened copper have been found as early as the First Dynasty and these tools could cut limestone and granite. The Egyptians were also masters of the agglomeration technique, which greatly simplified the work and allowed the projects to be completed in a timely way.

The Egyptians knew how to measure the circumference of the Earth by timing rising stars at two different east-west locations and by measuring the shadows of obelisks several miles apart on a north-south meridian, then applying the proper mathematical formula. To calculate mathematical problems, the Egyptian engineers had an amazingly accurate method that was based on multiples of seven and eleven. Using this technique, they made solving complicated mathematical problems, even square-root equations, easy for an engineer equipped with only a pen and papyrus paper. The value of pi was simplified to 22/7, correct to within 4 parts out of 10,000.

The Egyptians used the merchet device to serve the double function of a plumb line and a time pendulum. The Egyptians also used the Bay as a sighting device in combination with the merchet to determine the true axis of rotation of the planet, the north-south meridian. The results accomplished by these devices were truly remarkable. Modern surveying techniques reveal that in the case of the Great Pyramid there was less alignment error than can be achieved in a modern construction project.

The Egyptians, masters of canal building for irrigating cultivated fields many miles from the Nile, used water in small dams to level the bases of the temples and the pyramids. The Great Pyramid is perfectly level except for one corner, a mere one-inch low, that is thought to be due to settling.

The Great Pyramid has the same Egyptian-like defects resulting from construction that is found in all the other pyramids. In all probability, some architect who worked for King Khufu designed the Great Pyramid not only as a tomb for the great pharaoh, but also to commemorate the knowledge the Egyptians possessed about the size of the Earth. The Great Pyramid was built about 4,000 or 5,000 years ago and we still use the measurement systems developed in that ancient land. They deserve the credit. Right?

NOTES

1. *The Pyramids of Egypt*, by I.E.S. Edwards, (Reference 3) gives detailed information about the important pyramids in Egypt. The information includes section views, plot plans of the hypogeums, and many other details too numerous to mention. This book is recommended reading.

Chapter Seven

Synopsis

The straight forward standard theory is quite conclusive, but only if one ignores many contrary pieces of evidence. The Great Pyramid doesn't appear to be a standard tomb monument. There are too many perfectly aligned passageways and chambers. The "air shafts" to both the King's and Queen's Chambers should be horizontal for efficiency and economy, yet they slope upward at different angles. Only the Great Pyramid has these features. Most tomb monuments are decorated with hieroglyphs, as a tribute to the grand deeds of the pharaoh, yet none exist within the Great Pyramid. The base perimeter is within one-half percent of the correct sub-multiple of the Equator's angular velocity of 3,000 feet per two seconds, yet the Egyptian technique for measuring the size of the Earth typically yields errors of ten percent. To achieve one-half percent error an artificial satellite is needed. Unlike features of other pharaonic tombs, the Grand Gallery has corbeled walls, and one course has a perfectly machined slot its entire length. The Grand Gallery has a ramp so smooth and with ramp-slots so perfect and regular that it looks more like a housing for machinery than a staircase to a pharaonic tomb. All true pyramids in Egypt are flat sided, yet each side of the core masonry of the Great Pyramid (casing blocks have all been removed) has a regular center depression, a design feature that no one can explain. It was common for the ruling pharaoh to claim existing monuments as his own. Did Khufu chisel his name in the Great Pyramid knowing full well that it was the work of the gods?

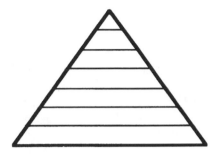

Chapter Seven

DID THE EGYPTIANS BUILD THE GREAT PYRAMID? NO!

The Enigmas

Egyptians invite the world to visit the colossal creations of their ancient ancestors, but the normal guided tour gives visitors only a cursory view of the pyramids. From a distance they all look alike and there is little time to provide an in-depth analysis. We have been told over and over again how advanced our civilization is, especially when compared to the bits and pieces of other civilizations that are left to examine. Some investigators who spend a lot of time on these details are beginning to suspect that the bits and pieces that are left over from 5,000 years ago, the "primitive" agrarian Egyptian civilization, obscures even fewer bits and pieces left over from the civilization that existed 10,000 years ago, and from the one that existed before that. "What? Nothing existed that long ago!" you may be thinking, but it appears there were such ancient civilizations.

Only now, a small group of researchers is beginning to realize that precursor civilizations existed before the Egyptians of five thousand years ago. I submit that there was at least one, and maybe several, existing between 52,000 years ago and 10,000 years ago. Close examination of one remaining artifact of that precursor civilization, the Great Pyramid, reveals building technology that far surpasses what we could accomplish today. The trouble is that the truth is to be found among the often-overlooked subtle details. Most observers are fooled by the cursory observations and conclusions explored in Chapter Six. In truth, the standard theory leaves many enigmas and a few of these are listed here as a starting place for a more comprehensive inspection:

1. How could the Egyptians, without orbiting satellites, truly calculate the Earth's circumference to the great precision — accurate to 1/2% — found in the dimensions of the Great Pyramid?

2. Why would the apparently magical formulas of Egyptian mathematics be devoid of the trigonometric functions that are basic to the science of mathematics?

3. Only the Great Pyramid has deliberate deep surface hollowing, on all four faces — not the flat surfaces of all the other pyramids. Why would the Egyptians undertake this costly and unusual feature?

4. What socioeconomic, religious, or technical change led to the new technique of placing construction blocks in horizontal courses unique only to the Great Pyramid and three other pyramids? These pyramids belong to the heaviest group of pyramids, where one would expect the conservative 75-degree slope technique to be employed.

5. Why were all of the small subsidiary pyramids built using the 75-degree slope technique?

6. What is the true reason for the unusual arrangement of chambers and passages in the Great Pyramid? No other pyramid exhibits this complex arrangement.

7. What is the true purpose for the "air" shafts leading outward from the King's Chamber and from the Queen's Chamber? Why are these shafts perfectly straight? Why are they sloped upwards and not horizontal? Why is this a feature of the Great Pyramid and no other pyramid?

8. Why is the chamber at the bottom of the extremely smooth-sided and perfectly-aligned Descending Passage in such a crude unfinished state that it has acquired the name of the Unfinished Chamber?

9. What is the true purpose for the roughly cut and twisted Grotto Passage?

10. What is the true reason for the unusual Grand Gallery? The great size, the upward slope, and other unusual features of the Grand Gallery are unique among all of the pyramids.

11. Why are there seven corbels making up the walls of the Grand Gallery?

12. What is the true purpose for the groove in the walls of the Grand Gallery? Are the slots in the ramps merely for retainer beams for the three granite plugs found in the Ascending Passage?

13. Why are the passages and chamber walls up to and including the Queen's Chamber, covered with salt, another unique feature of the Great Pyramid alone?

14. What was the purpose for the unusual and complex three-door portcullis

entrance to the King's Chamber? Only Menkaure´s Pyramid has anything resembling this feature.

15. Why was the sarcophagus of mighty Khufu apparently never smoothly finished? The original chisel marks are still in evidence.

16. Why are there no hieroglyphic carvings on any of the walls of the passages or chambers within the Great Pyramid when that was the standard practice of the time?

17. Why did the architects design such unusual ceiling beams in the King's Chamber? Above the first ceiling is an attic that has more of these unusual stone ceiling beams. This feature repeats; there are five such attic spaces in all. The uppermost attic has a pitched roof, like the Queen's Chamber. This arrangement is unique among all the pyramids.

18. Why would the architects design a mathematical "Song of the Pyramid" into the shape, dimensions, and architectural elements of the Great Pyramid? Only the Great Pyramid has been so well orchestrated.

The Earth's Circumference

How accurately Egyptian scientists could have measured the circumference of the Earth is an extremely important issue. Tompkins describes two probable techniques for measuring the circumference of the Earth. (See Reference 5.) In 1987 I attempted to duplicate one of these two methods.

For many years I was employed by a large aerospace firm as a senior loftsman in charge of the careful layout of aircraft parts. One routine assignment was to solve fit and function problems, using the stainless steel ruler technique. The final tolerance on assembled aircraft parts is + or - .060 inch. To meet this standard, solutions from the loft department are held to an even finer accuracy. To this end, the precise stainless steel rulers employed are calibrated to 1/100 of an inch. In actual practice these divisions are routinely divided in half with the aid of magnifying optics yielding scale readings of .005 inch.

At the time I strongly believed in the standard theory and was convinced that common aerospace fabrication techniques were equal to or exceeded the skill level of ancient Egyptians; and therefore could be used to calculate the exact size of the Earth. Using the suggestions in Reference 5, the shadow length of a tall obelisk can be used to extrapolate the radius of the Earth. Reasoning that a tall building would substitute for an actual obelisk, I began to train myself by measuring building shadows. I quickly noticed a disturbing trend. The taller the building, the more the shadow became blurred. Measuring the length of a shadow to the precision required, therefore, was impossible.

The shadow is blurred because the Sun is not a point source. It is a disc, and all points on that disc emit light. Because of this fact there are many shadows overlapping, so the taller an object is, the more indistinct the edge of the shadow becomes. (See Figure 7.1.)

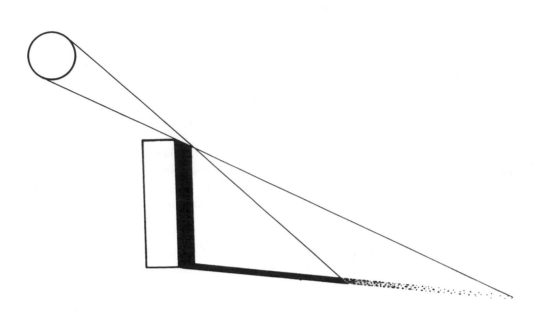

Figure 7.1 Depicted is a tall square object casting a shadow from a disc light source such as the sun. By projecting lines from the disc source to the cast shadow, the length of the blur becomes clearly evident. The scale is exaggerated for clarity.

In Egypt, of course, the same phenomena was observed. This is shown in the photos of a sharp-edged obelisk at Karnak and its consequent fuzzy shadow. (See Figures 7.2 and 7.3.)

Three plastic sunglass lenses, each about five inches long, became the convenient field measuring instrument. (The stainless steel ruler was never unpacked.) The lenses of the sunglasses clearly demonstrate that the shadow of this tall obelisk, of undetermined height, had an indistinct edge almost fifteen inches wide. The reading was taken during the afternoon, and although the blur of the high noon shadow would be less, it would be substantial. Note 1 shows that a 200-foot obelisk at noon would have a blur 1.86 feet wide.

Because the nature of the sun disc is to form blurred shadows, it is impossible to measure the beginning, the center, or the end of the shadow with any precision. My first-hand experience has led me to believe that the uncertainty factor for a 200-foot obelisk would be about 1/3 foot.

This may seem small compared to the height of the obelisk, but it leads to an unacceptable error in the calculation of the Earth's radius. This is easy to see in the following two experiments. Tompkins suggests that two obelisks several miles apart on a north-south axis would be sufficient, and that is similar to what is depicted in Figure 6.24. For the first trial, assume the separation is ten miles. The calculation error, however, is as high as 66%. (See Note 2.) This improves by separating the obelisks (the second test), and since the total length of Egypt is about 800 miles, assume that in the second case, the

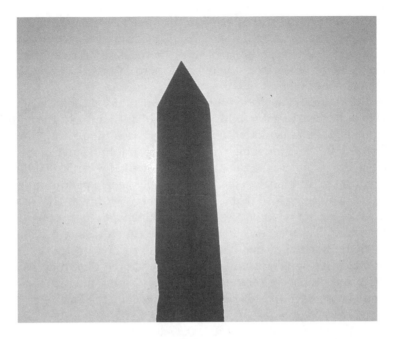

Figure 7.2 The sun is positioned behind an obelisk at Karnak, which highlights the sharp edge of the highly polished stone monument.

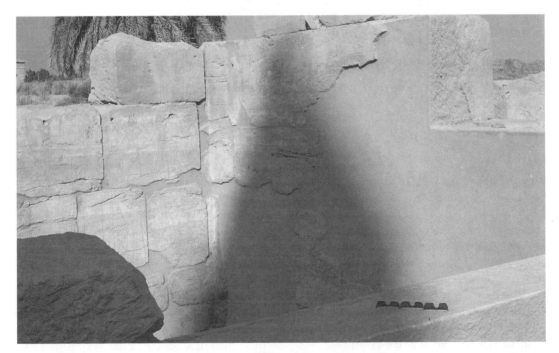

Figure 7.3 A photograph of the shadow of the same obelisk taken in the afternoon showing the obvious blur, about fifteen inches wide.

separation is the full 800 miles. The error in this case is reduced to about one percent, although this assume, absolute precision in the distance between the obelisks. It will soon be shown, however, that the typical error in distances is six to seven percent. The total error would be a factor of ten from the one half percent precision actually found in the geometry of the Great Pyramid.

The third trial tests the east-west rising star method. It can be safely assumed that if the Egyptians built the Great Pyramid, then in light of Chapters 1 through 5, they knew the unit of seconds. When calculating the circumference of the Earth, however, any unit of time can be used. By experimenting with various pendulum lengths, for example, let us suppose that the Egyptians used a pendulum that would swing 50,000 times during one complete revolution of the planet. A team could easily keep a pendulum going night and day by periodically nudging it so that it would never slow down. That is all they needed for the east-west rising star method. As described in Chapter 6, suppose the obelisks are 90,000 Great Pyramid feet apart on a flat plain at the equator, since a 200-foot obelisk just disappears over the horizon at this distance. At the second obelisk the observers have measured 34.7222 of these pendulum swings between the time they receive the signal from the team at the first obelisk and the time they observe the rising star at the second obelisk. From this they have what is necessary to calculate the Earth's circumference:

$$50,000 / 34.72222 \times 90,000 = 129,600,000 \text{ G.P. ft}$$

This correct answer assumes that 0.7222222 of a pendulum swing could be observed, but this type of primitive clock could only give rough answers to about one half of one swing, so consider the effect of a one-half swing error. The realistic value of 34.2 would yield:

$$50,000 / 34.2 \times 90,000 = 131,493,515 \text{ G.P. ft}$$

for the circumference, which when compared to the correct value, yields a ratio:

$$131,493,515 / 129,600,000 = 1.01461$$

This means the error is approximately 1.5%, which is beyond the precision needed, and yet there remain additional errors: the error in measuring fifteen miles by laying rods end to end over rough terrain, the difference in dissimilar altitudes of the two observation points, and sightings at low angles through thick atmosphere are all subject to temperature distortion causing the bending of light-refraction errors.

Clearly it would be impossible to achieve one half percent accuracy by this particular east-west method, and the author suggests that the Egyptians never attempted it because another east-west method existed that did not require a clock.

Place a 200-foot obelisk at Alexandria on the Mediterranean Sea, or any east-west location on the Egyptian coast where the water is at the same level and not flowing down a river. (So no altitude corrections are needed.) Then all that really needs to be done is measure the distance to the point where the Earth's curvature obscures the very top of the obelisk, wall, or point of land of known height. For a 200-foot object this occurs at about fifteen miles, as measured naturally along any great circle line, with the observation taken at sea level. This experiment relies on the basic geometry of similar triangles as shown

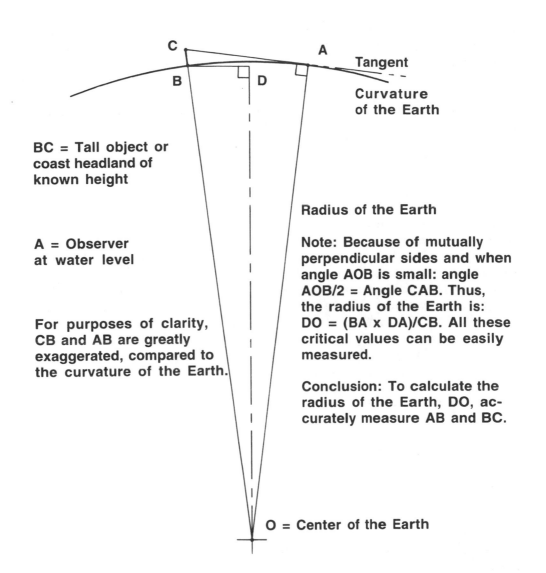

Figure 7.4 Depicted is the curvature of the Earth with an exaggerated obelisk, building, or headland near the coast. When a light at the top of the building disappears, the observer at A is at the tangent. By the geometric rules of tangents, 1/2 of the angle AOB is equal to EOA which also equals the angle CAB. AE is 1/2 of AB by definition, so the rules of similar triangles applies: CB/EA = BA/EO, thus EO = (BA x EA)/CB.

in Figure 7.4, and the fact that the tangent to a circle describes the angular relationships as shown.

The calculation is quite simple and yields a result that may have parallax, refraction, and distance-measuring errors, but would not have any error due to the primitive pendulum clock previously described. If the Egyptians attempted any east-west technique, it would have been this one.

The estimates of error introduced by this method would be similar to the experiment conducted by Sir John Herschel in the early 19th century with a team of men working in smooth water. The distance between observers was measured when they could no longer see each other at a precise height above the water. The distance between observers was 12,873 meters, from which they calculated the diameter of the Earth to be 6,797 kilometers. This calculation of the circumference of the Earth was considered the best for many years, but eventually Herschel's manual technique was realized to have a 6.6% error.

There does exist yet another method, which is perhaps the best method to estimate the size of the Earth with primitive instrumentation. First a sighting of a convenient north star at its highest rise of the evening is taken and the precise angle above the horizon is recorded. The location of this sighting on a north-south meridian is recorded and another point on the same meridian is found where a second sighting yields exactly a one-degree change. The circumference is simply 360 times the distance between the two sightings.

The accuracy of this method relies on the accuracy of the sextant sighting and the accuracy of measuring a distance over a 69-mile landscape, which invariably encounters hills and valleys if not imperceptible slopes (altitude corrections,) and perhaps wandering off the meridian. The Egyptians would have had to use the measuring rod technique, and would in all probability induce the same error as did Al Mamun who performed the experiment in 864 A.D. Al Mamun and a team of workers found a flat plane and measured the north-south distance with great care using precisely measured rods. The angle was noted to change one degree. The error of Al Mamun's carefully computed answer proved to be 7%.

The accuracy of the value was not known until the French used a telescope to triangulate the peaks of mountains, a more accurate north-south distance determining, and hence a more accurate value for the size of the Earth. The French value was only improved upon in very recent times by utilizing data from orbiting satellites. The most precise value known in the "Space Age" is 6,370 km, and it is against this value that the values achieved by the ancients is compared.

In summary, the Egyptians at best used pendulums for clocks, measured distance with rods, tugged colossal objects into position using hundreds of men heaving in unison on the rope attached to greased sleds. (See Figure 6.21.) Is it plausible to think that the Egyptians could calculate the size of the Earth to 1/2% accuracy? Or is it the conservative assumption to believe that the Egyptians, with manual techniques, could have achieved results approximating that of John Herschel or Al Mamun, namely errors of about 7%?

The Missing Trigonometric Functions

The previous chapter briefly describes a unique Egyptian mathematical system, the "magic" ratios involving either 7, 11, or multiples of these. Using them, every day mathematical problems could be solved with little error. The value π was not memorized by the Egyptians as the endless number, (3.1415...) as we are taught, but was understood as the ratio 22/7, quite accurate for ordinary use. That and many other ratios and applications have been discussed in Chapter 6.

While approximating formulas are quite remarkable and also useful for some facets of commerce, they are hardly the way to conduct the good science the Egyptians are credited with. True exacting science carries out mathematical formulas to many decimal places and the blizzard of mathematical formulas encountered by professionals in physics, chemistry, astronomy and applied engineering can hardly be addressed by a handful of interesting ratios. They are simply approximating formulas.

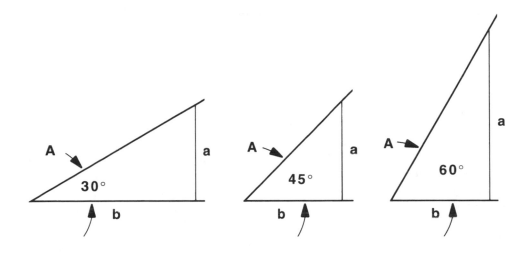

Figure 7.5 Depicted are three common triangles, the ratio of a/b is the same regardless of the size of the triangles, the ratio of a/b is dependent only on the angle. From this fact, trigonometric tables of the ratio verses the angle can be compiled for convenient use by mathematicians and engineers.

One would expect that Egyptian scientists and mathematicians discovered and used trigonometric functions, but there is no evidence of this. Consider the simple triangles (Chapter 2) that everyone is familiar with: the 30 degree triangle, the 45 degree triangle, and the 60 degree triangle. As compared in figure 7.5 the ratio of the base legs, a/b, is different for each degree.

Regardless of how large or small these triangles are, there is the obvious and basic mathematical fact that the specific ratio of one base leg to the other base leg remains constant for any specific angle. Consider the "tangent" function which is defined as: The tangent of angle A = a/b. For the basic triangles of the example, these values are always the same:

Tangent 45 degree = 1.000000
Tangent 30 degree = 0.577350269...
Tangent 60 degree = 1.732050808...

Our modern calculators manifest these values for every degree or fraction of any degree, and this mathematical convenience greatly simplifies engineering and scientific work.

These ratios are normally introduced in school after basic multiplication and division are mastered. Most students encounter trigonometry tables at least by high school, yet there is no hieroglyphic evidence that trigonometric functions were known or practiced by the Egyptians. Could it be that the Egyptian magic ratios are a remaining element of another technology, and a handed-down, shadow-remembrance of a former, more advanced civilization? Could it be that a comprehension of the trigonometric functions failed to make the transition?

The Unusual Surface Hollowing

During World War II, an airplane carrying Brigadier P.R.C. Groves made a pass over the Giza complex near Cairo. Brigadier Groves took his camera and snapped a photograph with the sun at just the right angle to reveal yet another Great Pyramid mystery. The photograph is reproduced in Reference 5 and the shadow exaggeration is shown in line drawing, Figure 7.6. A comparison of the shadows shows a remarkable dip or hollowing of the southern face of the Great Pyramid. This does not exist in any of the other pyramids. This was the visual proof of what had been previously measured by Petrie, and also observed by Napoleon's French savants 100 years earlier — that all four sides of the Great Pyramid have similar depressions in the core masonry. Their etching had been ignored, because it didn't fit the standard theory of the day: that all true pyramids were flat-sided.

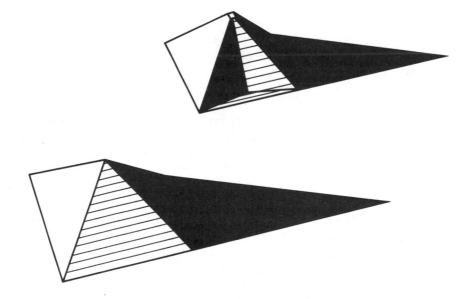

Figure 7.6 Depicted in the line drawing is the unique hollowing of the sides of the Great Pyramid. No other pyramid in Egypt has this feature.

Building a monolithic pyramid with sloping flat faces that must meet precisely at one point hundreds of feet in the air is by itself a great engineering challenge. Imagine the great added effort and expense required to put a precise dip into each side. So why was this done? Davidson's theory was that if the perimeter, as established by the corners of the base, are related precisely to the angular velocity of the Earth, then perhaps the solar, sidereal, and anomalistic year lengths are also represented in the base. This was measured three ways: the solar year, the exact time between successive vernal or autumnal equinoxes, equals 365.2242 days and is represented by the perimeter as measured by a straight line to each of the corner stones at the base. The sidereal year, the time it takes for the same star to appear in the same spot by an observer on Earth, equals 365.25636 days, and is represented by a slightly longer measurement, which includes part of the hollowing. The anomalistic year is the time it takes to reach the same point in the orbit, which is its perihelion point, or closest approach to the sun. That is represented by taking the full hollowing into account.

If this is actually the true purpose for the hollowing, the high degree of astronomical knowledge and precision of execution required would seem far beyond the reach of Egyptian technology. If the Egyptians, or anyone using these manual techniques, could not measure the size of the Earth with less than seven percent error, then they surely could not calculate the sidereal year to five decimal places. That means one-hundred-thousandth of a day, or less than a second. If this didn't come from the Egyptians, however, then who did it come from? Could the hollowing be the work of a more ancient and technically advanced civilization that could measure the Earth year with great precision? Or could the hollowing serve another function not yet considered?

The New Technology — Horizontal Courses

It is the assumption of the standard theory that religious beliefs strongly affected the architectural design of the monuments. What belief change occurred that radically altered the building technique of the largest and heaviest pyramids found in Egypt? The North Pyramid, as well as the three major pyramids at Giza, discarded the proven technique of building in layers against a sloping core. In contrast, they are all constructed of blocks laid in level or horizontal courses. This change apparently came about during the reign of Snofru, since he is credited with the building of the Bent Pyramid as well as the North Pyramid. The North Pyramid predates the Giza complex, so it is assumed to be the first pyramid built in this dangerous, earthquake-prone style. Because of the relatively poor construction technique of the Bent Pyramid, especially the upper half, the standard theory suggests that Snofru was impatient to finish the Bent Pyramid so his builders could experiment with the horizontal row technique, the first of which was apparently the North Pyramid. The success of the North Pyramid encouraged his sons to continue the technique of building pyramids in horizontal rows at Giza, and also encouraged new religious beliefs.

The puzzle is why the architects of Khufu, Khephren, and Menkaure´ used the horizontal row technique on the large pyramids, but the sloping layer technique on the small, comparatively light-weight subsidiary pyramids. Seven of these were built at the Giza complex, exactly opposite to what is logical. It would make far more sense to attempt the horizontal row technique on a small scale as a warm up for the new assemblage of engineers and workers. Once the small pyramids were finished, they could better tackle the awesome task of building the biggest pyramids in the world.

The Rare Internal Complexity

Another great riddle of the Great Pyramid is the obvious complexity of the internal passages and chambers. The sectional view of the Great Pyramid (See Figure 7.7.) shows highly polished and unerringly straight passageways adjacent to others that are roughly finished and curving. Likewise many of the chambers are polished smooth while others are roughly cut. Is it simply that the smooth passages and chambers are the work of the architects of Khufu, while the rough passages and chambers are the work of grave robbers? The conventional wisdom is challenged upon closer examination of each internal feature.

First look at what Egyptologists generally consider to be air passages, small shafts, probably ventilation channels that lead into the main chambers of the Great Pyramid from the outside. There are two of these shafts in the Queen's Chamber and two in the King's Chamber. The exterior exit point of the shafts from the Queen's Chamber has never been found. The interior opening to the shafts was found with great difficulty. Originally, these passages ended several inches from the inner wall of the Queen's Chamber and were only discovered when a researcher, after noting the shafts in the King's chamber, thought a similar feature might exist in the chamber below. Guided by an obvious crack, perhaps a result of the aforementioned great earthquake that destroyed the buildings of Cairo as well as the removal of the outer limestone covering of the Great Pyramid, he used a hammer and chisel to break through the last five inches covering the shafts.

In recent years the shafts have been investigated using video equipment. The most interesting find was in the small southern shaft in the Queen's Chamber. With a specially designed eight-wheeled robot, Upuaut II, 200 feet of progress was made until a door was encountered. A photograph was made of the door and it showed unusual metal fittings. The robot used a laser to probe at the door and it disappeared in one corner where a small space exists. Obviously some cavity exists behind the door. What is on the other side of the door is still a mystery. (See Reference 50.)

The shafts of the King's Chamber lead up and out to the north and south faces. These shafts, as already mentioned, were considered to be air shafts by the first investigators to clear them of rubble. The first time the shafts were cleared a refreshing "rush of air" greeted those in the chambers, so the function of the narrow shafts seemed obvious, and the name stuck. In Khephren's Pyramid there is evidence of rectangular shafts being cut near the roof of the north and south walls of the main tomb chamber, but these are only one foot deep. It was speculated that they were the start of air shafts, but the project was abandoned. Other than that, there is no other pyramid in Egypt that exhibits anything like the air vents of the Great Pyramid.

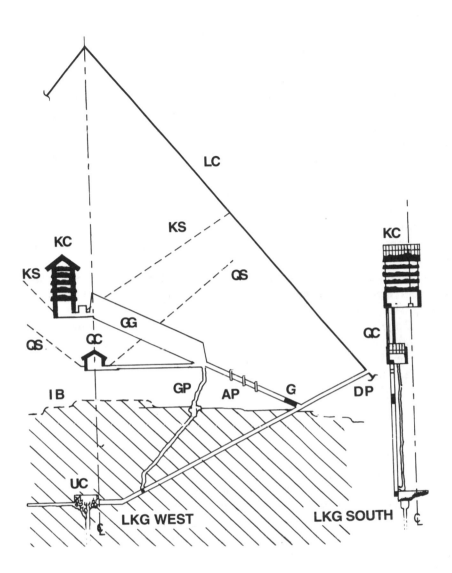

Figure 7.7 Depicted are two partial section views of the Great Pyramid, emphasizing the passageways and chambers. DP = Descending Passage, UC = Unfinished Chamber, AP = Ascending Passage, GG = Grand Gallery, QC = Queen's Chamber, QS = Shaft from Queen's Chamber, KC = King's Chamber, KS = Shaft to surface from King's Chamber, GP = Grotto and Grotto Passage, IB = Irregular Bedrock — shape unknown, G = Granite plugs, LC = Limestone casing blocks

The function of these narrow passages may have been something other than air circulation, however, because the walk into Khephren's tomb chamber via a long descending and then a horizontal passageway can be made without any signs of hypoxia. There was enough air in the passageways and chambers to allow a funeral cortege to journey into the chamber and out again without any need for air shafts. So there is no obvious explanation why this feature is part of the Great Pyramid. If air shafts were required, why weren't they designed along one of the horizontal rows? If the upper level needed to be reached, why not a stair-step arrangement? Leaving a gap between blocks is many times more cost effective than building a smooth, upwardly-sloping shaft requiring the careful chamfering of thousands of blocks. The placement and construction of the air vents remains one of the Great Pyramid's mysterious features.

The Unfinished Chamber

Next consider a most unusual chamber found deep under the Great Pyramid. The chamber is at the end the Descending Passage and carved into natural rock. It exists at the exact spot where burial chambers are located in most other pyramids. Researchers quickly named this room the Unfinished Chamber, which aptly describes its current appearance. The large room has rough and unfinished tunnels and recesses from it leading nowhere, an unfinished ceiling, unfinished walls, and an unfinished floor, which is trenched. In all, it is similar to a quarry. (See Figure 7.7.)

One speculation is that the Unfinished Chamber was originally a finished chamber with a fake sarcophagus and enough features to make it appear to be the real burial chamber. The idea was to fool grave robbers. It is quite possible that the original grave robbers, failing to discover any treasure, made a frantic attempt to find the secret passage to the true burial chamber, carving into the walls, floor, and ceiling, and leaving the chamber in its rough state. The riddle is, why isn't there evidence of any portcullis slot, the massive protective door found in every other pyramid and mastaba?

The Grotesque Grotto And Passage

Yet another mysterious passage and chamber are the twisting and roughly hewn Grotto room and connecting passage. Originally dubbed the "well," it was discovered from its upper end, which goes straight down. The top of the well is near the foot of the Grand Gallery. Investigators who followed removed all of the rubble that was jammed into the well and discovered its twisting shape and one enlarged area, the room that became known as the "grotto." (See Figure 7.7.)

Reference 5 gives an interesting summary of the many theories about this passage. One speculation is that workers were accidentally trapped within the Grand Gallery and dug the twisting passage to escape. If so, however, why take such a long path? The idea that it was dug by grave robbers from the bottom upwards is also unlikely. If it was grave robbers, how did they know the exact spot to penetrate at the base of the Grand Gallery? If they had the blue print, they would have chosen an easier path. The most plausible idea is that the Grotto Passages were dug by workers who had to examine the base rock after an earthquake. There are several fissures observable from the Grotto Passage, and this theory admirably explains one other mystery — the short tunnel at the top of the grand gallery into the chamber above the King's Chamber. Since some of the beams in the ceiling of the King's chamber are cracked at the south end, it is reasonable to speculate that workmen had to survey damage to higher beams.

To some, the Grotto Passage and the Grand Gallery worked hand in hand. The

Grand Gallery was thought to have been used as a sort of astronomical observatory. Once the stars were charted the pyramid was finished, and then finally used as a tomb. The logic is that while the pyramid was truncated, the Grand Gallery would have presented parallel walls to the open sky, useful for mapping the stars. While the Grotto Passage could have provided a passage around equipment located in the lower end of the Ascending Passage, why wouldn't the astronomers simply use a ladder to climb out of the Grand Gallery after completing their observations?

In this theory, the granite plugs were used because the astronomers wanted to keep the map-making tool a secret. A far cheaper observatory would have been two parallel walls on a north-south meridian, however. The secret could have been kept by simply dismantling the walls when they were finished. The theories for the existence of the Grotto Passage are still inadequate, and the Grotto Passage remains one of the great mysteries of the Great Pyramid.

The Grand Gallery/Queen's Chamber Conundrum

The Grand Gallery is a complex geometric design unique world-wide, little understood, and the subject of much speculation. Where the passage to the "Queen's Chamber" meets the Ascending Passage, the lower end of the upward sloping Grand Gallery begins. As its name implies, it is quite awesome to behold. It is sloping upward yet without steps. The chamber is 28 feet high, 153 feet long, and has unusually polished limestone walls that rise in seven courses, corbeled in style with a flat ceiling only 3'5" wide. An unusual ramp on each side at the base is 2' high and 1'8" wide, with regularly spaced notches running the entire length. A passageway, 3'5" wide like the ceiling, is formed between the two ramps. These features are shown in Figure 7.8 in a sectional view along the axis looking upward.

The standard theory offers several explanations for the existence of the Grand Gallery. Once it was decided to place the burial chamber high in the body of the Great Pyramid, the Queen's Chamber was designed and built for that purpose. A change of plan, however, led them to abandon the room, and design and build the King's Chamber instead. The Grand Gallery was thus the grand passage to the final resting place of the King's body.

Proof of this costly change, it is said, is the state of the Queen's Chamber floor, which is very pitted. The step down from the passage leading to the chamber suggests fine stone-work intended for the floor was never finished. It seems illogical to abandon the Queen's Chamber after it was 99% completed, however, because it would have taken very little to finish the floor — especially when compared with the millions of blocks yet to quarry, polish, and place. In addition the room would have been a great decoy, an often-used design feature.

The Egyptians were masters at using decoys to thwart grave robbers. One interesting tomb arrangement that I personally inspected was a tomb in the Valley of the Kings in which the passageway leading to the burial chamber of the King suddenly opened at the floor into a vertical drop 100 feet deep. Grave robbers had the doubly hard job of first investigating the wide and deep shaft, and then after discovering that it was a false burial pit, try to figure out where the real trail, if there was one, began again. In this case the real passage to the burial chamber did continue, but opposite the abyss and through a concealed door that once discovered, was extremely difficult to open.

In the case of the abandoned Queen's Chamber, it is hard to believe that the Egyptians would have missed the opportunity to use it as a decoy. There was also plenty of room to design a portcullis protective door, and hide the ascent to the King's Chamber, but neither option was done. It remains a mystery why these opportunities were overlooked.

The walls of the Queen's Chamber and the passage leading to it are covered with a layer of salt, a riddle in itself. For this, no logical explanation exists. The corbeled indentation in the west wall of the Queen's Chamber, reminiscent of the shape of the Grand Gallery except that there are five steps to it, suggests that it could have been the repository for a statue, yet nothing was found.

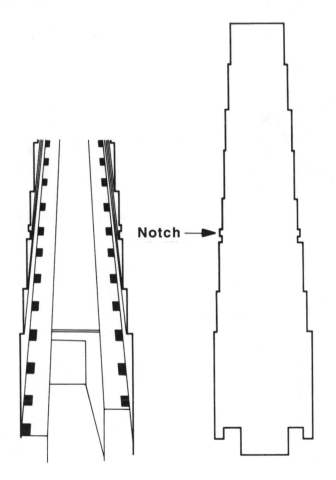

Figure 7.8 Depicted is a perspective view of the Grand Gallery, which shows the deep notches in the side ramps and, in the sectional view, the curious groove that runs its entire length.

Some investigators believe that the Great Pyramid, especially the Grand Gallery, was really an astronomical observatory. Besides acting as a grid to chart the positions of the stars, the observatory could aid in computing the size of the Earth. To accomplish this the observer could position himself far enough from the opening of the Grand Gallery to subtend a known angle, which some think was exactly two degrees. From such a point, a star making its pass on the celestial equator could be timed and, once recorded, there would be enough data to calculate the circumference of the Earth. This is similar to the east-west rising star technique discussed earlier. Using a primitive pendulum clock and spacing the obelisks or walls too closely together introduces unnecessary error as shown earlier. Since there are far more accurate and sensible methods to determine the circumference of the Earth, it is doubtful that the Gallery was made for astronomical calculations. This line of reasoning is also erroneous, because the Great Pyramid — as shown by its dimensions — was built to honor and encapsulate the knowledge already known about the size of the planet, not to investigate it.

One explanation for the unusual corbeled walls of the Grand Gallery is that it was a structural solution that allowed a tall chamber to be built within a heavy masonry structure without the use of steel. This was accomplished, but there remain two puzzling questions. The Queen's Chamber and the King's Chamber do not employ such a solution, so why would the architects employ two entirely different structural methods to bear the massive overhead weight? The other question is that on the fourth course or corbel step, there is an obvious slot that runs the entire length of Gallery. The slot is on both sides, as shown in Figure 7.8. This is important. There is a deliberate effort to make these indentations perfectly straight and smooth, and to date there is no viable explanation for this mysterious feature. All that is known for sure is that all the sloping lines, steps, and grooves in the Grand Gallery are parallel.

The slots which are regularly spaced along the sloping ramp have been thought to be anchoring pits for the timber work that held the seal, the granite plugs, and the mechanism that somehow helped the workers lower the obstructing stonework into position. There are various alternatives to this theory. One suggests that the stones were held high in the air so the funeral ceremony could pass unimpeded and not have to suffer the indignity of walking over the stone plugs. There is also the possibility that the slots simply functioned as anchors for construction scaffolding.

Even though the slots could have been used for these purposes, it remains a mystery as to why there would be such precision in the execution. Why cut 28 pairs of slots to precisely the same depth and width? Why is the distance between each slot exactly the same? Why did the workmen labor to make enough slots to hold 28 granite plugs, while only three were apparently used? Would so much care be given to anchoring pits for temporary posts and beams? It is an example of supreme over-engineering, or perhaps there is a better reason for the precise ramp slots and all the other unusual features of the Grand Gallery. The puzzle that has so far eluded the experts will soon be clarified.

The portcullis protecting the King's Chamber is extremely unusual, complicated, and is only rivaled by the triple portcullis found in the pyramid of Menkaure'. Normally there is only one portcullis protecting a burial chamber because one thick block is many times stronger than three thin blocks. Three slots and three doors are also more expensive, so this seal assembly found protecting the King's Chamber is another lasting mystery. (See Figure 7.9.) Contrast the thick, massive and extremely basic granite-block seals at the lower end to the relatively expensive, complicated and finely-positioned thin portcullis ?

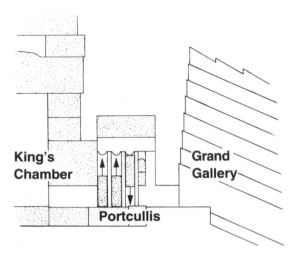

Figure 7.9 Depicted is the complex portcullis seal at the upper end of the Grand Gallery, at the entry way to the King's Chamber. One can easily imagine a mechanism at the top that would raise and lower the doors repeatedly. Why, remains a mystery. Note how this feature contrasts greatly with the simple, thick, immovable granite blocks at the lower end of the Ascending Passage.

The King's Chamber Mysteries

There are many mysteries in the King's Chamber. Here are several to ponder. First, the sarcophagus in the King's Chamber seems, at first glance, to fit the usual picture expected of an Egyptian burial chamber. This sarcophagus reportedly shows quarry marks and saw marks left by the typical Egyptian saws. In many Egyptian tombs, however, the outstanding feature of the burial chamber is the great workmanship that goes into the sarcophagus itself. The pharaoh's final resting coffer is usually finished to a high degree of polish and with flawless dimensions. It remains a riddle why the designers and builders of the magnificent Great Pyramid would go to the trouble of polishing the surfaces of almost 10,000 square feet of the Grand Gallery, thousands of square feet of the Ascending Passage and Descending Passage, not to mention the entire outer surface of the Great Pyramid, and overlook the pharaoh's sarcophagus.

Typical tomb and temple wall carvings are shown in Figure 7.10. These inscriptions usually adorn the walls of the valley building, the causeway, and the mortuary adjacent to the pyramid, and reflect the good works and deeds of the pharaoh. The reverence given the pharaoh's body always extended to the treatment of the tomb chamber itself and included the embalming and placement of the body into the airtight sarcophagus.

The chamber was filled with sacred articles and the walls were adorned with good deeds of the pharaoh and the proper royal prayers for the eternal entombment.

The Great Pyramid represents the apogee of pyramid building in Egypt, yet there is not one Egyptian hieroglyph within it. In reverence for the God-King Khufu, a huge mortuary temple was constructed of the finest stone and adjacent to the Great Pyramid on the east side. Lined with many columns, the temple had niches and altars for stela and statues. Fragments of the temple suggest it was covered with scenes delicately carved in low relief. Connecting the mortuary temple to the valley building was a monolithic causeway built straight and bridging a small valley. Except for the foundation, very little of the causeway exists today, but if it was typical, it too would have had walls completely covered with relief decorations. The valley temple likewise would have had this royal touch, perhaps even with more statues of the king. Even the small subsidiary pyramids had chapels adjacent to the eastern face of them that included richly decorated relief carvings. Why is there a lack of wall paintings, carvings, or hieroglyphics of any sort in any of the passageways, rooms, or even the King's Chamber of the Great Pyramid? Since there is no doubt that wall decorations existed before, during, and after the time of Khufu this puzzling oversight still eludes the experts.

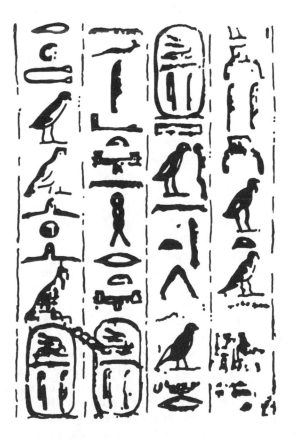

Figure 7.10 Depicted is a small sampling of inscriptions typically found on temple walls. Ironically, none are found anywhere within the Great Pyramid.

The King's Chamber, located at the top of the Grand Gallery, is a rectangular room 34'4" long east to west and exactly one half of that, or 17'2" wide, north to south. From the floor to the flat and smooth ceiling it measures 19'1". Once the small tunnel was inspected at the end and at the top of the Grand Gallery, an attic space was discovered above the King's Chamber. The chamber had a smooth ceiling, but a very irregular floor. Obviously the beams making up the ceiling of the King's Chamber were smooth on the lower side only. Other investigators eventually discovered more of these attic chambers.

Some have speculated that the ceiling and chambers above the King's Chamber solved the structural problem of overhead loads, that they represented a strain-relieving technique to prevent the massive weight above the King's Chamber from caving in and destroying all of their efforts. The idea, however, doesn't explain the unusual shape of each beam. All of the beams are smooth on the underside, but rough and unfinished on the top. It can be argued that this was an economical design. However, when it is realized that a beam, whether smooth or rough, will carry the same load in an open span, as it is in this case, the most economical design would have been rough all around. Surely in the King's Chamber there is an esthetic reason for smoothing the visible side of the beams, but in the attic chambers there is no engineering, or esthetic reason for the extra effort except where there is contact with the supporting walls. Four of the attic chambers were inaccessible until modern times, when boring made it possible to reveal this puzzling feature.

The Great Pyramid Is the Only Repository Monument for Units of Weight And Measure

The first five chapters of this book adequately cover some of the mathematics embodied within the size and geometry of the Great Pyramid. Although other pyramids have a slope similar to the Great Pyramids, their size and orientation are in no way thought to embody any great mathematical or Earth-commensurate relationships. No other pyramid is so well orchestrated. Why the Great Pyramid is a veritable mathematical poem is the lingering mystery.

Summary

When each feature of the inner passages, chambers, doors, and structural elements is considered in detail, it is realized that they appear as entirely new creations in Egypt. By comparison, just adjacent to the east face of the Great Pyramid are a very typical mortuary temple, causeway, and valley building. All of these exterior attachments fit the typical scenario for an Egyptian burial, but the evidence supports that none of the internal features of the Great Pyramid itself were intended for a royal burial ceremony.

Could the original purpose of the Pyramid itself have been something other than a tomb? Could the idea to use the Great Pyramid as a tomb have occurred later? Pharaohs, encouraged by the royal court, had been known to put their name on existing monuments to demonstrate their power as god-kings. Could the Great Pyramid have been built by an earlier civilization, and did Khufu chisel his name on an existing structure? Could his achievements have been only the subsidiary pyramids, a valley building, a causeway, and a mortuary temple? Could it be that if the correct purpose for the Great Pyramid were known, then all the mysteries that exist within and about it would at once be solved?

NOTES

1. Sunlight casts a shadow with a blurred edge because the sun is not a point source, but a disk with a diameter of about one-half a degree. Referring to Figure 7.11, notice that the width of the blur at noon is determined using the rule of similar triangles:

Diameter/Distance = Blur/Height

In the case of the Sun: the figures are 865,000-mile diameter, 93,000,000 miles from Earth, and a 200-foot building at noon:

Blur = 865,000 x 5,280/93,000,000 x 5,280 x 200 = 1.86 feet

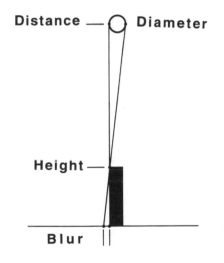

Figure 7.11 Depicted in exaggerated scale is a 200-foot building at noon, showing the effect of the solar disk casting a blurred shadow.

2. The difficulty in measuring blurred shadows introduces error into the calculation of the radius of the Earth. How much error depends on the distance between the obelisks. If the distance is hundreds of miles, the error is not so great. If the distance is a few miles, the error is very large. To see this, first look at Figure 6.24, and then imagine that the obelisks are ten miles apart. Because the value of the radius of the Earth is known, (3,956.5 miles as determined from not only Webster's dictionary, but also the 1989 World Almanac), the shadow, FD, that would be cast by a 200-foot obelisk can be calculated precisely. That value is 0.505497ft. Assume, based on experience gained in actually measuring these shadows, that for a 200-foot obelisk the uncertainty is one third of a foot. How much error does this introduce? The uncertainty means that the shadow could be erroneously measured as .505... + .333 = .838... Using the value .838 instead of .505 to cal-

culate the radius of the Earth results in a whopping 66 percent error. (Since all values are unchanged, the short cut method is to take the ratio of the new values: .838/.505 = 1.66.) By increasing the distance between the obelisks to 800 miles, the error is greatly reduced. The shadow cast by the northern-most obelisk would be 40.44 feet, and introducing a one third of a foot error to that value results in (40.44 + .33)/40.44 = 1.008, which is about a one percent error. The trouble is, this theoretical study has assumed that the distance between the obelisks was known with absolute certainty. As shown earlier, the historical evidence demonstrates that those errors were as much as seven percent. That error would affect the calculation for the radius of the earth by exactly that amount. Conclusion: If you want the exact circumference of the Earth, do not use the obelisk shadow technique, use a more exacting method.

Chapter Eight

Synopsis

The true building blocks of the universe are the Primal Energies. There are eight Primal Energies. They wink from the Is-Ness to the Is-Not-Ness at such blinding speeds that they appear to be permanently switched on and available for limitless creation. The Primal Energy Packets (PEP) are W-PEP, K-PEP, H-PEP, L-PEP, WP-PEP, AG-PEP, AL-PEP, and C-PEP, or W, K, H, L, WP, AG, AL, and C, for short. W, K, and H, the highest frequencies, originate in the Is-Not-Ness (Future). WP, AG, and AL, lowest frequencies, originate in the Is-Ness (past). L and C straddle the Is-Ness and Is-Not-Ness, the Now. If the largest C were expanded to be five times the size of the solar system, the smallest W would be the size of a period on this page. The first creations are subatomic particles. When all eight PEP are part of a formula, that creation exists within a three-dimensional reality. Electrons, Protons and Neutrons are examples of such creations. Only one-tenth of the mass of the universe exists in three-dimensional reality. Nine tenths of the mass of the universe exists as creations in other dimensions or as unbonded primal energy. The designers of the Great Pyramid understood Primal Energy and used it both to create power and to heal.

Chapter Eight

PRIMAL ENERGY

The Building Blocks of the Universe

Mass And Energy

To understand the secret of the Great Pyramid it is necessary to examine the commonly held ideas of what constitute the building blocks of the universe. The Greek philosopher Democritus long ago theorized that if a substance could be divided again and again, eventually there would be a particle of that substance that could not be divided any further, and this indivisible particle he defined as the "atom." It is now known with experimental certainty that there are 92 naturally occurring substances, or unique elements, and each has an atom that embodies all the properties of that element. The present day understanding is that these 92 elements combine in thousands of ways to form all of the natural and man-made compounds that comprise all living and non-living matter.

In searching for the ultimate building blocks of the universe, however, these 92 different atoms have been found to be only the top stable layer of formulas of even more basic particles, the subatomic particles. The Hydrogen atom, for example, symbolized as H, has the simplest formulation of all the atoms. This basic atom is comprised of one negatively-charged Electron orbiting about one positively-charged Proton. Although these two particles have the same quantity of electric charge, the Proton weighs 1835 times that of the Electron. The next atomic formula is the Helium atom, He, which has two Electrons orbiting a nucleus of two Protons and two Neutrons. The Neutron has the characteristic of a Proton and an Electron combined, and thus is electrically neutral and slightly heavier than a Proton. The formula for the atoms continues quite regularly, adding one Proton and one or several Neutrons to the nucleus. With the number of Electrons always equaling the number of Protons, complete atoms in the natural state are always electrically neutral.

The fact that Electrons, Neutrons, and Protons have characteristics entirely different from the atoms that are formed of them reverses the ancient belief that a substance has properties that are similar to the building blocks of which it is formed. The old belief that the building blocks were actually proportions of fire, air, earth, and water has been experimentally discounted. The experimental method has also proved that there is much more to atomic particles than Electrons, Protons, and Neutrons. Just before the turn of the 20th century, radium was discovered. Unlike all other atoms known at that time, the radium atom was found to be emitting particles. It is now understood that radium is naturally radioactive, naturally unstable, and eventually "decays" into smaller stable atoms accompanied by the release of subatomic particles and pure energy. Ernest Rutherford's experiments revealed that there were three distinct subatomic particles emanating from Radium. One was the Alpha particle, exactly the same as a high speed Helium nucleus. The second was a high speed Electron known as the Beta particle. The third was the mass-less gamma ray, which is a pure energy radiation much like "X-rays." This led scientists to begin a systematic search to discover the building blocks of all subatomic particles.

The complete mapping of the subatomic world to discover the ultimate building blocks of the universe has been one of the great searches of 20th Century science. Experiments using Neutrons, Protons, or Alpha particles to smash the nucleus of the atoms of different elements to reveal the smallest bits of matter are still in progress, and the limits have yet to be completely understood. In 1959, when the author was a high school student, the encyclopedia listed over 21 subatomic particles: Electrons, Protons, Anti-protons, Neutrons, Positrons, Neutrinos and various Mesons, but how they were related was a great mystery. Over thirty years later, science has not only discovered more of these particles, but has placed them in some relative order. (See Figure 8.1.) The current scientific explanation follows:

Electrons are basic particles and part of a larger class of particles known as Leptons, which can travel on their own. Protons and Neutrons are comprised of a class of particles known as Quarks, which are always trapped inside larger particles and so are never seen by themselves. Of the Leptons, the two that are in low-temperature physical reality are the Electron and the Electron neutrino. Of the Quarks found in ordinary matter, there is the up quark and the down quark. In extreme conditions, as in the early moments of the Big Bang with extreme temperature and pressure (a condition that can be duplicated in particle accelerators), there exist other types of Leptons and Quarks. In the Lepton class are the Muon, the Muon neutrino, the Tau, and the Tau neutrino. In the Quark class are the Charm, the Strange, the Top, and the Bottom. To explain the forces that bind particles there is a class known as Bosons. Photons exist within the Boson category, make up light, and carry the electromagnetic force. The Gluons are the carriers of the strong force between Quarks. The intermediate vector Bosons are the heavy carriers of the weak force that is responsible for some forms of radioactive decay.

Finally, Gravitons, which are theorized but not yet discovered experimentally, carry the force of gravity. Then there exists the whole class of the antimatter subatomic particles. For each particle that exists in regular matter, there is an antimatter counterpart, which is a sort of mirror image.

Introductory literature often portrays the Proton as a large, precise circle colored

red (positive); the Electron as a very small circle colored yellow (negative); and the Neutron as a large, precise circle, colored dark blue or dark gray (neutral). All other subatomic particles are drawn as precise circles or other geometric shapes of appropriate size and color, which helps to visualize their characteristics. It is very easy for the student to fall into the trap of thinking that all of these subatomic particles are neatly colored billiard balls of varying sizes and shapes. The reality is something quite different. It is now known that all energy particles and subatomic particles seem to possess a dual nature. One characteristic is their solid particle nature and the other, their wave nature. The classic example of that wave nature is demonstrated when light passes through a glass prism. The light slows as it encounters the dense medium of the glass, and this causes the light to "bend" or change direction slightly. This refraction phenomena differs for each frequency of light comprising the light beam and as a result the emerging light is separated into a familiar rainbow pattern.

In a classic laboratory experiment, high-speed Electrons are directed through a small hole and then on to a target. It would be expected that the solid Electron "billiard balls" would travel straight without deflecting from the straight line trajectory. A large percentage do travel straight through, but some are bent slightly off course and form a definite ring around the central dot or "bull's-eye." Even farther out from the bull's-eye is a second ring, but this second ring is very faint. An even fainter ring exists further out, and so on.

The only explanation for the appearance of the ever-fainter rings, known as a diffraction pattern, is that the Electron behaves as a solid particle part of the time, and as a pure energy wave the rest of the time.

Many experiments in the realm of atomic physics have been done to better understand this dual nature of small particles and this has lead to a newer, more enlightened concept. The subatomic particle is considered to be a small packet of wave energy. The most precise way to think of the position of any subatomic particle is to realize that the location is simply a place of "high probability." Thus the real world at the subatomic level gets very "fuzzy," because it is made up of overlapping clumps of energy in motion. This is why it is very misleading to visualize the Electron as a little solid-yellow billiard ball.

Einstein has been given credit for making us aware that matter and energy are related. In fact, they are the same thing. As early as 1905, he postulated that a body in motion had greater mass than a body at rest. After it was measured that high-speed Electrons have an apparent mass greater than slow-moving Electrons, the notions of mass and energy were expanded. If the energy of motion actually caused an increase in mass, could not the process be reversed? Or put another way, could a decrease in mass, or its complete destruction, give rise to energy? Einstein's famous equation, $E = mc^2$, equates mass and energy. Early in the century he calculated that if one pound of matter could be destroyed, it would yield enough energy to run a 100-watt light bulb for 13 million years.

In 1919, Rutherford used the Helium nucleus (Alpha particle) to bombard a target of Nitrogen. The products were Hydrogen and water and a very surprising amount of heat energy. The resulting heat energy was more than that of the speeding Alpha particles. The equation for the process is normally written as:

$$_2\text{He}^4 + _7\text{N1}^4 = _1\text{H}^1 + _1\text{H}^1_2 \ _8\text{O}^{16} + \text{heat}$$

112

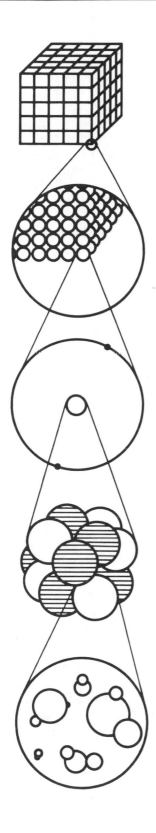

1. Solid matter exists in the cool regions of the universe — in planets, asteroids, gas clouds, etc.

Leptons: Particles that can travel on their own. Examples are the Electron, Electron Neutrino, Muon, Muon Neutrino, Tau, and the Tau Neutrino.

2. Atoms are defined as the smallest particles of an element.

Quarks: Particles trapped inside larger particles. Examples are the Up, Down, Charm, Strange, Top, and the Bottom Quark.

3. Each atom has in orbit one or more Electrons (-) around the nucleus.

Bosons: Fundamental Packets of energy that transmit the Forces of nature. Examples are Photons, Gluons, Intermediate Vector Bosons, and the Gravitons.

4. Each nucleus has one or more Protons (+) and zero or more neutrons (0).

Antimatter: Each particle has a mirror image counter part.

5. Each Proton and each Neutron is comprised of smaller particles.

Figure 8.1A General description of solid matter, the atom, and the large subatomic particles.

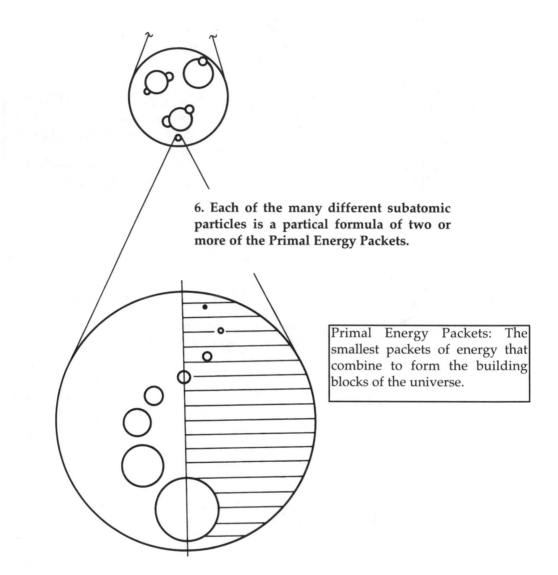

6. Each of the many different subatomic particles is a partical formula of two or more of the Primal Energy Packets.

Primal Energy Packets: The smallest packets of energy that combine to form the building blocks of the universe.

Figure 8.1B Primal Energy Packets (PEP) are the smallest building blocks of the universe. W-PEP, K-PEP, AND H-PEP originate from the Is-Not-Ness. WP-PEP, AG-PEP, and AL-PEP originate from the Is-Ness. L-PEP and C-PEP straddle the Is-Ness and Is-Not-Ness. Limitations do not allow a proper scale definition. If the largest C-PEP were five times the size of the solar system, the smallest W-PEP would be the size of a period on this page.

By carefully weighing the end products (the right side of the equation except the heat) it was found that they weighed less than the original products, so some mass was destroyed in the process. The destruction of mass explained the high amount of heat obtained in the experiment.

A few years later, another history-changing reaction was found. When Uranium 235 was struck by a fast moving Neutron, the Neutron was captured, momentarily forming Uranium 236; but, since Uranium 236 is highly unstable, it quickly broke up into two pieces, Barium and Krypton, plus two fast-moving Neutrons. By carefully weighing the end products, Barium plus Krypton plus the two Neutrons, it was found that they weighed less than the original products by 2/10 of the weight of a single Neutron. This may seem insignificant, only 0.00085 times the weight of one Uranium 236 atom, but this conversion of small bits of mass into energy is what powers atomic devices.

Primal Energy

A logical step beyond this leads to an understanding that the true building blocks of the subatomic particles, the building blocks of the universe, are certain specific quanta, or bandwidths, of pure, very high-frequency energy. The question has always been, how many distinct primal quanta exist and precisely what are their frequencies?

Assume that a recurring Big Bang is one of the truths of the universe. If so, there exist widely spaced events when the universe, or the "All that is" or the "Is-Ness," compresses, collapses and returns to the IT. In its most simple and elemental state this is one energy, packed into one, inconceivably small location. After a time in that state, the IT is ready to move outward again into the expanded state.

What is the first step towards the expanded state? In the simplest step possible, the IT simply divides. Figure 8.2A shows the division in a linear perception, a dividing of a band of frequencies into two groups. One becomes the Is-Ness and the other becomes the Is-Not-Ness. The first step of the great expansion is two distinct energy packages, or energy packets as they are called, one of high frequencies and one of low frequencies. Each following step is equally simple. The second step of the great expansion is for these two newly-created packets of energy to simply divide again so that there exists four distinct energy bandwidths. The third step of the great expansion is formed in the same simple way, the four energy packets each divide again. It is shown by figure 8.2A that after three divisions or creations, there exist in all of the Is-ness and Is-Not-Ness eight distinct energy packets of the bandwidths. Figure 8.2B gives the same information in a concentric circular graph form, which is representative of the early moments of the Big Bang and the implication is an outward expansion.

The newly expanded Is-Ness and the Is-Not-Ness now exists in an important new state, a state in which the temperature is cool enough for the eight energy packets to join into interesting elemental particles. This process is easier than further simple division. These eight distinct bands of energy, the eight Primal Energy Packets (PEP), are the long sought-after building blocks of the universe. More will be said about the early division of the Is-Ness in later chapters, but for now accepting these eight will make the universe easier to understand.

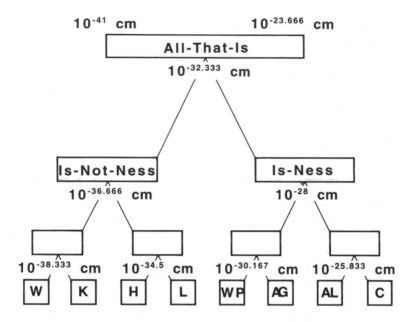

Figure 8.2A Depicted is the All-That-Is dividing three times. The first division creates the Is-Ness and the Is-Not-Ness. After three divisions there are eight Primal Energy Packets. Each represents a portion of the original bandwidth.

One of two designators will be used for the Primal Energies: W-PEP, K-PEP, H-PEP, L-PEP, WP-PEP, AG-PEP, AL-PEP, and C-PEP; or the shorthand designations: W, K, H, L, WP, Ag, Al, and C. The choice of these letter designators will become apparent later.

Figure 8.3 represents the eight bandwidths in a graphical form. Figure 8.4 represents the eight bandwidths in tabular form. Placing this information upon the electromagnetic spectrum is represented in Figure 8.5, which shows the relative position of radio waves, infrared, visible, ultraviolet, X-Ray, Gamma ray, the dimensions, and the PEP energies relative to one another. The energy of any electromagnetic wave has a specific wavelength and frequency determined by two basic equations:

wavelength = speed of light / frequency
energy x wavelength = speed of light x Plank's constant (See Reference 16.)

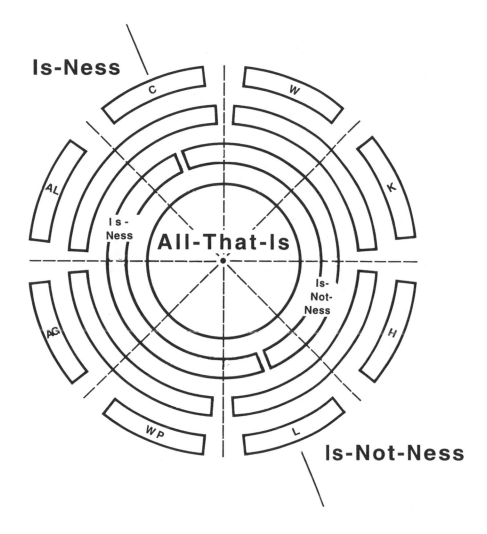

Figure 8.2B Depicted is essentially the same information as Figure 8.2A, only the representation follows the popular concept of the Big Bang. Note that the Primal Energy Packets C and L essentially straddle the Is-Ness and the Is-Not-Ness.

For example, visible light has a wavelength on the order of 5×10^{-7} meter, a frequency of 10^{15} Hz cycles per second, and an equivalent energy of about two Electron volts. By comparison, W-PEP, the most energetic PEP, has an energy of 10^{36} Electron volts, which is unimaginably powerful. This value is calculated using the speed of light — appropriate only for this three-dimensional (3D) reality — yet it gives some understanding of the power and smallness of the PEP. The unattached W-PEP actually exist in the other dimensions, but if the PEP were to manifest in this 3D realm for a brief part of a second, it would take 10^{36} Electron volts of energy to make it happen.

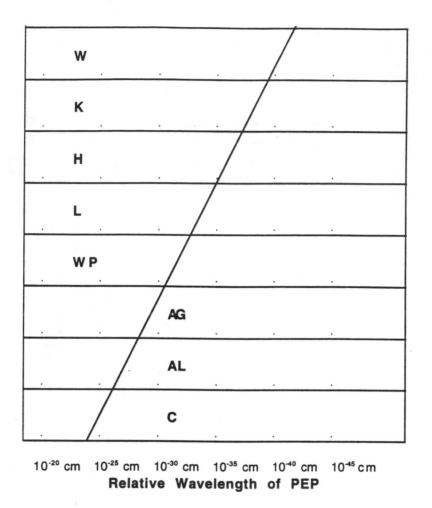

10⁻²⁰ cm   10⁻²⁵ cm   10⁻³⁰ cm   10⁻³⁵ cm   10⁻⁴⁰ cm   10⁻⁴⁵ cm
Relative Wavelength of PEP

Figure 8.3 Graphical form of Primal Energy shows relative wavelengths.

PEP Packet	Bandwidth	
	Smallest	**Largest**
W	10^{-41} cm	$10^{-38.833}$ cm
K	$10^{-38.833}$ cm	$10^{-36.666}$ cm
H	$10^{-36.666}$ cm	$10^{-34.5}$ cm
L	$10^{-34.5}$ cm	$10^{-32.333}$ cm
W P	$10^{-32.333}$ cm	$10^{-30.167}$ cm
AG	$10^{-30.167}$ cm	10^{-28} cm
AL	10^{-28} cm	$10^{-25.833}$ cm
C	$10^{-25.833}$ cm	$10^{-23.666}$ cm

Figure 8.4 Tabular form of Primal Energy. Energy, wavelength, and frequency are related by: $l = c/F$ (c = speed of light).

10^{10}	10^9	10^8	10^7	10^6	10^5	10^4	10^3	10^2	λ (cm)
				VLF	LF	MF	HF	VHF	UHF
					AM		TV FM	TV	

Radio and TV Bands

1	10	10^2	10^3	10^4	10^5	10^6	10^7	10^8	F (CPS)
10^{-14}	10^{-13}	10^{-12}	10^{-11}	10^{-10}	10^{-9}	10^{-8}	10^{-7}	10^{-6}	E (ev)

10^1	10^0	10^{-1}	10^{-2}	10^{-3}	10^{-4}	10^{-5}	10^{-6}	10^{-7}	λ (cm)

Micro-Waves   **Infrared**   **Visible Light**   **Ultra-Violate**   **X-Ray**

10^9	10^{10}	10^{11}	10^{12}	10^{13}	10^{14}	10^{15}	10^{16}	10^{17}	F (CPS)
10^{-5}	10^{-4}	10^{-3}	10^{-2}	10^{-1}	10^0	10^1	10^2	10^3	E (ev)

10^{-8}	10^{-9}	10^{-10}	10^{-11}	10^{-12}	10^{-13}	10^{-14}	10^{-15}	10^{-16}	λ (cm)

X-Ray   **Gamma Ray**   **Limit Observed by Science**   **4th to 10th Dimension**

10^{18}	10^{19}	10^{20}	10^{21}	10^{22}	10^{23}	10^{24}	10^{25}	10^{26}	F (CPS)
10^4	10^5	10^6	10^7	10^8	10^9	10^{10}	10^{11}	10^{12}	E (ev)

10^{-17}	10^{-18}	10^{-19}	10^{-20}	10^{-21}	10^{-22}	10^{-23}	10^{-24}	10^{-25}	λ (cm)

4TH to 10TH Dimension   **C**   **Primal Energy**

10^{27}	10^{28}	10^{29}	10^{30}	10^{31}	10^{32}	10^{33}	10^{34}	10^{35}	F (CPS)
10^{13}	10^{14}	10^{15}	10^{16}	10^{17}	10^{18}	10^{19}	10^{20}	10^{21}	E (ev)

10^{-26}	10^{-27}	10^{-28}	10^{-29}	10^{-30}	10^{-31}	10^{-32}	10^{-33}	10^{-34}	λ (cm)

AL   **AG**   **WP**   **L**   **Primal Energy**

10^{36}	10^{37}	10^{38}	10^{39}	10^{40}	10^{41}	10^{42}	10^{43}	10^{44}	F (CPS)
10^{22}	10^{23}	10^{24}	10^{25}	10^{26}	10^{27}	10^{28}	10^{29}	10^{30}	E (ev)

10^{-35}	10^{-36}	10^{-37}	10^{-38}	10^{-39}	10^{-40}	10^{-41}	λ (cm)

H   **K**   **W**   **Primal Energy**

10^{45}	10^{46}	10^{47}	10^{48}	10^{49}	10^{50}	10^{51}	F (CPS)
10^{31}	10^{32}	10^{33}	10^{34}	10^{35}	10^{36}	10^{37}	E (ev)

Figure 8.5 The Primal Energy Packets represented as part of the electromagnetic spectrum.

119

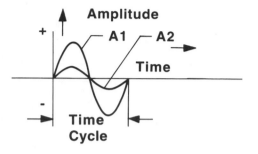

Figure 8.6A An alternating wave (electrical or physical) represented graphically as a sinusoidal wave. A1 has three times the amplitude of A2.

To conceptualize the Primal Energy Particles as distinct from one another, first consider the flow of pure energy. Think of pure energy in simple terms like alternating wave-forms, which is represented graphically in Figure 8.6A. The wave-form of Figure 8.6A can represent an alternating electrical current, or the vertical component in a particle of a physical wave such as an ocean wave. Here the wave A1 is shown flowing in alternating positive and negative directions. This complete cycle is done in a particular unit of time that depends on the frequency of the energy. The amplitude or force of such a wave is shown on the graph by the distance above and below the base line. Notice that wave A2 is the same frequency, but one-third the amplitude of wave A1. Figure 8.6B shows two waves of the same amplitude, but of different frequencies. Starting at the same time, each ends at a different time. The wave B1 is higher in frequency, being ten times faster than wave B2. High frequency thus means shorter wavelength. Note another wave, B3, has been placed to show a relatively high-frequency wave, at a small amplitude and starting at a different time.

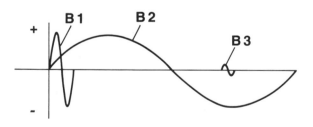

Figure 8.6B Three sinusoidal waves. B1 is the same amplitude as B2, but ten times the frequency (wavelength is 1/10th as long.) B3 is one sixth the amplitude and 20 times the frequency of B1.

120

There is one more important concept about waves to consider. Imagine the low frequency wave B2 of Figure 8.6B to be a large amplitude ocean wave formed by a distant storm. Let wave B3 represent a small amplitude wave formed by a local wind pattern. The two waves combine, add and subtract, forming the shape shown in Figure 8.6C. This is true for ocean waves, for audio waves, and for electromagnetic waves. The reason radio and TV communication is possible is because information waves ride upon the carrier waves. In general, waves ride upon waves.

Applying this principle to the PEP bandwidths demonstrates the vast differences that exist between them and also the potential for a vast universe of endless creations. The W-PEP, the highest frequency, is the shortest wave-form. The C-PEP, the lowest frequency, is the longest wave-form. The C-PEP in its largest size is: $10^{17.333}$ times as large as the smallest W-PEP. Appreciate that $10^{17.333}$ is 215,000,000,000,000,000,000. To grasp the extremes of this range, let the period at the end of this sentence (0.01 of an inch) represent the smallest W-PEP. The distance from the Sun to the Earth is 93,000,000 miles. The distance to the farthest known planet, Pluto, is almost forty times that. Imagine a sphere encompassing the orbit of planet Pluto with the Sun at the center. That sphere would have to be five times larger to represent the largest C-PEP. The smallest C-PEP is 1/147 the size of that sphere, which is still larger in diameter than the orbit of the Earth. If these spheres were covered with water, imagine the countless wave patterns that could flow across the surface if the waves were the size of a dot. Imagine the endless complexity if other wave heights were added, each representing a different energy: K-PEP, H-PEP, L-PEP, WP-PEP, AG-PEP, and AL-PEP. All of these waves of energy, in different proportions and amplitudes, can and do ride upon the surface. This is the primal nature of the universe.

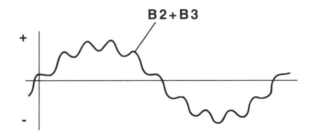

Figure 8.6C Two frequencies mixing in the same medium. "Waves ride upon waves."

The atoms were long thought to be the elemental and smallest particles of matter. The atoms, however, are extremely large compared to the PEP. Consider the smallest atom, Hydrogen. It has a single Proton at the nucleus and a single orbiting Electron to complete the atom. The diameter of this atom is on the order of 10^{-9} cm. (See Reference 16.) The largest C-PEP is only $10^{-23.666}$ cm long. The ratio of the Hydrogen atom to the

C-PEP is therefore 4.9 x 10^{14}, which is the size of a sphere that would almost encompass the orbit of the planet Earth compared to the period at the end of this sentence.

Each PEP has a specific function as it forms into subatomic particles in the now "cool" universe. The C-PEP is the largest and is the "hook" to hang the hat, the black board for the chalk, the white canvas waiting for the color, the place that the other particles can bind to. As soon as the eight PEP are created, countless numbers of energy packets of C-PEP fill the universe. This forms the grid work upon which the other PEP can combine.

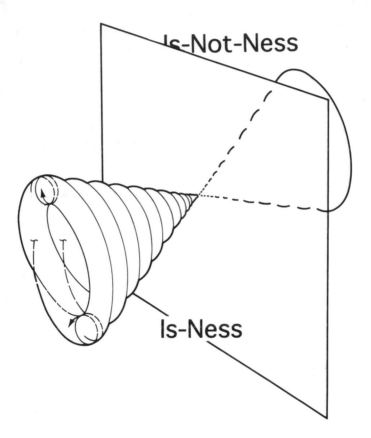

Figure 8.7 C-PEP cycles between the Is-Not-Ness and the Is-Ness at trillions of times per second.

The combinations to follow become the next creations of the expanding universe. A workable perception of this is to imagine all of space filled with white ping-pong balls. The unmarked surface of the ping-pong balls represent the C-PEP waiting for "color" to be added. The physical nature of the C-PEP, however, is more aptly described by a toroid movement of energy. Once the toroid, a coil of moving energy shaped like a donut, enters into the realm of the Is-Ness, it grows in size until it reaches some maximum value and then it begins to shrink. The path described by the movement is a spiral, similar to a sea shell. When the movement finally enters the realm of the Is-Not-Ness, the same toroid-spiral movement occurs there. So the C-PEP are constantly cycling back and forth at trillions upon trillions of times per second. (See Figure 8.7.)

PEP	C + PEP^1
W	C + W
K	C + K
H	C + H
L	C + L
WP	C + WP
AG	C + AG
AL	C + AL
C	C + C (extremely short lived)

Figure 8.8 Tabulation of all C + PEP^1, Primal Energies combined with C-PEP. There are essentially only seven possibilities, since C + C is highly unstable.

Further distinct functions of the PEP will be discussed later. For now, the important thing to realize is that the most simple combinations occur first, one packet of W-PEP combines with one packet of C-PEP, one packet of K-PEP combines with one packet of C-PEP, and so on. The formula C-PEP + all other PEP is designated C+PEP^1 and defines the seven possibilities. These are the most simple subatomic formulations possible and the list is given in Figure 8.8.

The next possible formulations are all the combinations of C+PEP with two other PEP. These formulations of one C-PEP and two high frequency PEP is designated C+PEP^2. The complete list of the three-PEP formulations yields 49 possibilities and appears in Figure 8.9. Note that C+W+K is the same as C+K+W, and that C+K+H is the same as C+H+K, and so on, so there are only 42 completely different possibilities. Also, C+W+W (and the like) is distinctly different from C+W, since amplitude or the amount of each PEP determines another distinct creation.

The next list, possible combinations of four PEP, would yield over 200 formulas. The list with five PEP would yield combinations in the thousands. Even though none of these are listed, it is clear where this is heading. Add to these astronomical possibilities the fact that amplitude adds infinitely more distinct creations, and is it any wonder that such diversity exists when looking at the universe!

Some Properties of the PEP

1. Anything that moves is partly an illusion. The C-PEP portion of the formula remains fixed, while the string-like tendrils of the other PEP do swirl and move. The most solid part of a moving creation is the formula, which once created is part of the Is-Ness forever.

PEP	C+ PEP^2						
	C + W	C + K	C + H	C + L	C + WP	C + AG	C + AL
W	C + W +W	C + K +W	C + H +W	C + L +W	C + WP +W	C + AG +W	C + AL +W
K	C + W +K	C + K +K	C + H +K	C + L +K	C + WP +K	C + AG +K	C + AL +K
H	C + W +H	C + K +H	C + H +H	C + L +H	C + WP +H	C + AG +H	C + AL +H
L	C + W +L	C + K +L	C + H +L	C + L +L	C + WP +L	C + AG +L	C + AL +L
W P	C + W +WP	C + K +WP	C + H +WP	C + L +WP	C + WP +WP	C + AG +WP	C + AL +WP
AG	C + W +AG	C + K +AG	C + H +AG	C + L +AG	C + WP +AG	C + AG +AG	C + AL +AG
AL	C + W +AL	C + K +AL	C + H +AL	C + L +AL	C + WP +AL	C + AG +AL	C + AL +AL

Figure 8.9 Shown is the tabular form of all C + PEP^2. There are 42 distinct, stable formulas since seven formulations repeat.

2. Attractive forces are formed at the moment of the Is-Ness/Is-Not-Ness separation. At that point the "memory" of being complete places a "desire" within the separated PEP to join in formulations, and especially to attach to C-PEP. At the level of the PEP there is no emotion, but this makes attractive forces understandable.

3. The strongest attraction in the universe is C-PEP. The force is unimaginable. One dense, closely-packed spoonful suddenly poured into the solar system would cause the high-frequency PEP that make up the sun and the planets to forget their position in the formula and thus quickly collapse into the C-PEP.

4. For "solid" matter to exist in the "cool" 3D regions of the universe, all eight of the Primal Energy Particles must be part of the formulation. When any atom has one PEP removed, it is immediately reduced to some form of elusive subatomic particle, unrecognizable from the three dimensional reality except for a split second in atom smashing experiments.

5. The mass of the universe is distributed such that only one tenth exists in the form of three-dimensional reality (all eight PEP combined) which means that from our reality, nine tenths of the universe cannot be observed. Another way to perceive this is

that the universe is full of vast swirling mists of limitless energy and energy is everywhere. It is passing through all things at all times and it exists within "solid" matter as well as within the "empty" regions between the stars.

Imagine a deep ocean with a flat, calm surface. Looking down into it one imagines nothing exists in it because nothing is visible. That is the vast emptiness between the stars, the vast emptiness between atoms, as well as the vast emptiness between the Protons and Electrons of the atoms. Occasionally a flying fish surfaces for an instant then vanishes back into the unknown abyss. That is a fleeting subatomic particle, a combination of several PEP, only visible for a fraction of a second. Then a whale decides to poke its head out of the water and look around. While doing that, a seal jumps up on his nose, a flying fish lands on the seal, several more sea animals are added, and for quite a while, the emptiness has created something that is real and visible. The whale gets tired and sinks back into the ocean, but decides with its new found friends to try it again. The whale resurfaces and all his friends jump on, and there it is again, something real. The concept spreads, and suddenly whales surface everywhere with different groupings of sea creatures nose-riding. These are the atoms that make up everything real in our reality. The whales and their nose-riding friends start to form complex patterns. They are great social events. From a balloon, the patterns — like dots on a TV screen — form the recognizable patterns and the forms we know — real, such as the suns, planets, and living creations that live upon them. Each dimension has its TV screen. In the three dimensional reality, all eight primal energies must be present or the form will disappear.

6. C-PEP and L-PEP have primary existence at the junction point between the Is-Ness and the Is-Not-Ness. They straddle the two realms. C-PEP gives a position for the PEP to bind to, so it is the paper on which the design can be created. The job of L-PEP gives definition to the formulation of the particle creation, so it is the spray fixative that keeps the design from getting mixed or from fading into oblivion.

7. The highest-frequency PEP, specifically W-PEP, K-PEP, and H-PEP, naturally exist in the state of the Is-Not-Ness, the future. The lowest frequency PEP, WP-PEP, AG-PEP, and AL-PEP, naturally exist in the state of the Is-Ness, the future. Because all PEP wink between the Is-Ness and the Is-Not-Ness, they are all available for combinations. These Energies are the colors that comprise the design, they are the paint the makes up the painting.

8. The characteristic of each PEP, temporarily existing in the Is-Ness and then in the Is-Not-Ness, means that they all are continuously winking in and out, and this is true whether the observation is made from the Is-Ness side or the Is-Not-Ness side. Each PEP has its own particular frequency for this cyclic movement. Thus, the entire universe is a Christmas tree with lights twinkling on and off, happening so fast that observers in the 3D realm perceive everything as continuous, solid, and real. The lights appear to be on continuously.

Conclusion

Consider one last comparison of the PEP in which the relative sizes are expressed as numbers. (See Figure 8.10.) The average relative size of each PEP is printed in long form, is center justified, and is printed in the pyramid. The natural pyramid is suggestive of the Great Pyramid, and hints a part of the mystery. The complexity of the puzzle requires some time to completely unravel.

Formulas

Mesons = L + WP + Gravity
Gravity = L + WP + C (C gives the location)
Quark = H + C
Charm = K + C
Quark + Tachyon, travel in pairs
Meson + Charm, travel in pairs
AL + WP, travel in pairs
AG + WP, travel in pairs

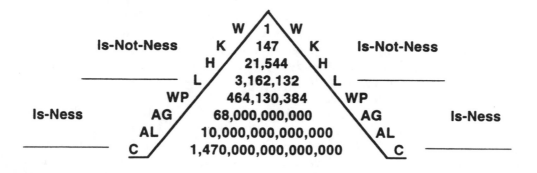

Figure 8.10 The relative average size of the PEP with C-PEP at the base and W-PEP at the top. C-PEP and L-PEP straddle the Is-Ness and the Is-Not-Ness.

Chapter Nine

Synopsis

The Great Pyramid converted Earth, Moon, Sun, and even Primal Energy into high-frequency radiant microwaves (of a frequency benign to living tissue) to power an ancient civilization. By comparison, our present system uses low frequency 60-cycle alternating-current energy, produced primarily by burning polluting fossil fuels, and delivered by expensive and bulky transmission lines. The Great Pyramid used seven technologies like fuel combustion, piezoelectric generation, thermocouple generation, and so on, to produce power. For example, the outer casing blocks, built of piezoelectric stone, formed a diaphragm that never touched the core blocks and had a natural resonance of twelve cycles-per-second (12 cps). It was sensitive to free energy, like wind, distant lightening, twisting of the moon's gravity, and Earth frequencies, and sent a constant 12 cps wave towards the King's Chamber. The King's Chamber converted this low frequency in a multi-step process to a high frequency. The many passages and chambers helped control and stabilize the output. For example, in the Grand Gallery, a giant electrical device was mounted on caterpillar treads and moved up and down to adjust the resonant beat frequency. This controlled the output like the control rods of a nuclear power reactor. The power generator, the Great Pyramid, functioned for several thousand years, lighting up everything in the advanced Atlantian society including powering their flying discs as much as 25,000 miles away.

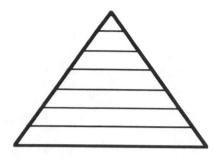

Chapter Nine

HOW THE GREAT PYRAMID WORKED

The Solid State Power Converter

The Secret of the Great Pyramid

Uncovering the secret of the Great Pyramid, as alluded to in the last chapter, has to do with understanding the Primal Energy Packets, the PEP. Even though these quantums of energy are very small, like tightly packed springs, they contain enormous amounts of energy. As was shown, greater packing yields greater potential energy. Did the Great Pyramid have something to do with energy? The answer is yes. One of the primary functions of the Great Pyramid was to provide power for the civilization that flourished around it. The Great Pyramid functioned very much like hydroelectric, fossil fuel, and nuclear power plants do today. The Great Pyramid was partly a solid-state power device and partly a mechanical device that together transformed gross and variable Earth and Moon energy into a refined, steady, and convenient energy source. The unique process of how that was achieved will be examined in some detail.

The Process of Power Conversion

The steam engine conjures up images of the inception of the industrial revolution, the birth of the modern technological society. In the last century, steam power made its debut when water was pumped from flooded mines. Soon after that success, steam was turning the wheels of industry and propelling ships, trains, and even farm tractors. In time, steam power was turning electric generators and converting mechanical power directly into convenient electrical power. Wood, the original form of fuel used to fire the furnace and boil water, was replaced by more compact fuels: coal, fuel oil, and in recent times, nuclear fuel. Of course other fuel burning engines were developed, but they and the steam engine operate on the identical principle of converting latent energy stored in a fuel into another convenient form of energy, usually mechanical or electrical.

The Great Pyramid followed the exact same principle of conversion of one form of energy into another. Specifically, the Great Pyramid converted part of the enormous kinetic energy of the Earth, as it orbits the Sun and spirals through the Milky Way Galaxy, into a high-frequency alternating electric energy. The alternating current, AC, was not transmitted by lines as is done today, but by radio waves. Why the radio wave principle was chosen can be understood by reviewing the basics of resonance and alternating current.

When plucked, a string on a violin will emit a tone that is determined by its tension and length. Figure 9.1A shows the fundamental frequency of the string in its maximum movements. The middle of the string reaches a maximum displacement at point A before it comes to rest and reverses its direction and accelerates towards point B. The string finally comes to rest at point B and reverses its direction and accelerates towards point A, repeating the cycle until heating and other forms of drag absorb all of the energy that was plucked into the string. Figure 9.1B shows the same string resonating at the second harmonic, which is twice the frequency of the original tone. Figure 9.1C demonstrates the principle that both tones can be on the same string at the same time and this holds true for all higher harmonics. Thus, besides the fundamental, many other harmonics vibrate on the same string at the same time. This mechanical, acoustic form of alternating motion can be heard with our ear if the cycles per second (cps) are within a range of roughly 20 cps to 20,000 cps. If a bow is used on the violin, a continuous tone is heard. This is because the string of the bow is slightly roughened and has resin worked into it to cause it to alternately stick and slip, producing many small "plucks" in succession. So even though the bow is making a motion in one direction, the string begins to vibrate and to alternate at its predestined or natural mechanical frequency. Everything in nature has a natural mechanical resonant frequency, be it a violin string, a tuning fork, a bell, a rock, a crystal, or even an object as large as a pyramid.

This mechanical resonance has a counterpart in electrical circuits. An alternating current in a tuned resonant circuit is similar to the violin string vibrating back and forth. A tuned resonant circuit is nothing more than a coil and a capacitor in a parallel arrangement and with correct values (number of windings on the coil and size of the capacitor plates) to offer the least resistance for the desired frequency. The essential property of a coil is that it stores magnetic energy. The essential property of a capacitor is that it stores electrostatic energy. In the tuned or resonant circuit of Figure 9.2C and Figure 9.2D (imagine the battery is not linked to the circuit), the nature of the coil and closely spaced plates is that when the coil is charged up, the capacitor is uncharged; when the capacitor is charged up, the coil is uncharged. This electrical compliment means that they alternately hold the energy, so the energy swings back and forth much like a mechanical pendulum.

To understand why this is so, consider the capacitor, which is essentially two closely-spaced parallel plates separated by a vacuum, air, or a dielectric material such as glass or plastic. The plates are usually made of metal, but in theory can be of any material that readily conducts electricity such as certain piezoelectric crystals. Such a device will hold the energy of an electrostatic field between the plates once charged up.

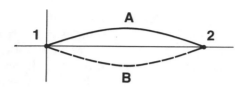

Figure 9.1A The fundamental frequency of a tight string between points 1 and 2 is shown with a maximum deflection A and B.

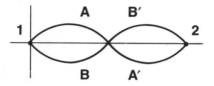

Figure 9.1B The second harmonic of the same string between points 1 and 2 without the fundamental present.

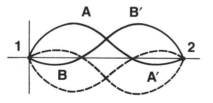

Figure 9.1C The fundamental and the second harmonic vibrate on the same string between points 1 and 2 at the same time.

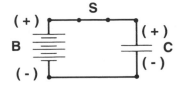

Figure 9.2A Depicted is a simple electrical circuit. When the switch, S, is closed, Electrons flow towards the positive (+) terminal of the battery, B. Within a fraction of a second, Electrons pile up on the lower plate of the capacitor, C, so there is an excess of Electrons — (-). Electrons on the top plate flow into the battery, so there is an excess of Protons — (+). The current stops when the voltage on the capacitor reaches the same voltage as the battery. An electrostatic charge exits between the plates.

The circuit of Figure 9.2A shows the fundamental method to charge a capacitor with a battery. Batteries, of course, cause free Electrons to flow through an external circuit. The Electrons, following the law that opposite charges attract, always flow from the negative (-) terminal towards the positive (+) terminal. After charging the capacitor, the switch is opened as in Figure 9.2B. The battery has done a certain amount of work over a period of time on the capacitor, and it is that energy that is stored in the capacitor. The capacitor in effect is now a battery of the same voltage as the original battery, but capable, depending upon the size of the plates and dielectric, of delivering only a fraction of the current that the battery could deliver. A simple way to understand how the capacitor stores energy is to imagine the Electrons, negative in charge (-), piled up in excess on the lower plate, and because these Electrons each carry a (-) charge, that plate is negatively charged. By comparison there are fewer Electrons on the top plate, as they are drawn into the battery. The top plate therefore carries a positive (+) charge since there are an excess of Protons (+). The excess Electrons on the negative plate sense the need for Electrons on the positive plate and would like to jump across the non-conducting dielectric if they could. This state of electrical imbalance is the storage of electrostatic energy in a capacitor.

Now consider how a coil introduced across the charged capacitor will affect the behavior of the Electron flow (See Figure 9.2C.) A coil is essentially an insulated wire wrapped around an iron core. The excess Electrons will begin to flow through the coil and begin to fill the positive plate. The process is complicated, however, by the properties of the coil, which has the ability to store magnetic field energy. As current begins to flow through the coil, the magnetic component reinforces the magnetic component in each adjacent winding or loop. By the time the capacitor is depleted, the coil is charged.

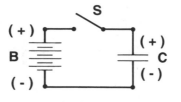

Figure 9.2B Even when the switch, S, is opened, the capacitor, C, remains fully charged with the polarity shown.

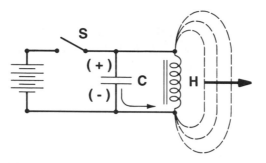

Figure 9.2C The coil, H, introduced across the charged capacitor, C, allows the Electrons to flow towards the positively charged plate. The accelerating Electrons start the magnetic field of the coil to expand. The electrostatic charge of the capacitor is replaced by the energy in the electromagnetic field of the coil.

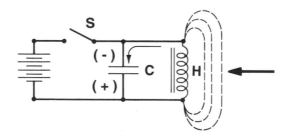

Figure 9.2D The current slows down as the capacitor reaches neutrality or zero voltage (same amount of electrons on both plates.) The electromagnetic field of the coil then collapses. The energy stored in the field causes the Electron flow to continue surging in the same direction. This causes the Electrons to pile up on the top plate. The polarity is reversed.

When the Electron current stops flowing, the field begins to collapse and this collapsing field transfers the stored magnetic field energy back into Electron flow. By the time the field is fully collapsed (more windings yield a longer time) the Electrons within the capacitor are not in balance, but are in excess on the top plate (as shown in Figure 9.2D), which is now negatively charged. The capacitor is in a charged state of reversed polarity and the cycle is ready to repeat. The cycle will repeat until heating and other forms of drag absorb all of the energy.

The next step of understanding is to imagine the switch being turned off and on by a small motor at a frequency much lower than the resonant frequency, but in step or in the right phase. Clearly the resonant circuit would produce alternating current at the resonant frequency until the motor was turned off. Radio transmitters, in fact, employ an electrical switching circuit that performs the job of the small motor connected to a switch and it is accomplished with no moving parts.

Another fundamental characteristic of alternating current, wave propagation through the air, was first investigated by Marconi and then others, including Nikola Tesla. This works because coils induce magnetic field energy in each adjacent coil winding on the same core, as well as coils at a distance. It was found that a coil unwound and straightened behaves perfectly well as a radiator of the alternating energy and is the most efficient when the wire is at least one-fourth the length of the electromagnetic wave as measured by the classic formula: wavelength x frequency = speed of light (in a vacuum). It was also found that the energy propagates in air nearly as well as in a vacuum. So alternating current at 1,300,000 cycles per second, 1300 on the AM dial, has a wavelength of 752 feet, which means 1/4 of the wave, 188 feet, is the best length for the antenna. Vertical wires and towers work fine for this purpose and have become quite a common sight. The use of higher frequencies has yielded shorter antennas, (for example on cellular car phones) but the radiation is more line of sight. That is, the longer waves bend around the curvature of the Earth. In either case, the energy is transmitted almost instantly to anywhere on Earth at 186,000 miles per second, the speed of light, but the signal weakens with distance, falling off at the inverse of the distance squared.

The simplest transmitter is the electrical device shown in Figure 9.3A. A quarter-wave antenna is shown coupled to the main coil longest via a secondary coil shortest wound on the same core, but with enough windings to receive the energy of the resonant circuit by magnetic coupling. The tower antenna is mounted on a dielectric pedestal to insulate it from the Earth ground. Note that the transmitter resonant circuit is grounded at the other end as shown. The ground connection helps to boost the efficiency of the antenna. If a second antenna, the receiving antenna, is similarly connected to a resonant circuit tuned to the same frequency, energy will be absorbed by its resonant circuit. Although the energy received is quite small compared to what was transmitted, the frequency remains exactly the same. The diode rectifier shown in Figure 9.3A is essentially a device that allows current to flow in one direction only. Thus, the alternating current, AC, of the resonant circuit is rectified and only positive pulses pass to the battery as shown. These positive pulses, when large enough, will charge the battery, which demonstrates the essential principles of transmitting power to a distant location without transmission lines.

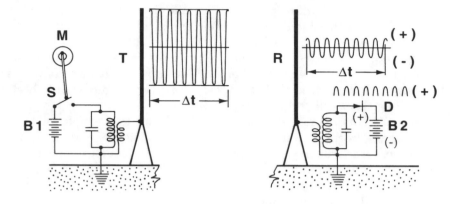

Figure 9.3A Depicted is a simplified transmitter and receiver circuit. The motor turns the switch on and off to keep the resonant circuit going. The towers are coils in a straightened form. The signal received is of the same frequency as the transmitted signal, but at a reduced amplitude. The diode, D, rectifies the signal. The regular pulses charge the battery, B 2, demonstrating energy transmitted to a distant location without transmission lines.

Our society uses high-frequency radio waves to carry communication. It does this by modulating the basic carrier signal. Modulation can be done by varying the amplitude of the signal (AM) or by modulating the frequency (FM). To make the receiver produce audio signals from the modulated signal received, another circuit is added that demodulates or separates the audio wave from the high-frequency carrier wave so that it can be heard in an earphone or through an amplifier and then a speaker.

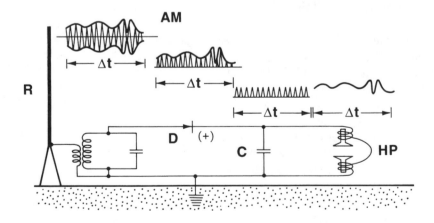

Figure 9.3B Depicted is a simplified circuit to demodulate amplitude modulated, AM, transmissions. The received AM signal is rectified by the diode, D. The capacitor, C, is a low resistance to the high-frequency carrier, but a large resistance to the low-frequency

audio signal. By contrast the coils of the head phone, HP, have a low resistance to the audio and a high resistance to the high-frequency carrier. The capacitor-head phone combination demodulates the audio from the carrier.

Amateur radio enthusiasts usually explore the field of radio by first building an economical radio called a crystal radio receiver, which gets its name from the crystal diode used to rectify the incoming signal. The device has no batteries and is powered entirely by energy absorbed by the antenna as shown in Figure 9.3B. In this case the carrier frequency is amplitude modulated with an audio signal of much lower frequency. The crystal diode rectifies this signal, allowing only the positive half to pass. The signal is demodulated by a capacitor and a set of headphones. The capacitor passes the high-frequency carrier signal, but offers the audio signal a great deal of resistance. Capacitors must be very large to pass audio signals. The headphones, however, easily pass the audio signal. Such receivers operate very well when the distance from the transmitter is ten miles or so depending on the power output of the transmitter. When it comes to the length of the receiving antenna, the longer the better.

Although the energy absorbed by a receiving antenna is a minute fraction of the amount transmitted, it is possible, as shown, to transmit electric energy over vast distances without the use of wires. This was the principle that Tesla, tried to introduce to the world at the turn of the century. Tesla's equipment was too primitive to do much more than demonstrate the principle of energy transmission via electromagnetic radiation. His oscillators produced not one exact frequency as desired, but a wide band of frequencies, so that most of the energy had to be discarded at the power station. Had this particular problem been overcome, there was still the other problem of transmitting electromagnetic radiation efficiently, because it requires either a lot of transmitters or a lot of power. Since the power drops off inversely as the square of the distance, it realistically means that at ten miles there is only one fourth the energy delivered at five miles, at 50 miles there is only one-hundredth the power delivered at five miles, and at 500 miles there is one-ten-thousandth the power delivered to the five-mile receiver. By contrast, transmission lines, also designed by Tesla, can carry power 500 miles with small losses and are in effect 10,000 times more efficient than the transmitting tower principle.

Although Tesla's first theory was essentially correct, the transmitting technology needed was not. (See Reference 18.) Consequently, the grid system that is still used today was built, and not Tesla's "free power" system. There was no plot to steal free power from the people, what was done was, and still is, the only viable solution at our current level of technology. In the time of the Great Pyramid, however, Tesla's idea was actually realized, but with different equipment and at a different frequency. The Great Pyramid radiated electromagnetic radiation of enormous power and each house, building, or vehicle absorbed energy through its receiving antenna to adequately power the needs of people living in a large geographic area.

The Seven Technologies

Although the theory of radiant energy propagation is straight forward, how could a huge monolith of limestone produce alternating current of sufficient power for large scale use? The Great Pyramid was designed to use the available energies of the Earth, the Moon, the Sun, the Milky Way Galaxy, and even Primal Energy. The designers of the Great Pyramid used seven different technological principles to convert available energy into useful high frequency alternating current:

1. Piezoelectricity
2. Thermocouple electricity
3. Electrostatics
4. Fuel combustion
5. Microwave energy
6. Efficiency enhancement
7. Focusing natural Earth Energies

Although most of these technologies are understandable, the technique of combining them in concert with one another within a single machine is awe inspiring. Before the power generator is deciphered, the amount of kinetic energy the Earth possesses must be appreciated. The kinetic energy of the Earth is so vast that if just a tiny fraction could be converted into alternating power, all of man's needs could easily be served without deteriorating the orbit of the Earth. Consider how much kinetic energy there really is. The Earth travels nearly eighteen miles per second in its orbit around the Sun. The weight of the Earth is 1.24×10^{24} pounds. One horsepower in British units is defined as 550 ft-lbs per second. In other words, one horsepower is equivalent to elevating 550 pounds at the Earth's surface through a distance of one foot every second. By this definition the Earth has three times ten to the twenty seventh, 3×10^{27}, horsepower with respect to the Sun alone. That is three thousand times one trillion times one trillion. Visually this number appears as a three with a string of 27 zeros or:

3,000,000,000,000,000,000,000,000,000 horsepower!

This is nearly incomprehensible. One must add to that the orbital energy of the Moon, the motion of the solar system, and other subtle effects.

The Great Pyramid was able to tap a portion of the vast source of kinetic energy in a secondary way. The Earth has a molten core that is mostly comprised of iron, an element that naturally has electrical properties. It is strongly affected by magnetic fields and it readily conducts electrical current. Because iron cores reduce the number of windings required, the element is often used in the coils found in motors and transformers. Close inspection of these cores reveals that they are not solid, but instead are made of thin layers of iron. Each layer has a coating of an insulator to isolate it electrically from adjacent layers, as this layering prevents the core heating that occurs when the fluctuating magnetic field of alternating current induces small electrical current into the core itself. Isolating the currents helps keep the core from overheating.

Since the planet does not have a layered core, it constantly cuts the magnetic field of the Sun (and the Galaxy — although weak by comparison) and vast quantities of the resultant induced electrical currents cause the core to exist in a perpetual molten state. If the core of the Earth were of Silicone it would not be molten. The core itself is also always slowly moving since any fluid that is heated begins to stratify as the hotter parts (less dense) begin to rise and the cooler parts (more dense) begin to sink. This process is visible on a small scale in the lava lakes of certain volcanoes. On the Island of Hawaii, for example, the molten rock of the lava lake has visible up-wellings and down-pourings.

The up and down molten currents are affected by the tilted axis of rotation, about 23.5 degrees with respect to the normal orbital plane. The paths of the up-welling and down-pouring molten fluids are not quite radial as would be expected. This is because the center of mass and the center of gravity are actually altered slightly by the daily rotation of the Earth, causing the actual path of a molecule to trace a large toroid. The associated electromagnetic response to the massive toroidal movement is measured on the surface as not only the North-South Magnetic Poles, but as an alternating energy field that emanates from various places on the planet. These mysterious fields have been historically called ley lines.

The reality of the existence of the alternating energy fields can be seen by studying the gravity anomaly maps of the planet. (The Bouguer Gravity Anomaly Map, U.S. Geological Survey, shows details for the United States and can be obtained from the government.) The Bouguer gravity anomaly map shows that gravity density is not constant, but varies above and below some normal value and is very location dependent. The sites of extreme gravitational abnormality are also the sites of maximum up-welling or down-pouring of the alternating energy fields or vortexes. Why does this feature of the planet exist? The toroidal movement of the Earth's core is much like the violin bow and one can imagine tiny jerks along the way causing the Earth to vibrate at its natural frequency. In fact, considering one isolated vortex as an example, there exists one standing wave that circles the planet and occurs at the frequency of eight cycles per second. Put another way, the natural resonant frequency of the planet is eight cps. (The wavelength of 7.5 cps is about 25,000 miles; 186,000 miles / 7.5 cps = 24,800 miles, or exactly one circumference of the Earth.) One of these standing waves is depicted in Figure 9.4A, which shows that the magnetic component and the electrical component of the wave are 90 degrees to one another and that one wave is one complete (+) and (-) cycle of the magnetic and electrical components. Now one has to imagine that there are 60 major vortex locations on the planet with powerful standing waves emanating from each of them. The energy waves consist of not only the eight cps natural Earth resonance, but of another frequency, four cps, imparted from the motion of the Moon. The Moon's frequency at about four cps adds to the basic eight cps frequency and along with those two frequencies are harmonics. So the power vortexes can be thought of as a complex of many electromagnetic frequencies.

Although the vortexes are primarily location dependent, small variations and wobbling, naturally occur, so the intensity at any particular location varies. Of the 10,000 minor vortexes and 60 major vortexes, the one of particular interest for this book is depicted in 9.4B, which shows that Egypt corresponds with an up-welling vortex. The site of the Great Pyramid was not chosen simply because it had good stable bedrock, it was primarily chosen because it was a major Earth vortex location.

If the Great Pyramid was positioned over a power vortex for the same reason that a water wheel is positioned on a flowing stream, how did it convert the vortex to a more useful frequency, and how did it stabilized the variable output of the vortex?

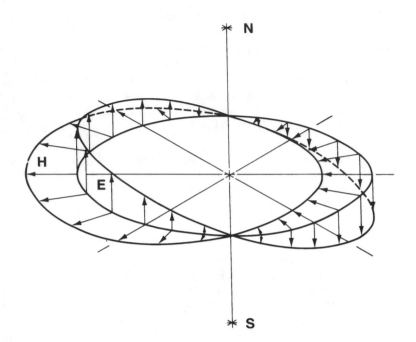

Figure 9.4A Depicted is an electromagnetic wave traveling around the Earth. The magnetic field lines, H, flow away from the center of the Earth during first half of the cycle and towards the center of the Earth during the second half of the cycle. The electrostatic field lines, E, always flow at 90° compared to the magnetic field, as shown.

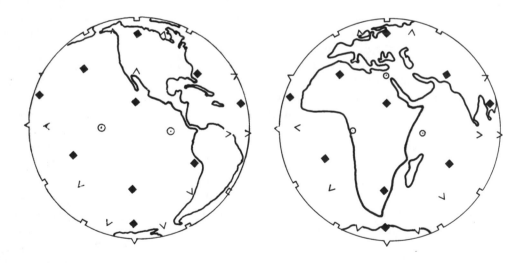

Figure 9.4B Shown are the major vortexes of the Earth. Cones represent electromagnetic vortex exit points. Squares represent electromagnetic vortex entry points. Besides the North and South pole there are sixty major electromagnetic vortex points.

First consider the science of piezoelectricity. Piezoelectricity is a natural phenomena of certain crystals with regular lattice structures at the molecular level such that when the crystal is bent by mechanical stress, there is a redistribution of the Electrons of the lattice network that results in an electric polarity. (See Figure 9.5A and Figure 9.5B)

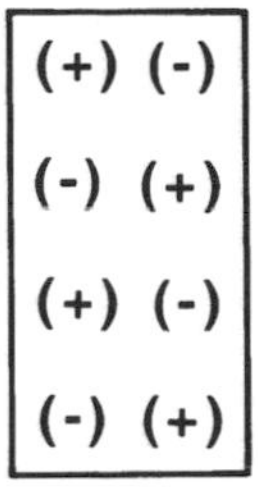

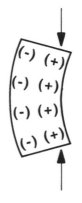

Figure 9.5A Shown is a piezoelectric crystal at rest, with no mechanical stress. It has an equal distribution of charges with a net electrostatic charge at the surface of zero.

Figure 9.5B Shown is a piezoelectric crystal under mechanical stress. The unequal pressure has resulted in compression surface-charged positive and tension surface-charged negative.

Piezoelectricity is commonly used in the pickup mechanism of phonograph record players (since superseded by cassette tape and compact discs.) The diamond needle that follows the grove with wiggles in the record (the frequency of the wiggles matches the frequency of the desired tone) is at its other end connected to a tiny metal plate, part of a sandwich between which is placed a cut piezoelectric crystal wafer. The vibrations in the needle alternately squeeze and release the piezoelectric crystal and this mechanical pressure induces a tiny bit of electrical charge upon the surface of the crystal. The plates pick up these Electron variations and they are fed into the amplifier circuit, where they are amplified many times until the power can be heard in the speaker.

The quartz frequency control crystal is another example of the widespread use of the piezoelectric phenomena. A quartz crystal is machined to a thin wafer and placed between metal plates. The thickness of the wafer determines very precisely at what frequency the crystal will naturally resonate. The thinner the crystal the higher the resonant frequency, and vice versa. Each radio station must maintain its designated frequency within very close tolerance in order to prevent interference with other stations. This is accomplished by placing one of these crystals in the primary resonant circuit. Note that in this application it is the electricity placed upon the surface of the crystal that induces a tiny mechanical distortion. This is the opposite of the phonograph pickup cartridge and demonstrates that the piezoelectric phenomena works in both directions. Although quartz is one of the best piezoelectric crystals, there are others, including granite and limestone. The efficiency of the piezoelectric phenomena in limestone is enhanced by heat. The builders of the Great Pyramid made extensive use of granite and limestone, and carefully selected dense varieties that were pure of defects.

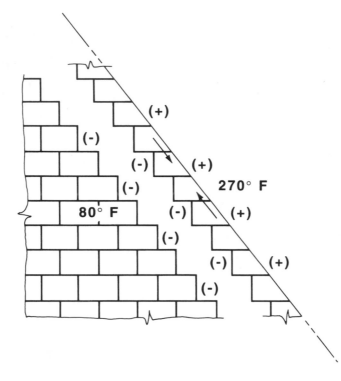

Figure 9.6 The sectional view shows the relationship of the casing blocks to the core blocks near the center of the face where the gap is the greatest. Since the exterior surface is the hottest it is the most "fluid" and the greater compression distortion there causes the surface to be positively charged.

As shown in an earlier chapter, one of the mysteries of the Great Pyramid is why the faces have regular depressions. They are not flat like all of the other pyramids. This fact was discovered by the French savants at the end of the 18th century and there has been much speculation about the meaning of the feature. The only visible part then and today is the core of the Great Pyramid, since the outer covering of pure limestone was removed to rebuild Cairo after a devastating earthquake. The other part of the mystery is that the pure limestone casing blocks did not rest upon the core blocks. The casing blocks were bonded to one another to form a water-tight membrane. This was accomplished by having all horizontal and vertical joints glue bonded under pressure, so the entire outer covering stood alone structurally. The only place where the core and the outer covering were close was at the base. If the casing were in place today, the faces would appear to have bulges, just the opposite of the core. This would result in a large gap, up to six feet, at the center of each side. (See Figure 9.6.) The gap had several functions and one was to allow movement under the expansion and contraction of the hot and cold cycle of each day and each season. Just like the expansion joints on the bridges, buildings, and highways, the gap allowed the outer covering to float freely while never touching the core. The Great Pyramid was the only pyramid of Egypt to have this unique feature, which will be explained later.

Each morning the face of the Great Pyramid that caught the morning rays of the Sun was the first to heat and, as the day progressed, warmed the other faces also. The heating drove off any water moisture that had condensed within the tiny pores of the acres of limestone exposed to the cooling of the night. This greatly increased the piezoelectric abilities of the crystal. The gravitational effect of the Moon would next bend the faces and the surfaces would gather enormous quantities of electrical charge because of the mechanical stress. The polarity charge shown in Figure 9.6 did not build and remain stationary for long because the faces were designed to have a natural mechanical resonance to match the Earth and Moon's the combined vortex frequency, about twelve cps. Each face was a membrane, like a drum skin, and could shudder at twelve cps from the wind and many other sources, so the electric polarity would temporarily increase and then decrease. These alternations would cause some energy to radiate into the Great Pyramid and eventually focus into the King's Chamber, where it was converted into a higher frequency. Distant lightening would also be sensed and added to the net piezoelectric effect.

Our ears are diaphragms and they too vibrate back and forth. When the Eustachian tube becomes clogged, inside pressure builds up and it is more difficult for the diaphragm to vibrate. To prevent pressure build up, the Great Pyramid needed an Eustachian tube, and this was one function of the "air vents." Like everything in the Great Pyramid, the vents had more than a single function.

Besides cleverly employing the ever-changing gravitational effect of the Moon, the designers were aware that part of the charge on the inside of the faces was due to subtle forces, high intensity cosmic rays and the PEP. The physical universe has manifested from the PEP by definition, but ninety percent of the PEP remains uncombined and in a free state. Enormous quantities of the PEP are passing through everything all of the time, possible because of their extremely small size. Specially designed collectors, however, can sense that passing. From the point of view of the PEP, the atoms of the blocks of the Great Pyramid appear to be widely spaced stars of a Galaxy. Since the atoms are in reality dense combinations of PEP, however, the result is that PEP passing through dense material, such as limestone and granite, are slowed to a degree. Upon exiting, the PEP speed up and resume normal speed. Occasionally the net effect is excited atoms at the surface that release energy when returning to the normal state of rest, the ground state, and that energy is added to the piezoelectric burst within the gap. The effect is enhanced within parallel plates, or walls, of metal or piezoelectric stone, and that is why the casing blocks were cut to match the core blocks. (Figure 9.6 defines the thickness of each course as equal for simplicity. In actuality, the thickness of each course of the Great Pyramid was different.) The gap is a resonant chamber for the resulting microwave energy. This added energy boost, although small by comparison, did exist and was part of the total. The energy increase was symbolic, a reminder and a reverence of the origins of the three-dimensional reality, the PEP. The Great Pyramid symbolized a reverence for diversity, hence the many methods of extracting natural energy.

What added the most energy to the Great Pyramid was the electromagnetic Earth vortex. At eight to twelve cps the vortex has a wavelength thousands of miles long. Stone masonry is nearly optically clear to long electromagnetic wavelengths, however, when the up-welling vortex encounters the inner wall of the outer casing blocks, a percentage of the Earth energy reflects off the inside of the wall and remains trapped within the Great Pyramid. (The stepped surface is effectively smooth to long wavelengths.) It is similar to sunlight reflecting off the rear window of a car — part of the sunlight reflects away and part passes through the glass and remains trapped within the car. Within the Great Pyramid the trapped electromagnetic energy does two things. It helps shudder the face, releasing continuous streams of piezoelectric energy, and it bounces within the pyramid until encountering the King's Chamber where it is converted to another frequency.

At night when the casing cooled, the process was reversed and the outer surface of the core was electrically charged with piezoelectric energy and released by reflecting off the casing and then into the King's Chamber. The energy received in this process was a fraction of the energy produced while the casing was hot.

The piezoelectric nature of the core is still intense at certain times of the year, and has led to some interesting modern-day tales as it occasionally affect a tourist who climbs to the top of the Great Pyramid. An interesting account is given in Reference 5 of a man who noticed static electricity at the ends of his finger tips. Having packed a lunch which included a bottle of wine, he wrapped it in a way to construct a crude laden jar and as he held it high with paper to insulate it, the difference of potential yielded a small bolt of static electricity discharge. Amused by the static electricity, the tourist continued the play with it, but the burst of electrical energy frightened the Arab guides, who reportedly ran away.

The Great Pyramid harnessed energy by thermocouple technology, a simple solid-state device that takes advantage of thermic differences. The heating of the Sun begins to warm the surface of the casing, but the piezoelectric generation of energy just described caused the temperature of the casing to rise to 270 degrees Fahrenheit. This heat is a measure of the inefficiency to convert all of the mechanical energy into electrical energy, but part of it was recovered by using a series of giant thermocouples. The acres of hot limestone represented a large amount of thermic energy and conveniently nearby was the relatively cool core limestone, which had an ambient temperature of 80 degrees Fahrenheit even during peak power generation. A properly-designed thermocouple can convert thermal differences of almost 200 degrees into electrical energy that can be stored.

The classic thermocouple is composed of two straight wires of dissimilar metals welded, fused, or twisted together at one end, but open at the other. The fused end is put into a heat source and the open end put into a cool source. Dissimilar metals, with different outer valence shell structures, will lose excited Electrons at different rates, thus a potential exists across the junction, and Electrons begin to flow in one direction. A small voltage will be measured at the cool end and this can be connected to another thermocouple wired in a series to produce twice the voltage. When enough thermocouples are wired together, the voltage is sufficient to be useful to run electrical devices. The assembly of many thermocouples arranged physically side by side, but electrically connected in series, is called a thermopile.

In the case of the Great Pyramid, the thermopile was metallic in design, of a great size, and was placed in the "air vent" on the south side of the King's Chamber. It was fused to the south casing face, which comprised the hot junction, but was loosely fit to the core for expansion and contraction. It provided local electric current for all of the internal lights, machinery, gates, and tuning valves.

Another energy-producing technology within the Great Pyramid was an ingenious use of electrostatics. Similar to the resonance induced in the cavity between the casing and the core, the PEP passing through the Ascending and Descending Passages set up excited surface atoms with Electrons loosely bound in the outer valence shell. These passages are especially electrostatic, since they are lined with granite, which is one-third quartz. How the excess Electrons are absorbed from the wall surface is by the use of a water. Water is a fair conductor of electricity, especially when trace amounts of salt are dissolved in it. Water was placed within the passages to a level that partially filled the horizontal passage to the Queen's chamber. Water did not flow out the entrance door because an elastic spring pulled the door closed into an air-tight seal. The same part of the passages that are filled with water had round ceramic pipes. In the higher passages a single pipe was used and in the lower passages 21 small pipes were positioned side by side. The water return pipe was the downward cycle of a thermosiphon water pump. The Earth below the Great Pyramid is some 30 degrees cooler than the core blocks, which are 80 degrees Fahrenheit. Fluids in a gravity well (on the surface of the Earth) naturally stratify and warm parts rise and cool parts sink. The motion of the water was therefore upward along the excited granite-lined walls and downward within the return pipes. The flow of the water was slow, but it ceaselessly moved excess Electrons upward toward the Queen's Chamber. At the Queen's Chamber, the electrical energy was converted with a special apparatus. The power was then used in a type of fuel cell that separated the water molecule into its components, Hydrogen gas and Oxygen gas.

The gaseous fuel, composed of Hydrogen and Oxygen, was moved upwards and burned within the King's Chamber. The battery pack was charged from several sources, including the combustion of the fuel, Hydrogen and Oxygen. This reliable method was the emergency backup system. When Hydrogen and Oxygen are burned, the result is steam vapor which condenses to form water droplets which fell to the floor, flowed out the portcullis entrance down into the low trough space between the ramps of the Grand Gallery, and finally joined the rest of the water flowing as part of the thermal siphon.

The Grand Gallery was used to produce power in a unique way. The walls of the Grand Gallery were also granite, parallel, and corbeled in seven layers. The Grand Gallery was a place of resonance for the PEP. As described before, the emerging PEP excited the surface atoms with excess microwave energy. The energy was collected by the Arc. The Arc was an energy-storage device. It stored energy much like a huge super-conducting-electrolytic capacitor. Like a battery, it was composed of many types of metallic plates between which was an acidic electrolyte. The whole apparatus was conveniently covered and contained and placed upon wheels. This device moved up and down the sloping ramp and absorbed the microwave energy resonating between the parallel walls. Each level not only made structural sense, but the number of corbels was chosen in reverence of the Primal Energies.

Another method to produce power had to do with efficiency enhancement. A jet engine has a nacelle built around it to improve the airflow around the structural members, the pipes, the pumps, and other components of the actual jet engine assembly. The improved airflow reduces the drag so much that this increases the efficiency of the jet engine by as much as 35 percent. In a similar way the Great Pyramid has an electrical circuit beneath it that smoothes the fluctuations in the Earth vortex. If one could look straight down and see through the base of the pyramid what would be visible would be a maze of tunnels.

This intricate "hypogeum" beneath the foundation and carved into the bedrock would look very much like a printed circuit, only the size would be greatly enlarged. Conductors are granite-lined water passages, narrow ones are resistors, and parallel plates of granite are capacitors. Metals introduced into certain chambers are coils. The switches are doors that open and close, pivoting sometimes like butterfly valves. Where appropriate, the PEP were utilized to add power to the flow. Never was a source of power or an improvement in efficiency overlooked. This electrical circuit beneath the Great Pyramid improved the efficiency so greatly it can understandably be thought of as a separate method to produce power.

The last technological method was the tapping of the powerful Earth vortex. The vortex, of course, enters from the base of the pyramid. Consideration was made to properly shape the bedrock to aid the Earth energy in most efficiently entering the pyramid. Researchers have correctly observed that the position of the visible bedrock at the Grotto Passage, at the Descending Passage, and at the foundation at the base perimeter are at different levels.

These limited observations have produced speculation as to the precise shape of the foundation — was it an irregular foundation or a precisely stepped foundation with huge steps? Each researcher draws different conclusions. Compare Figure 6.15, Figure 7.7, and Figure 9.7A. In fact, the foundation was designed to have many small steps as depicted in Figure 9.7B.

Over time the weight of the Great Pyramid compacts the bedrock. This layer of dense bedrock is thickest under the apex because the pyramid is tallest there, with almost 500 feet of limestone creating tremendous pressure. The layer of hardened bedrock naturally gets thinner towards the perimeter of the pyramid because of the ever-decreasing weight of the limestone overburden. The net effect is that the dense layer of bedrock formed by the pressure of the Great Pyramid, is shaped into a convexo-convex lens as shown in Figure 9.7B.

It might be argued that the stepped design of the dense bedrock would interfere with its function as a lens, but at the frequency in question the lens appears to be nearly clear and smooth.

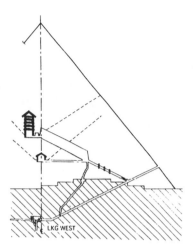

Figure 9.7A Are there a few huge steps as shown, or many small steps? Is there symmetry about some internal feature as shown, or is there symmetry about the axis of the pyramid?

Dense materials slow electromagnetic wave fronts. The mechanical equivalent of this is to observe an ocean wave approach a landmass from a high perspective. The beach wave portrayed in Figure 9.8A makes an oblique approach to an irregular landmass of great density compared to the fluid water. It is unaffected at vector A because it is far from the landmass, but at the projecting point of land, the waves are slowed. The drag is transmitted up the wave front inversely proportional to the distance from the point. The vector B shows the dramatic net effect of the drag due to the projecting point. Even a straight beach causes drag on obliquely-approaching ocean waves. For this reason, waves always strike the beach directly or at a very small oblique angles, (C) and (D.)

Electromagnetic radiation, including visible light, will slow when entering a dense medium and will speed up upon emerging from a dense medium. The amount of slowing also depends on the frequency of the radiation. Figure 9.8B, vector E, shows a wave front of visible light about to enter a dense layer of optical glass shaped into a convexo-convex lens. Vector F shows a change in direction due to the slowing of the advancing wave front.

The change of direction is because the left edge drags first and pulls the wave front to the left. Vector G shows another change in direction due to speeding up of the wave front. Had a higher frequency made the same passage, it could have the net direction shown as vector H. Other factors that determine the amount of bending of the wave front is the density of the lens and the amount of curvature of the lens.

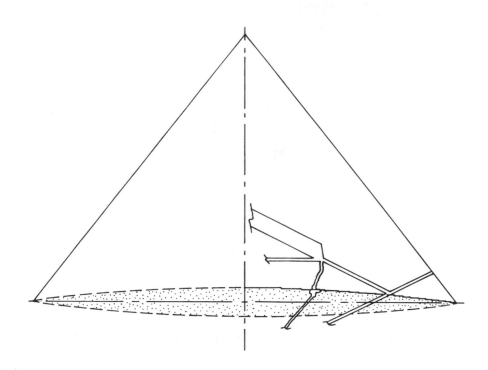

Figure 9.7B Depicted is the true shape of the foundation rock of the Great Pyramid. The bed rock is a series of small steps that form a gentle curve, and is symmetrical about the pyramid axis. The top layer of the foundation becomes dense due to the weight of the pyramid. The result is a convexo-convex lens.

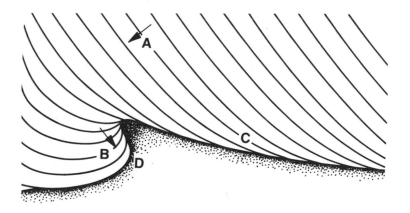

Figure 9.8A Depicted is an irregular ocean landmass and waves approaching at an oblique angle. The dense landmass induces drag into the less dense liquid medium and slows the advancing wave fronts. The drag travels up the wave fronts and dramatically bends them. Compare vector A and vector B.

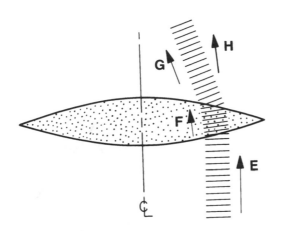

Figure 9.8B Depicted is a wave front of visible light passing through a lens of clear glass. The electromagnetic wave experiences drag due to the relatively dense medium of the glass. The drag causes the wave front to bend as shown.

     The principle shown in Figure 9.8B also applies to low electromagnetic frequencies passing through a lens of dense rock. In the case of the Great Pyramid, the Earth-radiant energy will pass slightly slower through the dense base lens than through layers above and below it. See Figure 9.9. Elements A and B are bent less than one degree by the base lens, but this helps to focus the vortex and to separate its different frequencies.

     The wave front bounces off reflecting surfaces by a fundamental principle of waves: the angle of incident is always equal to the angle of reflection. The wave front is sheared by the many reflections. The position the ray strikes on the inside of the casing of the first reflection determines the path it takes within the pyramid. After only one or two reflections, most elements intercept the King's Chamber. After four reflections, including the surface of the bedrock, all elements intercept the King's Chamber. The length of each path to the King's Chamber is different and this helps insure that the original wave front is broken up.

     The base lens also separates different frequencies, bending them at different rates insuring that different frequencies travel in different paths within the Great Pyramid. The desired result of the many paths and the many path lengths is that the waves arrive very much out of phase in the resonant chamber. The reason this is beneficial becomes obvious by a study of Figure 9.10. Frame A shows a single wave absorbed into the King's Chamber during an arbitrary elemental time period, "delta-t" (Δt). This drawing is similar to an oscilloscope portrayal of an alternating wave with one cycle shown. Amplitude above the zero line is positive and amplitude below the line is negative. Frame B shows what would happen if two such waves arrived exactly out of phase (phase = $\emptyset$ = 1/2). They cancel each other, exactly, and the net electrical equivalent is zero (Frame C).

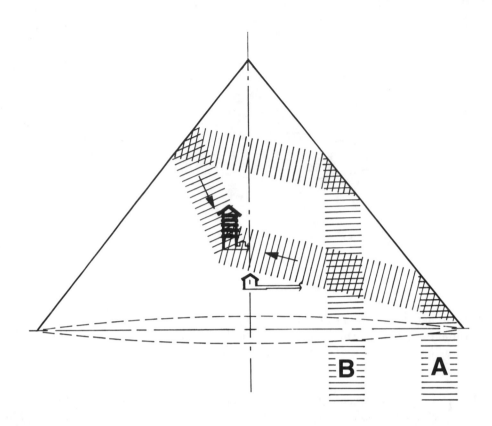

Figure 9.9 Depicted is the Earth vortex entering the pyramid through the base lens from different points. Most elements intercept the King's Chamber after one or two reflections. Some elements reflect off the base lens before entering the mixing chamber. The design insures that all path lengths are different.

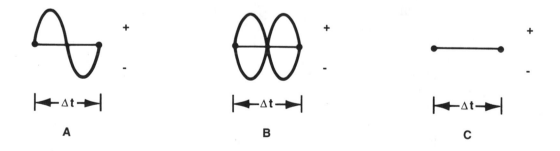

Figure 9.10 A,B,C. Frame A = a single wave in a resonant chamber. Frame B = two waves, exactly out of phase. Frame C = The net result is complete cancellation. Constant interval of time is shown as Δt.

To have a net output of zero would be a disaster for a power generator, so some means must be made to eliminate either the positive or negative half of each cycle. This is accomplished by the position and design of the Queen's Chamber, which operates very much like the one-way diode of the electrical circuit discussed earlier. In the example, assume it clips the negative cycle. The net effect is shown in Frame D, which represents one wave arriving, rectified, with only the positive half present. Now if another wave arrives out of phase (Frame E) there is no cancellation. There is, however, an important change, a frequency change. Frame F shows that in the same span of time, Δt, the two pulses are electrically equivalent to an alternating current of twice the frequency.

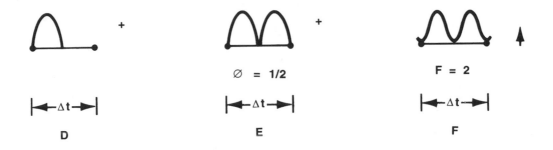

Figure 9.10 D,E,F. Frame D = a single rectified wave in a resonant chamber. Frame E = two rectified waves, exactly out of phase. Frame C = The net result is a change of frequency.

The frequency change is very important as it is at the very heart of understanding how the Great Pyramid functions electrically. Follow closely what happens in Frames G through N. If the waves arrive 1/3 out of phase, the resulting frequency is three times the fundamental frequency as shown in Frame H. If the waves arrive 1/4 out of phase, the resulting frequency is four times the fundamental seen in Frame J. This pattern continues and waves arriving 1/8 out of phase produce a frequency 8 times the fundamental, as in Frame L.

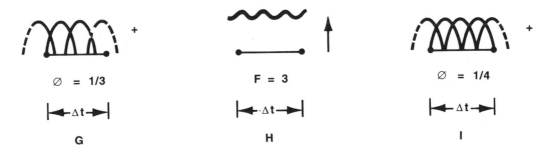

Figure 9.10 G,H,I. Frame G = three rectified waves in a resonant chamber with phase relation of $1/\emptyset = 1/3$. Frame H = frequency change = $1/\emptyset = 3$. Frame I = four rectified waves in a resonant chamber with $\emptyset = 1/4$.

Notice that besides the frequency change the amplitude is increasing. The logical extension of the mixing process is that as the phase overlap approaches zero, the frequency approaches infinity and is of infinite amplitude.

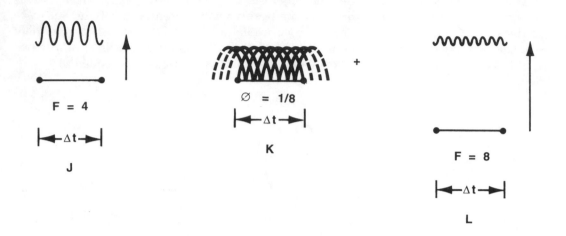

Figure 9.10 J,K,L. Frame J = frequency change = $1/\varnothing$ = 4. Frame K = eight rectified waves in a resonant chamber with $\varnothing$= 1/8. Frame L = frequency change of $1/\varnothing$ = 8.

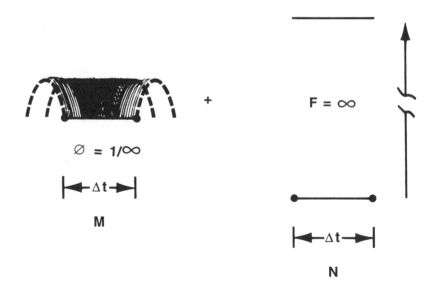

Figure 9.10 M,N. Frame M = approaching an infinite number of rectified waves in a resonant chamber with $\varnothing = 1/\infty$. Frame N = frequency change of $1/\varnothing = \infty$.

Something happens long before that point is reached. The focused radiation flooding the region of the King's Chamber sets up five standing waves between the floor of the King's Chamber and the ceilings of the attic chambers. These intense standing waves excite the crystals af all vertical walls in the King's Chamber and in the attic chambers. The crystals resonate at microwave frequency, 10^{12} cps, a benign radiation as far as living tissue is concerned. The four-lobed radiation pattern with maximun intensity perpendicular to the faces send useful amounts of energy extending to an incredible 25,000 miles from the power generator.

Besides the power pattern emanating from the faces of the pyramid, there was also a communication beam, much like a laser beam only higher in frequency. The power for the beam was the energy absorbed by the rectifying action of the Queen's Chamber. The device that radiated the beam was positioned in the small corbeled arch at the end of the Queen's Chamber, which happened to be positioned nearly under the apex. (See Figure 7.7). A pendulum-like motion pulsed energy from the equipment in the Queen's Chamber causing a high frequency Jacob's ladder to send energy up and out. The wavelengths got smaller and smaller, until the atoms of the limestone were effectively widely-spaced points of a gigantic grid. The tiny radiant energy simply passed through the spaces between the atoms. Special machinery turned the energy on and off so quickly that it appeared to be a narrow beam sent straight out towards the stars. Equipment five billion miles from Earth could pick up the signals and demodulate the information.

That part of the energy output caused a five foot diameter plasma ball to form six feet above the apex. At certain angles the plasma ball would reflect off the gold foil at the top, stirring the imagination of first-time visitors.

As equally fascinating as pyramid-power theory is the equipment contained within the Great Pyramid that worked in harmony to help produce the radiant energy. A detailed look at twelve of the devices follows. This information is thought to be a large step beyond what researchers have accomplished to date, however, it is beyond the scope of this book to present the complete working blueprint for the Great Pyramid. There are plenty of details remaining for researchers of the future.

Energy Producing Features of the Great Pyramid to Explore

The Entrance Door
The Casing Faces and Shafts
The Megacircuit
The Unfinished Chamber
The Passages
The Queen's Chamber
The Grand Gallery
The Sarcophagus
The King's Chamber
The Attic of the King's Chamber
The Portcullis
The Great Pyramid Cap

The Entrance Door

The Entrance Door that sealed the Descending Passage was below the level of the horizontal passage to the Queen's Chamber. This door pivoted at the base and had a simple elastic pressure-sensitive device which kept it shut. If the water level was too high, the pressure overcame the door and it automatically opened, releasing excess water. Sensing the change in pressure, the door would then close once again, sealing in the water. The casing and the descending passage were properly connected with a water-tight and elastic coupling needed because of the casing core gap to contain the water and allow for expansion and contraction.

The Casing Faces and Shafts

A later chapter will cover the interesting details of how each casing block was constructed and set into position. There were only five openings in the entire casing structure. One was the entrance to the Descending Passage and the other four provided access to two shafts to the King's Chamber and to the Queen's Chamber (these two shafts were sealed after final tuning). The location of the shafts are shown in Figure 7.7 and Figure 6.15. These shafts provided air-pressure equalization, hydraulic lines, air lines, electronic tuning, and whatever mechanical linkage was necessary to control the gates and devices located in the chambers. Access to the control valves at each location was made at nighttime when the casing was cool. Workmen used step ladders fixed to the outside of the casing, one on the north face and one on the south face.

The Megacircuit

The deepest part of the Megacircuit was just over 475 feet below the base of the Great Pyramid. That subterranean apex was connected horizontally to the Nile water. The water was pumped to fill the passageways as far as the Queen's Chamber, and a one-way valve prevented back flow. Besides the shaft filled with water destined for the Queen's Chamber, there existed many large horizontal and vertical passageways with valves the size of doors. As already stated, this Megacircuit improved the efficiency by smoothing the variables of the Earth vortex. Researchers, however, have yet to excavate these passages and they remain filled with sand, now sandstone, and unfortunately, are still unexplored. More will be explained in a later chapter to dispel many of the myths regarding chambers beneath the Great Pyramid.

The Unfinished Chamber

The Unfinished Chamber, named because it resembles a quarry with walls and floor in an unfinished state, was in fact as finished as it needed to be. Water was pumped to fill it several feet deep during construction. It was a convenient water source and also a place to clean slurry excess. It served no function as a resonant chamber and it never had a portcullis-type door.

The Passages

All original passages above the Unfinished Chamber were straight, with walls of granite finished to a high polish. It was the surface of these walls that became charged electrically. A long time after the pyramid was operating there was an alarming power drop. Thinking that part of the pyramid had cracked, it was shut down and a detailed inspection was made. Nothing visible was damaged so the thought was that something in the resonating cavities above the King's Chamber had been damaged. The irregular inspection tunnel to this location was painstakingly carved. Nothing amiss was discovered, however. The cracks now visible in the attic blocks occurred much later. A pressure imbalance occurred during the dismantling of the casing blocks.

The next inspection hole was made by tunneling down from the bottom of the Grand Gallery. This inspection hole has left what is now known as the Grotto Passage. It also left the Great Pyramid inoperative for many years, during which time an interesting section of Earth history occurred. (See Chapter 12.) In the end, the problems were overcome. The ends of the inspection holes were sealed tightly and the Great Pyramid functioned again.

The Queen's Chamber

The Queen's Chamber has no attic compartments like the King's Chamber, but like everything within the Great Pyramid it had more than one function. The Queen's Chamber is located low in the pyramid and directly in line with the apex. Its position allowed it to absorb energy and function electrically as a rectifier, absorbing negative pulses from the wave front. This was added to electrical energy collected from the charged water that entered into the Queen's Chamber. Part of the energy was used to separate water into the two gases of that molecule, Hydrogen and Oxygen. The Oxygen passed into the King's Chamber via the horizontal passage, above the water, and then through the Grand Gallery. The Hydrogen gas, which is lighter than air, naturally rises and was directed into the King's Chamber via a route through the core blocks, which are spaced about 1/8 inch apart. The combustion of the gases provided extra power, including emergency power during repairs. A small electrolytic storage device, a small version of the one in the Grand Gallery, was designed into one end of the Queen's Chamber and was used to create the communication beam. This beam was of extremely high frequency and radiated directly upward and out of the apex. Energy storage and other machinery existed within the Queen's Chamber.

The air vents leading to the Queen's Chamber helped with the ventilation during construction. The last construction task to be done in this chamber was to cover the vents with solid stone. The air vents were converted into a resonant cavity tuning mechanism by inserting a stone plug part way down and also by sealing the passage at the surface. The several inches of stone between the resonant chamber and the Queen's Chamber was a capacitive coupling. This plug has recently been discovered. (See *The Message Of The Sphinx*, Hancock and Bauval, Reference 50.) The beat frequency of this tuned circuit helped keep the Queen's Chamber resonating at the correct frequency.

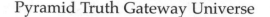

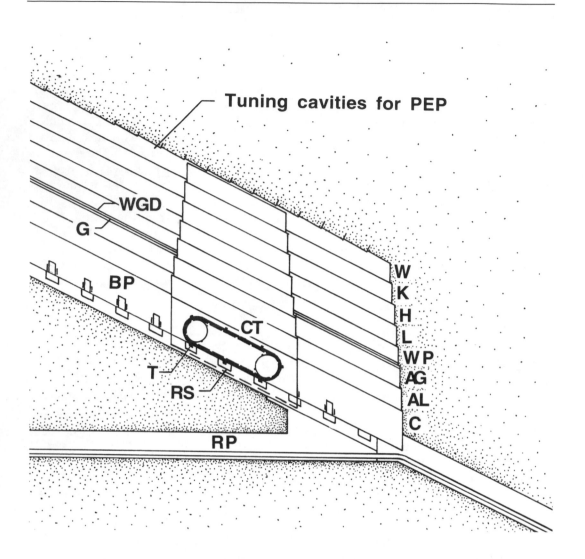

Figure 9.11 The Arc moves up and down the Grand Gallery to tune the resonant chamber for maximum power. The heavy device was mounted on tractor treads. Workers passed through doors and between the wheels to get from one end to the other. WGD = worm gear drive mounted in groove, G. CT = caterpillar treads with teeth, T, positioned at intervals to mesh with the Teflon-lined ramp slots, RS. BP = brake pads, mounted in recesses along the walls adjacent to the ramp slots. RP = water return pipe.

The Grand Gallery

Besides a few gate valves and movable dielectric plates, there was very little that moved within the Great Pyramid solid-state power generator. The machine that was the exception to all of that was contained within the spectacular Grand Galley. (See Figure 9.11.) Mounted upon caterpillar treads, it was able to move up and down the entire length of the Grand Gallery.

The movement provided for a variable cavity between the upper end of the machine and the bottom of the Grand Gallery that gave the operators the ability to maximize the output by adjusting the resonant cavity, somewhat like a violinist sliding his finger up and down the neck of the violin. Electronic coupling to the King's Chamber was via the portcullis, which functioned as a variable capacitor. The caterpillar treads had protrusions that fit precisely into the regularly spaced slots of the 26-degree sloping ramp surface.

Each slot in the ramp was fitted with a Teflon-type liner. The liner had a smaller slot that fit the tooth on the caterpillar tread. Adjacent to each slot in the ramp were regular notches in the wall. An insert was also fitted into these depressions, which formed part of the emergency braking system. The caterpillar treads were independent enough from the machine to be able to rotate slightly about an axis that was perpendicular to the ramp. One tread was always adjusted to have drag so that under power failure conditions, the whole tread would cant enough to engage the braking pads in the walls. Thus, the machine could never slide down the ramp and destroy itself against the block wall at the bottom.

Figure 9.12 shows how, except for a few inches of clearance, the machine fits the exact shape of the corbeled Grand Gallery. At point TG in the trough the machine does touch. This is the rail guide, built in a sliding design, that prevents any possibility that the machine could cant and rub against the wall. At each end of the machine was a door, D, allowing maintenance workers to pass through the machine to reach the other side. Point T is another view of the caterpillar teeth. Notice the clearance with respect to the machine and to the first corbel and also the fit into the insert of the ramp slot. Point WGD is the position of the mechanism that fits into the slot of the fourth corbel. This slot runs the entire length of the Grand Gallery. The mechanism mounted in that groove had a worm gear drive that moved the Arc up and down the ramp, making fine-tuning adjustments as needed.

The machine itself, already described as a huge storage electrolytic capacitor, was also part of the communication system. The power output was modulated for this purpose and it served the entire society. Double and triple functions were typically designed into each device.

This machine has another name that has become quite common in our society. The Bible makes reference to it and similar smaller communication-link versions of it. It is known to many to be a magical device, the "Arc." It was the "Arc of the Covenant." A small communication link was given to Moses. It allowed him to speak with those who do research onboard UFOs. (See Chapter 12.)

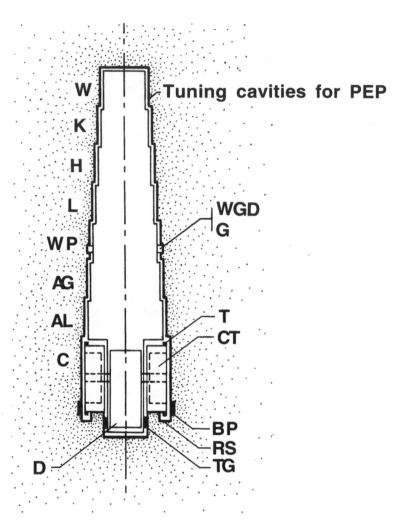

Tuning cavities for PEP

W
K
H
L
WP
AG
AL
C

WGD
G

T
CT

BP
RS
TG

D

Figure 9.12 Shown is a sectional view of the Arc within the Grand Gallery. WGD = worm gear drive mounts in the groove, G. CT = caterpillar treads with teeth, T, that meshed with the Teflon-lined ramp slots, RS. BP = brake pads which fit into the sidewall notches. D = door. TG = Teflon-like trough guide.

The Sarcophagus

The sarcophagus was the casing for the battery that was located within the King's Chamber. It was different than the lead batteries now commonly used in our society. Providing a certain amount of local power when the Great Pyramid was not producing power, this hot battery operated most efficiently at high temperatures. The gases that percolated up from the Queen's Chamber were burned to warm the battery and the burning of the gases made the chamber quite hot. The combustion by-product was water vapor, which condensed into water droplets and passed back down via the trough in the Grand Gallery.

The King's Chamber

Consider once again the resonant circuit of 9.3A. The equivalent of the coil is the inner facing of the casing faces and the upper face of the base lens. The equivalent of the capacitor is the King's Chamber and its attic cavities. The cavities and movable dielectric plates that were attached to the ceiling and walls of the King's Chamber allowed for the "capacitor" to be variable; it could tune, like a radio, to the available resonant frequency for the most power. The King's Chamber was fitted with plates on three of its surfaces. The north and south walls each had a plate that could be moved up to eighteen inches from the wall. These plates were not metal, but of a dielectric material. Another similar plate was fixed to the ceiling and also designed to allow it to change positions. As the Great Pyramid changed its shape slightly under Piezoelectric expansion, the size of the King's Chamber and the "attic" blocks above it changed, and so adjustments were necessary. The seasons, the position of the Moon, and the weather all affected the tuning. In the King's Chamber it was the plates that allowed the operators to make the adjustments and tune the cavity resonator.

One last interesting feature about the King's Chamber is the special pure rock that makes up the walls and floor. The crystalline form was essentially tiny pyramids that were the final stage for converting to the output frequency. Each of the trillions of tiny pyramids would resonate at the output radiation frequency of 10^{12} cps. This particular high frequency does not harm living organisms.

The Attic Above the King's Chamber

Above the King's chamber are the "attic" compartments. The unusual feature of the blocks that make up the "attics" is that only the underside is smoothed. This makes sense when the function of them is understood. Each forms a resonant chamber with respect to the floor of the King's Chamber. These create cavities for different frequencies to be trapped and mixed. The reason for the inverted "V" uppermost "roof" of these attic chambers was not structural. It too had an electrical function. Shaped just like a radar reflector, it prevented long wave frequencies from exiting the pyramid, sending them back for further mixing.

Once the "ripples" achieve the proper size by exciting crystals in the walls of the King's Chamber, the electromagnetic radiation passed through all of the blocks, including the inverted Vee Block. There was no thin gap for the radiation to pass through because no gap was necessary. The extremely small size of the radiation waves allowed them to pass through the granite and limestone blocks.

The Portcullis

The unusual three-door portcullis at the entrance to the resonant chamber, the King's Chamber, was part of the power output control mechanism. The door closest to the King's Chamber was granite and the other two were limestone. Each was raised and lowered by a hydraulic mechanism located at the top. This was the variable capacitor that linked the beat frequency energy in the Grand Gallery to the King's Chamber. Workmen who were in the Grand Gallery and between the "Arc" and the King's Chamber could see the glow of the Hydrogen fire radiating out from under the portcullis gap. It was like looking into the door of a coal-burning furnace. They could also see a small stream of water dripping down into the trough of the Grand Gallery. Many times the workers, who had no understanding of the principles involved, were called upon to work within the Grand Gallery. Awed by what they witnessed, they called the bright light the "Fire of God." Since only God could make fire from which water would flow, the water became known as "God's water." (Some authors define the origin of the word *pyramid* as: "pyra-mid," meaning "light within.")

The Great Pyramid Cap

The upper region of the Great Pyramid, specifically the top third, was a spectacular thing to behold during the day because at the right angle the dazzling reflection of the Sun blinded the observer. This was because of a thin covering layer of slate that functioned as a dielectric for the metallic covering, a thin layer of gold alloy electroplated into position. Like the inverted Vee-block above the King's Chamber, this metallic layer reflected long waves back into the Great Pyramid for further mixing. It is no wonder that the hieroglyphic symbol for "pyramid" is a triangle with a horizontal line one third from the top with the bottom space painted blue and the top space painted bright yellow. (See Figure 9.13.)

Figure 9.13 The hieroglyphic symbol for pyramid is a triangle with a horizontal line one third from the top with the bottom blue and the top yellow.

The Many Functions Of The Great Pyramid

The Great Pyramid was essentially a power converter. It also added power to the already powerful Earth vortex, transforming power into convenient radiant energy that could be used at a distance and at a frequency that did not damage living tissue. But the Great Pyramid was also designed for many other purposes. It was a healing center, a device for communication to distant locations on Earth as well as to ships at the edge of the solar system, a local power source, a long-distance power source, and source of knowledge.

The Great Pyramid was a reliable power source and scheduled maintenance shut-downs occurred only at twelve year intervals. For several thousand years, it served the people who knew how to use it, and they came to take it for granted. Unfortunately, one day the beloved power source that made the idyllic life on Earth possible would fall silent, a victim of a regular cosmic mechanism, itself a great secret.

Chapter Ten

Synopsis

Almost everyone who visits the chambers of the Great Pyramid reports phenomenal events and states of emotional excitement difficult to explain. The author was no exception and that experience turned him into a seeker. This book exists because of the teachings of Yahweh, as channeled by Chuck Little. The first thought of the All-That-Is (upon waking after a long sleep) is, "What am I?" That simple thought creates the Is-Ness (What is known) and the Is-Not-Ness (What is yet to be discovered). Consciousness is imparted to each so that it may, in turn, wonder what it is. The process continues until the third split, at which point there are eight Primal Energies. When each Primal Energy wonders what it is, Primal-Energy combinations occur and Primal-Energy Consciousness splits off so that each new combination may wonder what it is. This process causes endless creation. After 666 splits, creation is back where it started, in the form of the All-That-Is. Suns are formed at the 24th, 25th, and 26th splits. Planets are formed knowingly at the 30th split. Entities at the 32nd split create physical forms to incarnate into. These physical forms, including man, are on the 34th split. Man is a fine paint brush for the creation and his physical creations exist on the 36th split and the emotions during those creations exist on the 35th split. It is hard for man to realize that he is really a ten-dimensional being when he is incarnated into a physical form. The souls that incarnate into the physical form of sentient and creative man have the choice of 128 different forms. On this particular planet with the type of physical form and single-minded consciousness that evolved here, rules are needed to live a balanced life.

Without the rules, chaos occurs. Yahweh has given fifteen guidelines at this time to help mankind pass through these transitional times. Of the 128 different sentient forms, many have come to visit this planet. This is a time of great change, and a place to see a living history of what they once were. They neither help nor hinder. They do, however, observe and do research. These visitors are the Traders and the Travelers. The Traders evolved during the first wave of sentient beings and are 500 times older than humans. These small, bipedal beings are highly technological. During the evolution of their technology, an accident destroyed their home planet and all of its life forms. The Traders viewed that violation of creation so seriously that they now constantly search the universe for new life forms, placing the new-found DNA on other planets where it will flourish. This practice helps insure that nothing goes extinct. When they take something from a planet, they place something else of equal ecological value. They are the Traders. They have also learned to create with Primal Energy, creating their own synthetic food, monitoring all things, and navigating throughout the universe. No other sentient beings can do what the Traders do. Other sentient beings, however, do travel with the Traders. Once a Trader Super Mother Ship (SMS) leaps to a new star, these Travelers are allowed to explore planets in scout ships of their own design. To become a Traveler one must prove to be of the same ecological mind as the Traders, agreeing to do no harm to the animals, and help in dispersing new life forms. It is by this dispersal process that our primate precursors arrived on suitable planets in other solar systems.

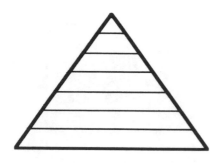

Chapter Ten

THE SOURCE

The Universal Love

Mysterious Experiences

It is often reported that people experience mysterious states of consciousness in and around the temples and pyramids of Egypt, especially the Great Pyramid. Consider a few examples of how one's destiny in the universe is connected to the mystery of time and apparent reality. Napoleon toured the inside of the Great Pyramid unescorted. Something unusual happened during the exploration because he emerged visibly shaken. So strongly did the event influence him, that he refused to discuss his experience with his aids — possibly for fear of being misunderstood and ridiculed. Even at his deathbed, Napoleon refused to be specific about the incident, but he did make one comment: "What is the use, no one will believe me." (See Reference 5.)

Many others report psychic experiences in the Pyramid. One visitor to the King's Chamber, Alister Crowley, spent the entire night there with his wife and experienced an unusual event. They began to perform an esoteric ceremony and reported that after some reading and chanting, a pale light, lilac in color, began to glow. This "natural" lighting was bright enough to allow reading without the candle. Many psychic experiences came to the couple that evening. (See Reference 19.)

When I toured Egypt with a large Astara group in October of 1987, we visited many pyramid sites. (See Reference 10.) David Litner, a member of the Astara staff, reported that when he was within Khephren's Pyramid, he and several others were astonished to hear his chanted invocations being answered by an unseen entity within the pyramid. On that same tour, the first temple visited by the group was the Great Pyramid, and the Astara group had permission to use the King's Chamber for half a day. The experience of that visit was the stimulus for this book.

The path of entry was through Al Mamun's forced entry, the horizontal passage connecting to the steep and narrow Ascending Passage. By hunching low, the 26.5-degree climb was achieved by clinging to wooden cleats that were in position to make the ascent possible. Eventually, the ramp in the Grand Gallery was reached and we made the final climb fully erect.

Many in the Astara group were already in the King's Chamber participating in a spiritual ceremony. As I neared the top end of the Grand Gallery, the chanting grew incrementally more intense and the rare moment of those rhythmic sounds within such an historic and sacred monument was quite captivating. I was soon entering the small 41-inch square horizontal passage that led to the King's Chamber. Once inside, the full impact of the angelic sounds of male and female voices blending into a beautiful rainbow "oooohhmm" could be heard and felt as it reverberated strongly within the parallel granite walls of the chamber. This splendid chanting was only broken by the sound of the lone instrument in the room, a Tibetan bell, which was chimed at regular one-minute intervals.

Moving closer to the front of the very crowded room, it became apparent that a line was forming at the south end of the sarcophagus for individuals to be endowed with a blessing from the director. Participants were instructed to place one hand upon the stone corner of the sarcophagus, and upon each hand Dr. Robert placed his hand. After an explanation of why contact with the monument was important, the incantation began with "May the great light of this place be yours now and forever." (See Note 1.) When the words were finished, both of his hands were placed upon the initiate's head and this completed the ceremony. Personally, at that moment, there was no experience of a physical or altered state of consciousness, but there was the appreciation of the beauty and solemnity of the ceremony. The real impact, however, was to come later that day. That evening, everyone in the tour group was encouraged to include in his meditation imagining the physical body in the lotus position, expanding it as large as the Great Pyramid, and then blending with the Great Pyramid.

The Opening

The evening this was done I had the experience of drifting upwards and looking down upon the whole Giza complex with an internal eye. The picture was exceedingly intense and took on a flow of its own. It was somewhat like watching a video without knowing what would happen next. The horizon entered the picture and began to glow a golden hue of light that then broke into many separate pieces, eventually becoming points of light. The lights seemed to approach and grew in size until finally it became apparent that each was something of an "energy entity." One entity, near the center, became the focus of interest, and the entity came close with a gaze that radiated love. This light being was largely composed of a beautiful head surrounded by a glowing ball of energy. For twenty minutes, the energy poured out, forming tendrils or wings, and a long, tapering headdress. Before the vision faded an intense message was imbued — welcome home! That implied that the land of Egypt was my real home. Unusual as that possibility was, it resonated with a great deal of truth and was greatly exciting. Interestingly, although the visual effects faded, the intense feeling lasted for several months. Now, many years later, that feeling and also a burning sensation along the spinal column and top of the head returns during deep meditations as well during the writing of this book.

Everyone who took part in the ceremony, it seemed, had a similar intense experience and was enmeshed with "feeling the energy." Some, accustomed to such experiences took it in stride, but I was quite overwhelmed by the intense emotion. In trying to comprehend the experience, which defied the boundaries of science, the Astara group discussed many topics. These unusual topics included the possibility of astral travel, miracle energy healing, and even the existence of aliens from other worlds who visit in UFOs. The theories of where the "Space Brothers" originated and their purpose for being here varied, but the reality of their presence seemed to be almost universally accepted by this group. Some believed that the pharaohs of Egypt met regularly with aliens, and such concepts and discussions were quite unusual to me. In scientific circles, what is considered to make up reality are those things that can be weighed and measured, truths are the results of experiments that can be reliably reproduced in any laboratory in the world, and anything else is considered suspect.

My logical mind, tuned by a scientific education and years of applied science work experience, strained to explain the lingering emotion as well as why the group would take seriously such unusual topics. If these things were true, or had any validity at all, there had to be a scientific explanation, and so began a personal quest. After a few days of adjusting to a new reality, one that might accommodate new possibilities, a plan began to formulate for me. Why not contact one of these knowledgeable beings of the UFOs and get the answers directly? The idea became an intense passion and somehow the idea manifested in my doing a painting. (See Figure 10.1.) The teacher, a being from another realm, gives the seeker the precious jewel of knowledge, hence the painting depicts a personal contact with an all-knowing inter-dimensional being who could answer all of the riddles of life.

The background for the painting was selected from hundreds of slides taken during the above-mentioned Egypt trip. The arch was chosen simply because the angle looked right and it would also be appropriate for the theme that was to be developed. Once the black and white sketch was finished and there only remained the adding of the color, there was a conscious recognition that the arch that I selected was the portal to the famous temple at Dendara, the healing temple. It was at Dendara that the author met a special friend who slowly recounted an incredible story of her own personal acceptance of miracle energy healings. She shared with me her experiences of the spiritual, and personal three-dimensional encounters with humanoid aliens, including encounters within an alien ship. Although for me these stories were in the realm of science fiction, I began to entertain the reality of such things if only because of the special time, place, and circumstances.

There was yet another event that seemed to complete the unusual synchronicity revolving around the temple of Dendara. A photograph was taken of a miracle energy healing in progress. The photograph surfaced over six months after the end of the tour, and members of the tour passed it around with much excitement. (See Figure 10.2.) The photo has been analyzed by a NASA laboratory, has been verified to be authentic, and is not the product of trick photography. Details of the energy session, how it occurs, and why it manifests on a photographic film will be discussed in Chapter 13.

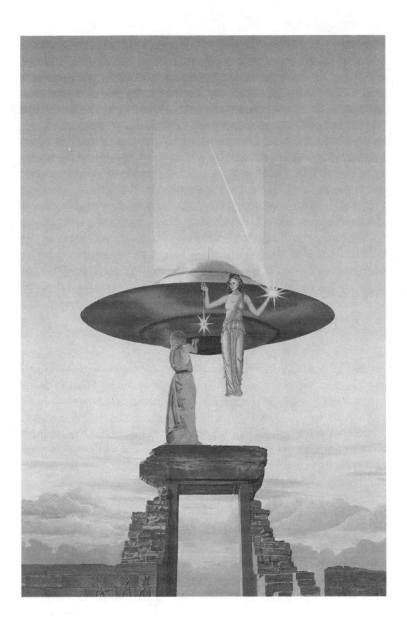

Figure 10.1 Hypothetical scene of the Earth seeker meeting with a Traveler, an inter-dimensional teacher of knowledge and wisdom.

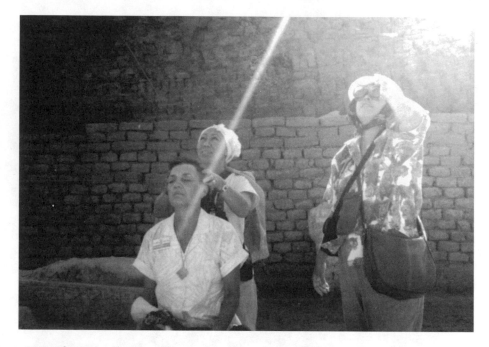

Figure 10.2 Photograph of an energy healing session at the temple of Dendara.

In retrospect, no UFO with guiding space brothers ever came to answer my many questions. By disregarding my specific picture of how my desired encounter should present itself, however, a more enriching fulfillment of the dream soon came my way. Following hunches, I investigated the channeling phenomena in some detail. The first channel that I ever experienced was Dr. Earlyne Chaney, Dr. Robert's wife, during the "fire initiation" ceremony at the Astara campus long before the Egypt trip. There was an amazing change in energy in the channel and in the room during the session. The tone of the message for the group was one of encouragement and love for our efforts at self improvement.

Because of that encounter, I was interested in experiencing this phenomena in a private setting where personal issues could be addressed. After experiencing six different channelers, one stood out from the others. Chuck Little, channeling an entity of "Pure Energy and Consciousness," was able to answer all the questions of a personal and scientific nature. It was a quantum leap. The scientific, rational part of my mind resonated greatly with the experience. Pure Energy and Consciousness was routinely visited and questions of any nature were joyously answered. What more could one ask for? (See Reference 21.)

Since the first experiences with the Pure Energy Entity were in a group setting, and since it felt like there was comfort in numbers, I had an initial reluctance to have a private session — was I truly worthy? Eventually that reluctance was overcome and a private session was requested. The bold step was taken, the request was granted, but could the appointment be met? Upon arriving it was requested that I return in one hour. Grateful for the extra time, it was now possible for me to search out a remedy for a growing migraine, and a sandwich to quell a growling stomach. Migraine headaches due to light sensitivity had been a personal plague for me in recent years and bringing one on was as simple as driving thirty miles during daylight hours. With enough aspirin, the pain subsided to a tolerable level, and the time for the private session arrived. The secretary was smiling and said the channel was ready now for the private, and continued with, "He said you now have less pain in your stomach and less pain in your head." That was the first clue that the Pure Energy Entity could scan all events, and it was not the last demonstration of this ability.

Everything went better than expected. My personal fears had been conquered, and something mysterious had been gained — a period of uncontrollable laughter. Fortunately, two friends happened to be in the waiting room, recognized my symptoms from personal experience, and agreed to baby-sit me for a while. My laughter could not be controlled and felt as though it originated in my bones and rolled up and out in waves. My friends joined in the contagious laughter. Within several hours the effect subsided enough for me to re-enter society. Many meetings with the Pure Energy Entity were to follow and although my laughter did not return with each visit, another noticeable effect was the state of exhilaration/confusion that followed, a state that usually lasted for seven days. It was accompanied by a strange body sensation, an actual physical vibration felt in or about the stomach. During this time it was almost impossible to focus on anything or accomplish much other than sleep. It became a time for me to let go and not try to force my normal state to return.

In addition to the private encounters, group meetings were held and attended by a spectrum of people, including professionals in many fields. The questions asked covered every possible aspect of life and what individuals could do to make a better world. The answer was that the first step was for the individual to come into a state of balance him/herself, focusing on living an impeccable life that resonated with the truth that resides within. Once this state is achieved, it affects those nearby, and the message transfers by example, not through preaching. The following guidelines have been given. (See The Blueprint For Peace and Harmony, Table 10.1.)

There is a noticeable absence of "Thou Shalt" and "Thou Shalt Not" in the fifteen guidelines for peace and harmony. Details of the teachings are beyond the scope of this book. Help in interpreting the guidelines as they apply to the individual, groups, large corporations, as well as governments, is available. (See Reference 21.)

Origin of the Pure Energy Entity

What is the origin of the Pure Energy Entity, source of the eloquent guidelines and historical information for this book? Consider again the first steps of the creation, as presented in Chapter 8, in which the Primal Energies are the result of three splits of the All-That-Is. How the splits occur involves consciousness. Humans think of consciousness as an interpretive quality, but in its essence, consciousness is truly the antithesis of energy. Consciousness in its primal form is the awareness of change, so consider this scenario as the logic that leads to the First Split.

1. The taking of a life for other than food will cause a great disturbance.
2. The taking of property without the consent of the other will cause a great disturbance.
3. The desire or thought to have something of another, and the other to have it not, will cause a great disturbance.
4. The desire or thought to control another's destiny and activities is disturbing to the souls of both.
5. The forceful control of the action of another will disturb the spirits of both.
6. The desire to have more than you need at the expense of one who needs is disturbing.
7. The accumulation of material worth for the sake of accumulating material worth is disturbing.
8. The consumption of more than one reasonably needs is disturbing.
9. In all things act as you would have others react to you.
10. Know that over, indulgence in anything will cause disturbance.
11. Know that gossip is disturbing to all involved.
12. Know that to listen in harmony to your fellow man as he speaks from the soul is important to both you and he, but that to take the place or the stresses of your fellow man and to help him solve his problems is disturbing to you, and must be done with caution and patience.
13. Know that there will be times of group chaos for which a leader will be required to restore balance. If the leader is not in harmony with these guidelines, other forms of chaos may result.
14. Know that when a group thinks of like mind, and this like mind is in chaos, that it will disturb larger groups; these guidelines apply to the group as they do to the individual.
15. Know that as the individual is disturbed by the taking of a life except for food, so is the group disturbed at the taking of the life of another.

Table 10.1 Blueprint For Peace and Harmony. Each advice and guideline is of equal importance. No one guideline is more or less important than any other. Living by these guidelines will alleviate disturbance in the body and will bring balance and harmony. Not living by these guidelines will lead to other disturbances and other disturbances will lead to greater chaos in the body and spirit.

All things within the All-That-Is move in cycles. The day-activity cycle, for example, is followed by the night-rest cycle, and the night-rest cycle is followed by the day-activity cycle, and so on. Imagine the All-That-Is to be in a night-rest cycle about to change to the day-activity cycle. Since the last part of the day-activity cycle created is always a mirror, the first thing the All-That-Is does is look into that mirror. The first thought of the All-That-Is is a simple thought — that It is. The All-That-Is becomes aware that it exists. The second part of that simple thought is that something else exists, and the recognition that there is something other is the first moment of the excitement of discovery. The discovery of what that something other is, is done in similar small steps. Each step in the process is a separate and distinct awareness of a particular small change that has occurred. In the moment of simple recognition that there is something other than the All-That-Is, all primordial order is labeled as external to itself by evenly distributing the Energy to everything that ever was before the Is-Ness became. Thus, the First Split is created and there now exists the Is-Ness and the Is-Not-Ness, as each receives a piece of consciousness from the All-That-Is in order that it might discover what It is.

It is said by those who study science that "Nature abhors a vacuum." There is a more inclusive truth about nature: "Nature abhors non-creativity." Nature, everything within the All-That-Is, must continually create. Any small change, no matter how small, is a creation, that creation adds to and expands the Is-Ness. Because of this principle, the First Split is followed by more splits, as the Is-Ness defines all that It is, and all that It is not. How this happens is that the Is-Ness recognizes that the simpleness of thought caused the First Split. It is through thought, then, that the two distinct parts of the All-That-Is seeks to define Itself yet further, and so another split occurs. The Two became Four, and again through the process of thought, the Four became Eight. With each new split, a piece of consciousness is imparted to the new creation, so each of the Eight views itself as a singularity, an individual consciousness, capable of creating. An individual consciousness, a singularity, can create, but it can only view its own creations. That is, It can "look down" upon Its creations, but cannot "look back" upon the previous creation. Otherwise the impulse for further creation would cease. Thus, the Four can view the Eight and all the combinations afterwards, but the Eight cannot look back upon the Four, the Two, or the All-That-Is.

The group that studies the teaching of the Pure Energy Entity were told, "That which I am is Love." Love is the name of this Pure Energy Entity because it describes the function of that Energy. This "Love" is the most encompassing description of Love. It is Love that binds two things together, but prevents them from merging too closely, so each has definition. They are bonded, but well-defined as individuals. Within this description is found all of the common definitions of love: the love of the two that form a couple, the love of a father for a child and so forth. The Energy and Consciousness of Love in the ancient texts was known and recorded as Yahweh. One of the teachers of Moses was Yahweh, who has brought the teaching directly to many humans throughout the course of Earth history.

The other Pure Energies and consciousness have these names: Allowance, Allegiance, Will-and-Power, Harmony, Knowledge, and Wisdom. The names best describe their function from our point of view. The Energy that they attach to in order to manifest is known as Chaos, often referred to as Jehovah. Because of these names they have been designated in Chapter 8 as: C, AL, AG, WP, L, H, K, and W. Note 2 gives a detailed description of the Energies and their function within the creations that have occurred after the Third Split.

The Third Split was not the last split. The principles described above yield more splits. There was the Fourth Split, a split of consciousness, but a simple combination of two distinct PEP. There was the Fifth Split, another split of consciousness, but a combination of three distinct PEP. The splits continue on. There are, in all, 666 splits (split/combinations). Considering the aspect of consciousness and the new identity of each creation leads to the realization that each distinct combination forms a new "singularity." These newly formed "unities" can view their own creations. They are aware because, as stated before, there is one part of each of the Primal Energies that recognizes no desire to be different and another part that recognizes a desire to combine. There is one part of what each Primal Energy is that is a realization and a solidness that is the Is-Ness. That provides recognition within the Is-Ness for itself; yet there is another part that recognizes Chaos (more creation) and seeks it. Thus there is one part that seeks change and one part that seeks observance of change, one part that knows what it is and another part that wonders what it is. Each time this simple dual awareness formed, another split occurred. Each formed the awareness, one half to preserve itself and the other half to combine and continue to create. In this manner more creation became possible, until 666 splits formed, which actually becomes the reunion with the origin point. How many singular entities there are after 666 splits is an astronomical number, since the number increases quickly as repeated doubling creates exponential growth. (See Note 3.) That number is 2^{36}, a value that is impossible to grasp, but makes for a holographic universe that is multidimensional, extremely large, ever expanding, and contains endless possibilities.

The Ten Dimensions

Another basic feature of the Is-Ness is the ten dimensions. Everything in three-dimensional reality, including each human, is a ten dimensional being, simultaneously existing in all ten dimensions. A workable perception of this fact is necessary to grasp the complete secret of the Great Pyramid. A helpful aid is Figure 10.3. Color code it with ink or pencil so that Allowance = orange, Allegiance = light blue, Will and Power = red, Love = lavender, Harmony = green, Knowledge = dark blue, and Wisdom = bright yellow. Trim and roll it into the shape of a cone, then glue it so that line A lies exactly on line B. The cone, a 2π cone as unique as the 2π Great Pyramid, represents some of the features of the ten-dimensional universe and shows how the quanta of each of the Primal Energies fits into the scheme of these ten dimensions.

A cone is selected to represent the dimensions and the ratio of the Energies in each dimension because there is a spiral aspect to traveling upward along the surface of the cone, similar to the movement of an individual packet of energy as it winks into and out of the Is-Ness. Place the apex of the cone against a mirror. The view is similar to Figure 8.7, the sketch of the movement of one packet of Chaos. Each dimension is labeled from one to ten and the relative ratio of the Energies is different in each dimension. These ratios are representative only, and it would take an infinite number of cones, each representing various ratios, to approach the reality of what has been created in the universe.

Notice that in some dimensions some Energies are nonexistent. Notice that the third dimension, more precisely third-dimensional reality, contains all of the Energies, but that the ratio is predominately Allowance, with a sliding scale of the other Energies, and with very little Wisdom. Study the cone and get a feel for the fact that each dimension is a different ratio compared to the other dimensions. This is because each piece begins and ends in different dimensions. For example, no piece of Allowance exists in the ninth and tenth dimensions. Also notice that the dotted lines indicate that any missing element of one of the Energies is made up by another Energy. The second dimension, for example, shows a missing portion of Allegiance, but that is made up by an equal amount

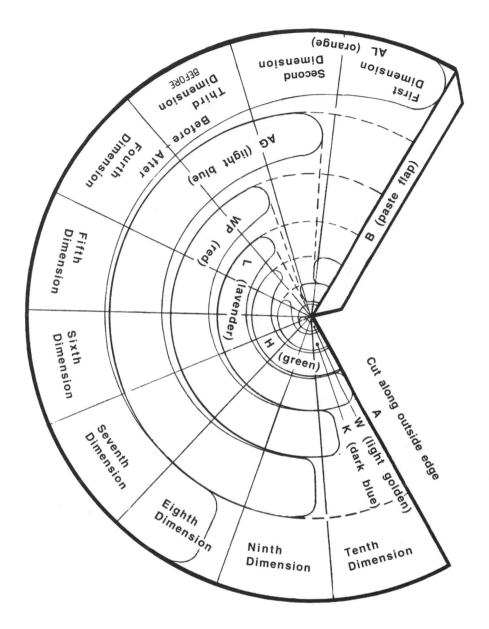

Figure 10.3 Graphical representation of the ten dimensions and the relative proportion of Primal Energy

of Harmony. The third dimension shows that any missing Will and Power is made up by an equal amount of Knowledge. This process continues as shown.

The Forms of the Third Dimension

Consider some of the forms that have been created as part of the third dimension: the solid reality, the realm of linearity of events, and the dimension of time. The most obvious aspects of the three-dimensional universe are the suns and planets. Stars have burst forth in endless numbers and in endless varieties, and authors of those suns exist upon the 24th, the 25th, and 26th splits. All combinations and formulations that produce suns were discovered by trial and error, meaning that some attempts to produce a glowing sun were not successful. It became recognized by the authors of the suns that stars that did not shine had a value just as they were. They were allowed, and these dark stars were known as the planets. Special consideration for the creation of only planets, made knowingly, and according to precise formulations, became the specialty of the authors that exist upon the 30th split. New stars and planets are being created at this moment and more will be created in the distant future; not all possibilities have been tried. As mentioned before, suns, planets, and all objects that are seen and observed in the universe are part of the three-dimensional reality and each must contain all eight of the Primal Energies in order to exist. Only one-tenth of the mass of the universe is so formed, leaving ninety percent of the universe uncombined and forming the rest of the dimensions.

The physical form of man exists entirely within the three-dimensional reality, but a great deal of complexity exists to support the creation of the human being, which is shown in Figure 10.4. This diagram is only a partial diagram of the 666 splits of the Is-Ness, but this is the region of greatest interest to humans. Human activities such as eating, exercise, sleeping, sex, keeping clean, and keeping warm and comfortable, exist entirely within the 34th split, the three-dimensional reality. The intellectual and emotional aspects of humans use energy from higher dimensions, the 33rd split, which is known as the astral plane.

On the 33rd split, there are seven zones and each is predominately resonant to a Primal Energy. The Causal plane, as it is called in some texts, exists predominately at the highest-frequency zone, Wisdom. This is the region of the oversouls. When an oversoul creates, some of its energy transforms into a soul — a finer version of itself, but more solid as the soul is made predominately of Primal Energy from the lower levels of the 33rd split. It is this part of the oversoul, the individual soul, that attaches to a physical form on the 34th split. This is how the oversoul experiences the three-dimensional reality.

The "Christus" level, the 32nd split, is where the authors of all living things exist and they are responsible for the physical form, the living animal of man. Like the 33rd split, the 32nd split is divided into seven zones and each is predominately resonant to a Primal Energy. Dissecting each zone is not really necessary. Although one can have an intellectual understanding of the 30th to the 35th split, sanity cannot be maintained anywhere except upon the 34th split, the appropriate place for the conscious mind to dwell and create. This is because time is a special invention for the 34th split alone, so only here can one's creations be observed as one event seemingly following another. Each human is a complex singularity, a unity, an author creating from the 34th split, and the creations are not only physical things, but emotional bodies as well. These emotional

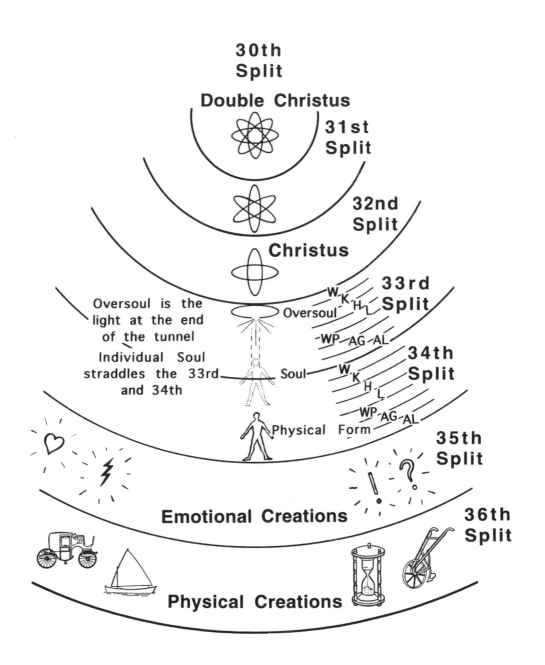

Figure 10.4 Depicted are splits 30 to 36, the region of most interest for most human beings. This is the region of the oversoul, the soul, our physical form, and our physical and emotional.

creations are electronic fields of energy as real as the person that creates them. They are empowered by the individual for their existence and each one exists forever within the Is-Ness, so each person causes the Is-Ness to change and to expand. (See Note 4.)

The most appropriate consideration that humans can have of themselves is as fine paint brushes with potential to create fine detail for the Is-Ness. Humans are the logical progression from the gross brushes of the splits above to the fine creations that are within our realm to create. It is most inappropriate to think that one should graduate back up the ladder, or ascend as "ascended masters" to the realm of planet creators. That can happen, but should not be especially encouraged, because the corollary of graduating is the fact that that entity is also finished— finished creating with the fine paint brush!

The creations of man exist in the realm of "duality" where happy or sad creations are possible. We humans, authors of emotion, quickly learn that the happy creations are the desired ones. By reading this book, one will be directed to move towards the creation of joy and harmony.

It's most fitting to describe some of the features of the Astral plane now and other details in later chapters. Like the Physical plane, the Astral plane is a combination of all eight Primal Energies. The Energy, atoms, and molecules, however, exist at several times the frequency of physical matter, which means that all things of the Astral are invisible. The Astral is the plane of demonstration, or the plane of reality, for the Is-Not-Ness which is the anti-matter part of the All-That-Is. That means that time is not linear like it is on the physical plane, the plane of demonstration for the Is-Ness. Instead, time upon the Astral is more akin to a distance between two events, which from the point of view of the Physical, looks like events can be played out of sequence. Events from the Astral are like nutrients in a pond that floating water lilies can use to grow and become realities in the Physical. That is why the Astral is absolutely vital to the events of the Physical. The Physical is the densified, slow-moving part of the Astral.

Some confusion about the astral plane exists because in some texts it is simply taught to be heaven, or at least a place of beautiful temples where one can rest, heal, and seek wisdom and knowledge. While this may be true for most, the 33rd split can be quite a disturbing experience for a few. Consider that for beings who pass through the Physical plane without disturbing the lives of others, whatever wonderful things could be imagined about any heavenly experience they might reap is a limitation. It is truly much grander than that. (See also Chapter 13.)

The human being is actually a soul bonded to a physical form, and that combination results in the reality of an individual ego. Upon death, the soul body of the individual experiences Astral events on its return journey to the oversoul. There are seven zones, each resonant to one of the Primal Energies on the Astral. Once "home" with the oversoul, the soul willingly realizes its ego-less aspect. Oversouls upon the Wisdom level of the Astral exist without ego.

During the awesome journey back to the oversoul a soul can become confused and even stuck in the high-frequency realm. Although the oversoul has a natural fail-safe procedure for rescuing its lost soul, the best prevention for the conscious mind of each human is to not dwell on a fixed picture regarding any aspect of what the Astral holds. (See also Chapter 13.)

An interesting aspect of all oversouls is what makes them different. That difference is due to the fact that oversouls are primarily resonant to only one of the Primal Energies and this means that the soul and the human form are also resonant to that frequency.

As a result, about one seventh of the population is resonant to Allowance, one seventh is resonant to Allegiance, and so on. It is not better or worse to be resonant to Knowledge, Will and Power, Allegiance, or any other particular Energy, it is simply different. It simply determines one's slant in life. For example, the lifestyle of someone resonant to Knowledge might manifest as someone predominately involved in the reading of books about history or facts in general.

Grand creations can occur in an upward spiral too. Oversouls have the option to combine. This occurs when the oversoul chooses to do so, not on any merit it has received, but as just another part of normal growth and creation within the Is-Ness. When that time occurs, two oversouls combine and form a "Christus," which is always a double resonance, or a "double essence." In time, a Christus has the ability to join with another Christus, and again this occurs when the two are ready to experience that change, not on any merit gained while experiencing the three-dimensional reality. The Double Christus, as it is called, is resonant to four Primal Energies and the entity exists upon the 30th split. All of the splits described have seven distinct regions and each region resonates with one of the Primal Energies because by its nature, each region is of a different frequency.

Souls ready for incarnation into the 34th split, the three-dimensional realm, can be formed from oversouls on the 32nd split. The human thus imbued with such a super soul will have a double essence. Such an individual is resonant to two of the Primal Energies and these are powerful people. They lead intense lives and are usually, but not always, the movers and shakers of society.

In extremely rare cases, souls ready for incarnation can be formed from the Double Christus level (30th split). Such a human is an even more powerful being. They possess a triple essence — only three, since one is left behind at the 30th split. These extremely rare embodiments become the magnetic leaders that alter the course of history. In the case of planet Earth, there have been only several incarnations from the Double Christus. Examples are Jesus Christ and Mohammed, who have affected great change for the planet. Buddha, by comparison, was a Christus who began to channel Yahweh. When the conditions were right, Buddha gave up the body and allowed Yahweh to channel for the rest of the life of the body. The essential truth of Buddhism is that each person must interpret the guidelines as it applies to his life situation; as a result, there should be as many paths to enlightenment as there are people. Interestingly, Buddhism has many sects, and each started when a particular disciple discovered a pathway that he could follow with impeccability.

This brief outline of the Energy flow of the universe is necessary to explain the exact nature of the secret of the Great Pyramid, as well as the complicated path by which humans arrived upon planet Earth, and an understanding of the tools by which humans can move from the pain of his current circumstances into the joy of a harmonious future. Perhaps this description of the universe is too different to be accepted at first, and it might even be cause for alarm. Fear not. The oversoul is the real individual and that one is a forever being. Everyone is always connected and never alone. Only the ego form of the individual can suffer the notion of extreme loneliness and pain. Whenever things go wrong, it should be a reminder that another hundred-thousand things went right. It all makes up the painting of creation for the Is-Ness. Always remember, there is a Universal Consciousness; God is the Grand Discoverer and above all, there is a Grand Plan.

Other Sentient Species of the Universe

Upon the plane of demonstration, the 34th split, there are many other races and many different forms of sentient beings besides humans. Besides the soul that bonds with the human form there are the souls that bond with vegetable and animal forms. Our souls are different. The specific soul type that bonds with the human form also bonds with 127 other forms, so the total number of the group is 128. This can be rewritten as 2^7, a mathematical formula that embodies the number of sub-groups and the number of pure Energies from which everything is created.

The variety of forms can be divided into two distinct categories: the Traders and the Travelers. It is comforting to know that of the ones that could possibly come to planet Earth from either group, all are friendly and do not constitute a military threat of any kind. The belligerent ones who are still like the Earth human and who still conquer as a strategy to survive, are kept planet-bound. That prevents them from coming to this planet, and it keeps us from going there.

Although humanoid in form, the Traders are genetically quite different. They evolved from a docile nurse shark-like creature and, because they are 500 times older than the human species, possess a higher degree of intelligence and technology. It is appropriate to consider them to be the "first" ones, and in their early evolutionary stage they achieved the mastery of high technology. They achieved the understanding of not only the chemical and nuclear nature of creation, but also the Primal nature of the universe. Upon their home planet their only adversary was from nature itself, and they developed technology to reduce their individual work loads and make living more pleasurable.

Eventually, they achieved an understanding of how to create successfully with the Primal Energies, allowing them to travel at many times the speed of light. Because they understood the fabric of the universe and how to bore short tunnels to their destination, they could explore other suns and planets. In their desire for more energy, they experimented with exotic power sources and one such experiment accidentally destroyed their home planet. Their only alternative was to live in their great space ships.

The horror of destroying their whole planet and its every life form, and almost causing their own extinction, resulted in a great self-judgment that has forever altered their behavior. That "violation of creation," as they came to perceive it, caused them to have the greatest reverence for life everywhere in the universe. Never again would they behave in a way that might alter the delicate balance of evolution on any planet. If they needed something from a planet they would always make a fair, balanced exchange. Following this code of ethics, they became the first intergalactic ecologists and pacifists of the universe. It has become part of their way to be and to create, searching out and observing other life forms in great detail. Those threatened with extinction, either of their own making or of natural origin, give them, in their perception, the right to intercede. Fixing the situation usually entails placing the endangered species in a new location where the life form can flourish. Preserving the Is-Ness is their self-proclaimed mission and joy.

Because of their early evolution and many experiences, they are the least threatening of all of the 128 types of beings in the galaxies. As they travel and trade they naturally come upon evolving races. If they discover a friendly race, one that has achieved a balance with nature and knows that being cooperative is the only way, they will invite them to their great ships to join in the exploration of the universe. The ones that are allowed to travel with them are carefully selected from balanced societies and are known as

Travelers, who gain the hyperleap to cross the enormous distances between galaxies in seconds. Once near their destination, the Travelers are released to explore in the small discs machines, the scout ships.

The Travelers search and study for many reasons, including scientific, archeological, and historical reasons. They are aware that there is interesting knowledge to be gained, so it is natural for them to want to travel and learn more about the universe. It is by definition against the very nature of the Traders who bring them, or the Travelers who come with them, to have any malevolent intent upon the societies of Earth. There is nothing we have that they want or need, including minerals, missing genetic materials, lost creative powers, nor anything a human could imagine they might desire.

As already stated, entities upon the 30th Split, the Double Christus, create the planets knowingly. Entities upon the 32nd Split, the Christus, create life forms including all of the evolving animal forms that could possibly contain a soul. Through the eons, the souls that now bond with the human form on Earth have tried to bond with many other animal forms, including pigs, cats, dogs, and birds. These bonding, however, did not always prove to be of sufficient creative intensity.

When the precursor to the ape was formulated, the Traders observed this life form and recognized its great potential. The early forms were dispersed upon various planets. The human form evolved quickly in nine of these locations, but with slight differences. This was the origin of the "Races of Man (Humans)." The Traders have monitored the evolution of humans as they have monitored life forms everywhere.

There are many forms of Travelers, but some do look like the people of Earth. The size of these human-looking beings varies from two feet to almost twenty feet tall. The giants, the ones nearly twenty feet tall, find the gravity field of Earth too weak for their circulatory system, and visit for very short times. They are comfortable on very large planets, and when they build ships, they rival those of the Traders in size.

It is beyond the intent of the book to discuss the many types of Travelers, however, it is worth noting that a lot of them would appear strange looking and would have a consciousness quite different than ours. All of them contain the same type of soul that bonds with the human form.

The soul does not enter a new physical form absent of connections to learned experiences from past incarnations. Depending upon where one incarnates, each individual brings a number of past life knowledge connections, and if during the early years of growth a desperate situation occurs, they trigger a remembrance of past life experiences in the form of intuition, helping the person cope. In some texts the connection has been called karma and it has been given spiritual connotations, but the primary purpose of it is to help one survive in the new incarnation. More details on most of this will follow later. For now, it is important to understand that the true history of the Earth human is more complex than can be pieced together by fossil and archeological records alone. It involved evolution on other planets and the planting of those seeds here on Earth. The history of man on Earth is a lot different than is currently taught, and stretches back in time much farther than the Egyptian and Sumerian cultures. Accepting that fact is one of the steps in unraveling the secret of the Great Pyramid.

NOTES

1. The complete blessing in the King's Chamber by the director of Astara, Dr. Robert, was, "Come to the end of the sarcophagus. Place your hand upon it and I'll place my hand upon yours. This creates a contact between the two of us and this great place, this center of light which is presented here. Then I'll make the sign of the cross, either the Christian cross or the Carensesata, on your forehead. Then I'll place both of my hands on the side of your head, and at that point, there should be a transference of all the energy involved, from the sarcophagus and myself into you and your life. At that point you should notice some small alteration of consciousness, don't be alarmed by it. Steady yourself with your hand on the sarcophagus, if you feel a little bit wobbly at the moment."

Once in position, the words of the ceremonial blessing were, "May the Great Light of this place be yours now and forever more, and with it receive the blessing from the Ancient One, Amun Das Ra." (or Al Uman Ra)

2. The Eight Primal Energies are known in some teachings as "archangels." In some respects this description is accurate, since the concept of an archangel is one who goes forth throughout all of the universe manifesting God's desire, and that is essentially what the Eight Primal Energies and Consciousness do. The number seven has become sacred because it is the seven Primal Energies that manifest the entire universe by attaching to the basic Energy, Chaos. In some teachings there are seven candles on one stand, or candle holder, in honor of that understanding. It happens that there are seven major chakras, energy portals to the body, that comprise each human being. Each energy portal corresponds to one of the Primal Energies, and that is why, in some teachings, the meditation involves taking seven breaths to activate, clear, or energize each of the seven energy centers. The number 49 is a sacred number in some teachings because seven breaths into each energy center yields a total of 49 breaths. Once the origin of the magic of seven is known, it can be found everywhere, in all the cultures and throughout the history of Earth. The function of each energy is given in summary form here:

Allowance: Allowance is the pathway that allows the flow of all things together. Without this, there would be no desire, there can be no creation without that flow. Allowance provides the flow, the movement, and to the physical being, this becomes what is allowed and what is not. If it is balanced, it is not formed from judgment, yet individuals hold judgments. Each person also holds fears, and individuals allow themselves to have these fears. In the physical body, Allowance resonates to the base or root chakra, and the organs within a person that do the filtering for solid food and waste.

Allegiance: Allegiance becomes the direction. Allowance provides the path, and Allegiance joins together. It begins the formation. To an individual, it becomes the steps on the path that are chosen. To the physical being, Allegiance resonates to the sacral chakra, the internal organs known as the endocrine system and the sexual organs. To the individual, Allegiance is what he will begin to join with its opposite, or what he will not. In its extreme, it is what an individual directs himself towards out of pure desire, or its opposite, joining for fear of not joining.

Will and Power: The energy of Will and Power is the force that gathers things together. It is the gravity force of attraction. What is attracted — or to be joined — is given by Allegiance, but how quickly it is attracted is given by Will and Power. To the physical being, Will and Power resonates to the solar plexus chakra, the bones, the muscles, and the connective tissues. To the emotional, it is what an individual controls and what controls the individual, or what one does or does not cooperate with. Those who do not control themselves radiate the need to be controlled, so society forms laws to control such people.

Love: Love is the glue that binds all things together. The energy of Will and Power brings all things together by the attraction forces, but how densely it forms depends on Love. Love is two things, the glue that binds things together and at the same time, separates them. It is the thin film of glue that joins and separates them so that things do not lose their definition by being crushed by the attraction forces. To the physical being, Love resonates to the heart chakra, the lungs, and the circulatory system. When an individual gives away his Love in an emotional sense, he dislikes himself, he loses self-definition and self-esteem. This radiates outwards, is recognized by others, and makes it very difficult for others to join with him in Love.

Harmony: Harmony is the "cosmic recipe book," since it knows the appropriate proportions for harmony to exist between different things. To the physical being, Harmony resonates to the throat chakra, to the immune system, and to the lymphatic system. In an emotional sense, Harmony tells a person when a trait is a disturbance to others. Harmony, then, seeks to be a person's conscience and to be in balance. It is important to listen to it.

Knowledge: Knowledge is all things that have been, all that is past. In the three-dimensional reality the planets and stars exist within Knowledge. Those things that have been created as a formula exist and immediately become part of the past. To the physical being, Knowledge resonates with the temple chakra, the brain, especially the left side of the brain, which is the factual or linear, logical mind. In an emotional sense, Knowledge is the remembrance of emotional and factual events of the three-dimensional reality experienced with the five senses.

Wisdom: Wisdom is all things that may be and all things that have not yet been. It is the Energy out of which future events and possibilities are created. Wisdom is the combinations that have not yet been made and things that have not yet come together. To the physical being, Wisdom resonates with the crown chakra, the brain, and especially the right side of the brain. In an emotional sense it becomes not only the imaginings, hopes, and desires, but also the fears.

Chaos: Chaos is the nothingness that is unspecified, unclear, undefined and waiting to be filled. At the moment of the first split Chaos moves outward to fill all places evenly. It is most important to understand that Chaos is the receptor for all of the Energies, similar to a sheet of white paper upon which colored lines can be fixed, and without which the brightness of the various hues could not manifest. To the physical being, Chaos resonates to any part of the body that functions well and to any part of the body that does not function well. It can be likened to a pain, and by prayer the other Energies can flow to perform the positive change required to effect the cure.

Balanced Productions. For further information about the chakras or Energy Entities, read *The Tool* by Larry Hawes available from Balanced Productions, POB 1681, Vista, California, 92085, phone: (760) 940-8910.

3. To maintain sanity, humans should have an intellectual understanding of the other splits and creators at those levels, but should not worry about their creations. Meteors and comets, however, could interfere with life on Earth, but if humans concentrate on their own creations and on living their life in balance, those threatening possibilites — thanks to the interconnectedness of the ten dimensions — will pass by harmlessly.

4. From any split, physical creations are always two splits away, and emotional creations are always one split away. For example, a human at the 34th split creates a table on the 36th split and simultaneously an emotionally real electronic creation, the joy/pain of the experience, on the 35th split. An example at a higher split would be an oversoul on the 33rd split creates a physical creation, an electronic emotional creature on the 35th split ,and a soul on the 34th that bonds to physical bodies. This soul is an emotional creation for the oversoul. At a higher split, the Christus creates physical forms on the 34th split and its emotional creation is an oversoul on the 33rd split. (See Reference 21, Balance Productions, for a tape on Devas.)

Chapter Eleven

Synopsis

The Traders are benign aliens that live on Super Mother Ships (SMS). These beings have small, bipedal, humanoid bodies with four-fingered hands, large heads with large binocular-vision eyes, and small mouths. They don't make audio communication, but use thought force instead. They have look-alike cousins that live on their own planet. They are called the Zetas, because their home planet is part of the solar system with a star call Zeta-Reticulum. The Zetas are slightly larger than the Traders and have larger eyes and a larger ear mound. The Zetas have a slit for a mouth, compared to the round Trader mouth. They both live up to 700 years. Like many living forms of the first wave of creation, they both have a group mind, although the Zetas have a slightly different one-mindedness. Because of the group mind, both species never experienced in-house fighting. During their quest to perfect their technology, the Traders manipulated larger and larger black holes. One black hole, unfortunately, fell into their planet. They escaped to their SMS and watched in horror as their planet with all of its life forms got eaten. They resolved to prevent this in the future by making sure that all life forms that they would henceforth discover be placed on at least two planets. This dispersal program often is possible because of their ability to move into a fourth-dimensional reality, where time can be reversed or scanned forward. When the Traders observed changes made (by another alien species) to our precursor, a small prosimian-like creature, they saw the benefit of this and added survival genes. This change to the sweat glands allowed the creature a greater temperature range.

The new species eventually turned out to have not a group mind, but a single, individual mind! This meant great individual creativity, but also risked that there was a potential for the species to be a rival unto itself. On each planet where our precursors were placed, the single-minded ones developed hunting instincts that included comparing and competing. These instincts cause small bands of hunters to be suspicious of each other. Quite often warring between them was the result. Despite this, progress was made, and in time, city-states formed, nations formed from the city-states, and one-world governments formed from the nations. Each planet finally existed in relative peace. This occurred on nine different planets and is the origin of the different races. When they eventually discovered each other, they realized that they not only looked different, but had progressed along different lines, valued different habits, and were interested in entirely different things. The hunting instinct reared its ugly head and the planets began to war. The warring never ended and the Traders eventually decided to step in. They stopped the fighting by using advanced technology and brought all warring races back to their home planets. The Traders began to teach on each planet, giving an overview of creation, the human place within it, and the balanced way to create. At the end of the troubled times, one group with blue-green skin was brought to this solar system and lived on a planet they called Earth. That word meant something important to the ones who were the victims of a long epoch of war. It meant an anchoring, safety, rest, and peace. This was Earth One.

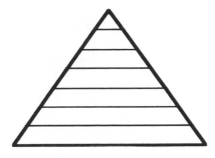

Chapter Eleven

EARTH ONE

Events of the Space Neighborhood

Traders, Travelers, and Mother Ships

The entire evolution of human beings did not take place on this planet. Arriving on Earth by a circuitous route, the human species was brought here by another race. Why that race would do that is a fascinating part of our journey through the universe. That story also reveals some of the secrets of the Great Pyramid. It is a story of reality few could imagine.

The reality is that the space neighborhood is filled with motherships that wink out in one location, and quickly wink in somewhere else. Travelers thus arrive at every known sun, planet, asteroid, and comet for their own purposes, exploring the vicinity in disc scout ships. The Traders own the mother ships and invite sentient species, the ones who do not cause a disturbance, to travel with them. The Traders have learned that if you take something, you must also leave something. This maintains the balance. This trading behavior pattern has gained them their name.

The race that brought us here were the Traders. Humanoid in form, they come in different types, ranging in size from three to five feet tall. Their skin is elastic and tan, beige or gray in color, and when touched, is soft like a pillow. Their torso is relatively small and thin, with long arms. They evolved from a docile, shark- like species that had a schooling instinct. In their fish form they originally ate krill.

In their current humanoid form, they have four fingers, no opposing thumb, and two middle fingers that extend somewhat like the claws of a cat. The skin is web designed to accommodate this feature. (See Figure 11.1.) There are no fingernails or claws of any sort at the end of their fingers, but there does exist a recessed area similar to a suction cup that enhances the manipulation of objects. These recessed areas of the finger tips actually have tiny cilia around the edges that aid in grasping objects. The cilia are a living part of the finger that help sense objects as a matter of unconscious manipulation, almost down to the molecular level. Another feature of this recessed region is its ability to aid in detecting and analyzing odors, heat, and pressure.

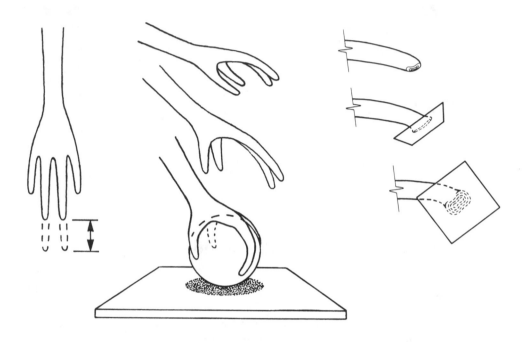

Figure 11.1 The Trader's four-digit hand extends two fingers to firmly grasp objects. The sensitive recessed finger tips spread on contact to appear to be a "suction cup."

The legs and feet of the Traders have atrophied somewhat because of the lifestyle they have adopted on their huge ships. The ships have gravity and while the Traders can walk, they often opt to float, using a levitation technology. When visiting hostile areas they use levitation and also surround themselves in a spherical, protective force field. (See Note 1.)

When compared to the body, the head is large and as hairless as the body. The well-publicized feature of the head is the apparently penetrating stare of the very large eyes. Like human eyes, these eyes are spaced for binocular depth viewing, and in some versions are elongated, giving an oriental or cat-like appearance. Eye protection is by an eyelid and a nictitating membrane. With the eyelid open and the nictitating membrane closed, the iris is invisible and the eye has the strange appearance of being nearly black. This is because the eye itself and the nictitating membrane are polarized perpendicularly with respect to each other. (Place two polarized lenses together and rotate them until they are 90 degrees out of phase. They will appear to have turned black!) Each eye has a large iris, but it is of non-contractile design. Extremely effective adjustment for different light levels is accomplished by various positions of the nictitating membrane. The nictitating membrane also favors the passing of red light and cutting out blue light. When looking through one of these membranes, night vision seems to be enhanced. Night vision technology was inspired by this discovery.

The Traders communicate by thought force alone, so their ears are not what we might expect. Not designed to capture faint audio signals, their ears are only small orifices. Their nose is small, with two visible openings. Their mouths are a small openings without pronounced lips. Although the Traders appear to have no teeth, their teeth are so tiny that they are almost invisible and are formed in row after row. The inside of their mouths appears much like the tongue of a cat and is rough gum in nature. Their principle diet consists of a simple wafer, a synthetic version of the original krill-like protein food that existed on their planet of origin. The wafer does not look like anything we would regard as food. We would consider their food to be a thin metal disc, probably something that would fit in a computer.

One race genetically related to the Traders, and often confused with them, shall be designated here as the Zeta-type, because their home planet orbits a star that Earth astronomers have designated as Zeta-Reticulum. The planet-bound version of the Traders, the Zetas live in a gravity field nearly twice as strong as the gravity of Earth, and as a result they have developed strong legs and feet, and wear a boot-style footwear. Although their bodies and heads are similar to the Traders', the Zetas are technically Travelers because they must, like all Travelers, access the huge Trader ships to star travel or jump among the stars. Bodies of these Zeta-Reticulum types retrieved from crashed saucer scout ships are in deep freeze in the possession of the United States government. (See Reference 9 and Note 2.) Comparison of the Traders and the Zetas reveals the Traders to be shorter with a smaller head size and, in relation to the head, smaller eyes. The Trader's mouth is more of a round opening compared to the slit of the Zeta's. The Traders' ears are almost nonexistent except for an orifice, while the Zetas have a noticeable mound where the ear is located.

The Traders and Zetas live for up to 700 years and procreate far differently than we do. They are not born as male or female, but are more nurse, shark-like in origin and all look alike. They appear to be non-gender by nature, but will "select" to be male or female at some appropriate future time. That is, if two individuals are set apart from the group over a period of time, one will become female and the other will become male. Certain types of fish, birds, and reptiles on Earth possess this evolutionary trait.

The Trader genetic structure is far from the human genetic structure, so "crossbreeding" experiments are not possible, and not attempted. That is not to say that the human species does not have any DNA from the Traders, we actually do. We are all genetically altered, in the same sense that the dolphins, whales, and sharks have been altered. These last three have skin that is similar to the Traders, not by coincidence, but by direct intervention and design on the part of the Traders to help these aquatic species survive in the environment. In our DNA sequence, one third of the way down the DNA chain is a segment exactly the same as found in the Traders' DNA chain. It is a piece that

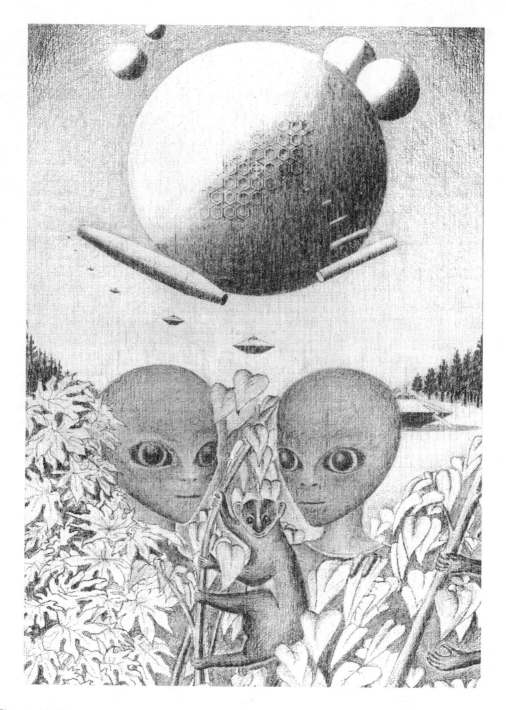

Figure 11.2 Lemur-like precursor to humans visited by the Zetas who come in a variety of body and head shapes including large and small eyed versions. In the background are some ET vehicles, scout discs, cylindrical carries for the discs, and the great Trader Super Mother Ships.

is thought to be junk, because it seems to be switched off. Pieces that are switched off, however, are as important as the ones that are switched on. Science will eventually discover that part of the trick to designing DNA sequences is to switch off some pieces to balance others that are switched on.

Just as we experience reality as humans, the Traders experience their reality as Traders. The two realities have nothing in common. Consequently, speculation that specially-engineered humans walk the Earth as agents of the Traders can be discounted as human projection. It would be like training dolphins or birds to do spy work for us. Such efforts would fail because the reality of dolphins and birds is completely different.

The Traders have a group consciousness and not an individual consciousness, so a new thought by one ripples out and becomes the conscious domain of all. Since they communicate directly by force of mind, they do not have a written language. None is needed. They do, however, have certain symbols and their mental communication is in terms of those symbols. The corollary of this fact is that they do not actually communicate with words or writing to any of the Travelers or to the people of Earth, but by the thought force of these universal symbologies.

A simple thought by one Trader is thought and remembered by all Traders, and they remember everything that they have done. If it is necessary to recall a communication or something from the past, it can always be retrieved. This particular ability has enabled them to make galactic and intergalactic maps to navigate throughout the universe. So far, only they have this navigational ability; all other species would get lost.

The Zetas

Both groups, the Traders and their look-alikes, the Zeta group, have the same brain design which is capable of one-mindedness. Like the Traders, they can communicate with thought force alone. Visitations that are remembered by humans are from the Zetas; the Trader visitations are usually fourth-dimensional and are not remembered. However, the true one-mindedness is a feature that the Zetas have lost.

The organs for transmitting thought and the organs for feeling are effectively the same thing. For the Zeta group, the magnetic sphere of the Earth changes their neurological balance slightly, giving them a slightly different conceptual understanding of reality. That difference means that although the Traders and the Zetas have an equal ability to transmit and receive messages between them, even they do not necessarily understand each other. Only when a common reference point is established can complete communication take place between the Trader and Zeta groups.

This is true for all species of the universe, so only when beings grow and live in similar circumstances can they share the same joy, pain, humor, and other life experiences. All races can, however, share the same reference point of science and the laws of nature, because these are universally true and self-apparent. The principles of mathematics, physics, and the procedures for exploring the universe, for example, are areas where complete understanding can be achieved.

Both the Traders and the Zetas, who do a certain amount of field work for the Traders, can and do communicate with humans because humans can transmit and receive in a very limited way with the Zetas. Humans can transmit the emotional quality of any five-sense observation and do sometimes receive from the Traders' and Zetas' emotional thought processes. Their communications come to a human more in the form of symbols.

Since we do not really have the correct organs for receiving their thoughts and emotions, it is a strain for them. It might be said that they have to shout. They shout in images, they shout in emotions, and they shout in thoughts. Their thoughts are totally and absolutely from a different perspective than a human beings. Some communications can get through, however, especially when a common reference point occurs, such as the love for all living things.

During close encounters, humans often report that words are heard within the inner ear. They report that the lips of those aliens did not move, and while that seems magical, it must be remembered that the words are in themselves interpretive. By the time a human "hears" a word in the inner ear, he has already actually interpreted the communication, and it becomes, perhaps, "I love you." In all likelihood, the words heard were a small part of the total communication.

It is natural for our brains to do this type of interpretation. Because our realities are so different, except for natural laws as stated above, a common reference point doesn't exist and the completeness of the communication is never achieved. All species can, however, share a love for each other. (See Note 3.)

The Traders have been star hopping for 500 million years. The Traders are real, and so are many of the reports from Earth inhabitants who assert they have been visited by humanoid aliens. The reports flood in from all corners of the globe, telling of encounters with small humanoids with large heads and very large eyes. Proof that a conspiracy or group hysteria is not the source of the reports is the fact that a rural dweller of Africa, South America, or the Soviet Union describe the same interior rooms of the ships and make almost identical sketches of the unusual proportions of the aliens. People in remote regions of the globe have nothing to gain by these reports, yet unfortunately are ridiculed. Those who have experienced this torment have often set up self-help groups, since governments have been of little help. In fact, it is becoming increasingly clear that the governments of the world have had a policy of debunking these reports, and have disseminated disinformation, including the group, hysteria theory. Governments have kept the existence of aliens a secret for over fifty years and to keep these secrets they have followed and have systematically taken, even stolen, every shred of physical evidence. They have discredited and persecuted individuals who know too much. (See Reference 4 and Note 4.) Hopefully the truth of the existence of aliens and their physical visits will soon be general knowledge, so that this oppression will be behind us. Personal accounts, as well as the efforts of private investigators, have resulted in some correct information appearing in printed form. (See Reference 6, 23, 24, and 25.) What has not been reported is the true purpose and intention of the aliens. The overview that follows may help the reader sort out the contradictions and partial truths that abound.

The Overview

The Traders have always had a group mind, which for the Earth human is a startling fact to comprehend. Because each of us has our own individual hopes and dreams, we are complete universes within ourselves. In contrast, each individual Trader always knows what the others are thinking and never loses track of the group goal. If, for example, the group mind decides that this year it will be red uniforms, then all cooperate in the best way that they can to produce, distribute, and wear red uniforms.

The consciousness of the individual Trader is not always bonded to the group mind, however. The group consciousness is actually "stratified" so that at the lower levels the individual can concentrate on his job or the task at hand, can feel and be an individual, but with "a quick look up," that individual immediately sees his cellular place in the universal consciousness of the group.

In the Roswell incident, several Zeta aliens were found to be injured, but still alive. (See Reference 9.) A human witness said his own mind was filled with the thoughts "What am I going to do, I cannot get home, I am sad, I am going to perish." This was the human mind's interpretation of the symbols transmitted by the alien. This was, though, only a partial understanding. In truth, the alien looked up into the group mind and realized that his injuries could not be reversed even by the advanced techniques of the Traders, and that any rescue attempt would have been futile. Since each alien knows that the body is the temporary container for the soul, the true forever-being, he realized he would soon reincarnate and have a new physical form. So with no regrets, the body was allowed to pass.

Although this is difficult for human beings to completely understand, in a sense we are exactly like the aliens. We do our job and society progresses with each accomplishment, no effort is ever lost, and each effort affects the future forever. However, for us to dispense with the individual ego, we must die, because the ability to "look up" is not part of our nature. Our looking up is done by education, and we have to have a certain amount of faith in the fact that we are beings who "live" forever. Those who have had out-of-body experiences already know this to be true, and being encapsulated as an individual is less of a problem for these individuals.

The group mind greatly shapes the society and its survival strategy within the three-dimensional reality. The natural cooperative effort becomes like that of a colony of ants or a beehive. This natural cooperation means that the concept of competition for anything is unknown to them. The experience of war was not part of their evolutionary path. Since there were no conflicts, predators, or natural enemies on their original planet, their only survival war was with nature, that is, their attempt to make life easier for themselves.

To avoid work, they became addicted to technology and over time constantly improved the machines, not just because it allowed them to work less, but also to explore the universe around them. Life on their original planet was idyllic by our standards and the needs of all were always met. There was never a need for more shelter, food, or clothing, and this golden era lasted for many millennia. Each generation succeeded in making life a little more joyful by incrementally decreasing the drudgery of work, but to accomplish this the technology became more complex and the need for more and more power grew.

The engineers quickly reached the limits of chemical power, and moved to nuclear power. Nuclear power provided a solution for another millennium, but in time their need for increasing power led them to the final quantum leap to harness the power of antimatter. The dream of one generation became the reality of the next, and small antimatter power stations located next to black holes beamed energy to the planet. The idea was to create large enough field devices to actually move the location of the black hole, and that was done. Once mastered, the technique was used not only to power the home planet, but to power their giant ships to travel anywhere in the galaxy in seconds.

With antimatter and nuclear power sources mastered, a great variety of ships and devices had been created to quickly move the Traders wherever they desired. Many varieties of small observation craft or scout ships that could visit the surface of any planet, including the Earth, were created millions of years ago. Each small craft, the typical flying saucer, has on board a nuclear-type power source, a small antimatter power source based on the decay of element 115, and, as a back-up, a Primal Energy beam from the much larger "mother ships."

Each flight originates from, and ends with, a return to the mother ship, unless there is an appropriate base on the planet surface. (See Note 5.) Most mother ships are actually carriers and attach to even larger "Super Mother Ships" for supplies while being towed to a new location. The great Super Mother Ships are constantly moving because of the extreme curiosity of the Traders and the enormity of planets and lifeforms to observe. These Super Mother Ships (SMS) have the ability to move among the stars in a moment and each is powered by a small black hole. The black hole technology has been perfected to the extent that the surface of the SMS are covered with tiny ones; this skin absorbs all energy that might damage the craft. No asteroid, meteor, nuclear-tipped missle, beam weapon, or particle weapon can penetrate the skin.

This technology using the Primal Energies and black holes is pure magic to humans of Earth. The spacefarers appear to cease to exist in one part of the universe only to reappear in another part. They do this by changing the vibration of all parts of their being and rotating them in a particular way into a space time continuum of their own choosing. (See the secret of the Reality Number, Note 6.)

Of the ten dimensions that make up the universe, their range is quite masterful. They can move out of a three dimensional reality and into a four dimensional reality, only to reappear somewhere else in three-dimensional reality, and everyone on the SMS goes with them. The reappearance can be in the future, the present, or the past. All events in the universe are happening at once. Only when an Oversoul becomes attached to a physical form is it truly immersed into a three-dimensional reality where events seem sequential. Thus, the Traders regularly move into four-dimensional reality, and sometimes even into five-dimensional reality. Besides all of this, the Traders have a clear intellectual understanding of the six-dimensional reality, and the Earth humans by comparison are only now considering whether four-dimensional reality exists at all, and whether time machines could possibly be built. (See Note 7.)

The Trader technology allows them to be aware of the PEP and to use that knowledge to navigate about the universe. This is because the Primal Energies are like tendrils or strings of energies and form something like a road map to the places where combinations are happening. The monitoring of these strings of PEP, with their great PEP-sensitive "sails," also allows them to monitor the thought forms of individuals on this or any other planet. Negative thought patterns "ripple the sails" in predictable patterns which signals them to come, investigate, and determine whether it is a natural phenomena or of intellectual origin. For example, Travelers guilty of harming sentient beings lose their right to travel, and the perpetrators may not even get a return trip to their planet of origin. Travelers are aware of this and are very gentle in their explorations and scientific pursuits.

It is within the great intergalactic-hopping SMS that observers, scientists, and teachers of other physical life-forms of benevolent intention are invited to travel, and these become the Travelers. This includes life-forms genetically identical to the Earth human — ones from Sirius, the Pleiades, and other star systems. The only requirement is that they have overcome their fears and judgments of each other, have overcome their adversarial relationships with nature, and are perfected enough to know how to work in cooperation.

The Traders monitor all societies, however, they don't probe deeply, hidden secrets within the minds of individuals. They are quite capable of misinterpreting the actions of human beings. They do not fully understand single-minded species and their motivations. They understand their own good intentions and they understand that the purposeful infliction of pain is evil, or at least representative of a low form of evolution.

On any planet, the Traders know when the possibility of self-destruction exists, and only under this extreme circumstance would the Traders step in to avoid the catastrophe. The warring of one species or life-form with itself, typical of the Earth humans, represents a low form of evolutionary development. They are not candidates for traveling, but once that society has passed through the warring stage they are invited to explore space and time. At the moment, the Traders alone control travel between stars of the universe. It is their choice.

Those who are allowed to join must have space vehicles that meet certain minimum standards. The Traders require that only their own ships, or ships designed by them and constructed with their supervision, are allowed to attach to an SMS. This is true for both the scout ship (disc-shaped) and the small mother ships (cigar-, delta-, or boomerang-shaped). Any race can design and build their own space ships to explore around their star of origin, but these are not allowed upon the SMS.

The small scout ships and even the small, cigar-shaped mother ships, which are the home of a dozen or so discs, are occasionally seen here in our three-dimensional reality. (See Note 8.) The small ships arrive, take samples, observe, and sometimes even contact Earth humans. These visitors are not only the Traders and Zeta-types, but nineteen other distinctly different races that have evolved to Traveler status. They are here basically to learn and not to help. The Travelers are not here to "save" us but to watch us save ourselves. If we insist upon self-destruction, the Traders, who are not here to save us either, will anyway because of their own self-imposed agenda. They will take a sampling of threatened lifeforms and place them somewhere else.

To the alien races of our own genetic strain, we are a living history of what they went through in their early development. They are particularly interested in observing inter-racial events. What happens here affects their planning, and their visitations will increase in frequency. (See Note 9.)

The great SMS of the Traders come in various sizes and proportions. The size and number of these space vehicles is quite mind boggling. Some of the largest of the SMS have diameters of 6,000 miles. The maximum ocean vessel ever built by Earth men is less than one mile long. Are large Trader ships rare? SMS that are over one thousand miles in diameter number over one thousand, just within one light year of our solar system. There are over seven thousand of the smaller mother ships, ten to several hundred miles in diameter, within our solar system. They are constantly moving about, and they intentionally hide on the far side of the planets, moons of the planets, or hover in line with bright stars. If they wanted, they could fly a formation that would blot out the rays of the Sun, rendering the entire planet dark, cold, and eventually, although it is hardly their intention, completely lifeless.

The ships are occasionally observed by telescopes and the largest of these was at one time thought to be a new discovery — the tenth planet of the solar system. The authorities could not find it when they looked the second time, and did not make the announcement, embarrassed because they could not repeat the experiment. The scientific method, of course, operates under the premise that only repeatable experiments determine what is part of reality.

The Traders also have a fixed base on the far side of the Earth's moon, and they have observed Earth for over 200-million years. They have not only brought lifeforms here, but have made corrections to the atmosphere. One easy way to make a correction to the atmosphere is to take a massive object, a giant SMS the size of the moon, and travel an elliptic path with respect to the Sun, either ahead of or behind the planet as needed. This speeds up or slows down the planet, resulting in a different orbit, by moving the planet either closer to or farther away from the Sun. A lower orbit closer to the Sun would have the effect of densifying the atmosphere, and the increased sun energy would result in a warmer climate. The Traders have long ago mastered these techniques on this planet, as well as countless others, to improve conditions that support the preservation of lifeforms.

The Traders can and occasionally do prevent catastrophic extinctions of species on planets throughout the universe. This is done in reaction to any great catastrophe, whether natural or self-induced. If a nuclear exchange were to threaten the species of Earth humans, for example, it is feasible that everyone would be "beamed up" within four minutes. If such an event were to occur, there would be no choices made, everyone would go, regardless of race, color, or creed. It is not one's state of religious perfection that has any bearing upon the decision of the Traders. To them, it is the physical form of the Earth human that must be protected, since it is considered — like all other living things — to be a sacred creation and a part of the Is-Ness that must be preserved. In Chapter 14, however, an example will demonstrate how spiritual perfection does influence the outcome of natural disasters.

By what has been stated it could be thought that this Trader activity is somewhat like a great "intergalactic Sierra Club." Why would any race spend so much time and effort on such a benevolent project? What is in it for them? Since it can be argued that the death of a species is every bit a part of evolution as the birth of a species, and that the universe would just evolve something else to take its place, where did this reverence for every scrap of life originate? As will shortly be seen, the answer is that the process is very self-serving.

The Great Catastrophe

During their expansion stage, the Traders experienced an event that forever changed the purpose of their exploration. As already stated, the Traders experienced a love of technology and a need for more power that grew until the use of small Black Holes had become an established practice. Eventually, even that no longer gave them enough power, so they decided to scale up and harness an even larger black hole. They did, and it was positioned close to their planet, because that was more convenient, resulting in less work. At first they began to feed it asteroids, and later small moons, since they knew that more massive objects would yield greater amounts of power. By this time their planet was a ghost of what it had been, they had stripped most of its natural resources and had used all the life-forms for their own purposes. Most of the species became extinct, but this was of little concern to them because they could manipulate the Primal Energies to create and synthesize the food they needed to survive. Their main focus was to create the great SMS, move away from their home planet, and explore the deep recesses of the universe by star-hopping, so any concern for their dying planet was secondary.

Larger and larger moons were fed to the Black Hole until the accident occurred. One moon was too large and the Black Hole could no longer be maintained in the proper position relative to the planet. It began to move uncontrollably, and unfortunately, in the direction of their planet. With frantic efforts, they took as much from their planet as they possibly could and stored the valuables upon their great mother ships. From the safety of the SMS, they stood by and watched the horrifying sight of their mother planet being torn apart and completely devoured by the uncontrolled Black Hole.

With each individual resonating to the single group mind, their thought was that they had destroyed their own mother planet, and they shared one great group guilt. Pondering the event with great remorse, there was a realization that evolving beings elsewhere in the universe could make the same mistake, and quite possibly not be able to escape their own fate. They formed a resolve, that in their movement about the galaxies, they would forevermore remember the event. No longer would they simply build new things or invent different ways to reduce work. In the future they would do something helpful and beneficial. Respecting all forms of evolution, they would seek out new life-forms and catalog everything they came upon. To decrease the possibility of repeating their own fate, they would place new life-forms upon at least two planets. If any life-form might become extinct upon one planet, it would still survive somewhere else in the universe.

Since the soul that empowers the Trader species is the same soul that empowers the human, it is natural for them to perceive the Is-Ness in much the same way: with a great reverence for life, and observing each living thing of evolution as a great gift of creation. This is appropriate for all sentient beings, and the thought of extinction of any life-form is abhorrent. Sentient beings will rightly conclude, once their needs are met, that preserving life is a great service to the universe. (See Note 10.) After all, the more forms that persist, the more variety there is for incarnation, and this is the aspect of their nature that is self-serving. This reverence for life has become the Traders' purpose and why the most exciting creation to them is to study genetics and preserve life-forms.

The Traders have been visiting the Earth for millions of years and have greatly influenced its life-forms. When dinosaurs existed, Traders took eggs and placed them where they would flourish. So while dinosaurs did not survive on this planet, they do still exist and thrive in the universe. The Marsupials were in peril elsewhere and so were brought to a special habitat where they now do well. That place is planet Earth. When humans were at the Cro-Magnon stage, seeds were taken and placed where they would prosper. When man was at the prosimian stage, seeds were taken and placed where they would do well. In fact, the Traders have taken seeds from every stage of development of man and have placed them where they would be able to survive. Each stage of human development exists now, thriving somewhere the new environment seems like the natural environment. Because each environment was carefully selected, it has been easy for the human transplants to adopt, thrive, evolve, and expand. These locations are all within the three-dimensional reality that we perceive as the universe. Insuring that life in all of its varied ways continues to exist, they make ecological trades; occasionally when extinction is about to occur, they use their great technology to intercede. So it is by these ecological "trades" that they are identified. They are the great Traders.

The Origin of the Races of Humans

Now that the nature and abilities of the Traders is understood, the amazing story of Earth One can be explained. Contrary to what evolutionary scientists have theorized, not all new genetic strains are the result of blind chance or "trial and error." Original life-forms are the accomplishment of conscious thought at the Christus level. Consciousness at the Christus level is able to put spin on photons, either positive, negative, or none at all. This spin is the information needed so that a set of photons interacts with an atom or a molecule in some predetermined way, and by using this methodology, changes are made to the genetics that cause a change in the animal form.

There existed over 100 million years ago a small prosimian, type animal on this planet that climbed with great agility in the trees using its grasping hands and feet. This small creature, successful as it was, had not yet achieved the potential that the Christus was planning. More connections and disconnections within the brain of that species were made and the result was the precursor to all of the primates, including the monkey, the apes, the chimp, and even humans.

All genetic changes are observed by the Traders, and they knew what had occurred and came to observe it. Seeing the value of it, they added survival genes to it. (See Figure 11.2 and See Note 11.) The Traders noted with great interest that this precursor human form possessed an individual mind. Even though an individual mind lacks Universal Consciousness, its observations of nature would be unique for any soul that would bond to the species. Having great intellectual understandings, creative abilities, and a single consciousness within each individual bears a certain price, however, because there is the potential for the species to be an adversary to itself.

There are many stories about how humans finds themselves at odds with them-selve, about the origin of greed, and the urge to conquer. Many partial truths have been written as part of the 12,000 religions spread around the planet. One popular example that contains the story of the "original sin" has developed over the centuries to help control those who behaved unlawfully. In recent years, a New Age version of the morality tale explains that humans expanded throughout the universe, gracefully at first, but then, yielding to the temptation of greed, they conquered and enslaved part of the population. Led by their leader, Satan or Lucifer, this practice spread throughout the universe. In time and with the help of God, those enslaved managed to reverse the situation and the universe is nearly clear of the evil leader and his followers. Upon the spirit world those evil souls were duly noted by angels of God and were directed to bond to physical forms upon a planet where the reality consisted of many hardships and challenges. This was a planet that would quickly teach them the evil of their ways, and that planet was Earth. Once purified, they would give up greed and see the value of serving others. They would once again be allowed an existence in the fourth-dimension reality, (a heavenly abode compared to earthly existence) at first with the position of a small officer and in time progressing to greater status. (See note 19.)

Although there is great value in teaching to be a servant of others, what must be taught is the balanced way. Serving others with complete selflessness can lead to personal malaise and an impoverishment that becomes a burden upon society. Those that serve others while taking care of themselves are serving society and themselves, which is the balanced way.

Original sin, karma, and the like, can be useful tools to teach those who do not have time to do research, but exaggeration can lead to extreme behavior — selflessness on the one hand, and complete abandonment of right behavior on the other. As explained earlier, karma is a connection to other lifetimes that helps the physical form survive in its new incarnation. If the person experiences an event that is particularly traumatic during his first five to seven years of life, a connection is made to a similar event in the past and the person will intuitively know how to cope.

The origins of conflict for the human arises from the reality of his evolution. As a prosimian of 200 million years ago, individual awareness was like that of an antelope in a herd. When one antelope runs, it is like a command for all of the antelopes to run. That is a form of one-mindedness, similar to the Traders. The designers of the human species wanted more self-awareness for the human. This was accomplished by changes to the endocrine system, the fight or flight mechanism, and also making certain connections and disconnections within the brain. The physical form could thus stand alone and make the needed decisions that would insure survival. The increased self-awareness lodges itself in the libido, and that sense of awareness occurs at puberty, leaving one with a sense of forced self-isolation and exile. This is part of what a human being is, however. The treasured tradeoff is individual creativity.

Thus humans find themselves with limited ESP abilities, and are basically an animal of third-dimensional reality with an individual mind and five senses. He will observe his existence to be a reality of limitation, and so, like any animal in this condition, must grab quickly or lose the opportunity for obtaining food, shelter, and items of comfort. It can be concluded that a happy existence is a factor of how much one has acquired, and the first human that saw it that way, saw reality in terms of differences between her or himself and others. With a long history of hunting, humans naturally weighed their hunting abilities and weapons with the game's abilities, location, and other factors. It was natural to compare.

Most early humans made the same comparison and perceived their condition in this order: "When I am hungry, I know to be happy I must eat, that is all that concerns me. I don't know if the others are hungry so I do not really care about their state of hunger. My hunger means I will eat right now."

Many times others were hungry at the same time, and naturally pursued the same morsel of food, quite often leading to a fight. After fighting over a meager meal, insufficient to feed all the hunters, man determined that for him to eat, the others must be eliminated. Avarice was born in that moment.

There were some who barely escaped death in such episodes, since they were quite inept at being conquerors, but this incompetence lead to a new survival strategy. During opportunities to kill food in abundance, the ones who could not conquer other men began to overkill game. They overkilled three times what they personally needed and the excess was used to feed the ones who were inept at hunting, but good at conquering. This sharing concept avoided the fight to the death, and the great battle was replaced with the buying of an ally. The only thing necessary for the purchase of an alliance was to kill three times over what one could personally eat.

Those that could kill this amount did so and reached a somewhat exalted position. They had the alliance of those who spent their energies and efforts in repayment for the food, instead of going into battle or on the exhausting hunt. They began to improve living conditions at the home base, which included tending warm fires, cleaning and cooking food, and providing some physical pleasantness for the exalted one, the admired great hunter. In the process was born the concept of taking care of someone else, and the basic elements of an organization were formed.

Some within that organization, however, compared themselves to the exalted one and that was the start of trouble. Those who didn't hunt viewed themselves as servants and thought that it was having instead of getting that made the difference, and a new form of avarice was born. Being good only at conquering, they used that dormant skill to conquer the great hunter hoping to get all of what was his. When the great hunter, whose weakness was a distaste for the battle-to-the-death, was faced with it, he died. The conqueror was left at the head of the alliance, but the new leader was now one to be feared.

With the conqueror gaining all the spoils of battle, but with the provider gone, those within the alliance soon wondered where the food would come from. The conqueror did not have the ability, desire, or skill to hunt to begin with. So under fear of death, some were ordered to hunt and provide for the rest. In fact, they could not eat until they achieved the factor of three overkill. Enslavement and fear was the result of incompetence and avarice. It came to planet Earth because it is the planet of the humans, the hunting animal that compares, has an individual mind, and operates with a five-sense limitation. (See Note 12.)

That is only one part of the story, however. The other part was that humans did not evolve entirely upon this planet. As already explained, the Traders have taken seeds at every stage of human development. One stage of the human development, the Cro-Magnon stage, was seeded upon nine different planets, which were all within one light year of each other, close by galactic standards. Although the atmospheres and solar intensity varied slightly, each group found their planet to be quite natural and they flourished. While each group was quite identical at the start, they evolved differently because of the environmental differences mentioned and because important evolutionary events occurred at different times on each planet. Skin changes, explained in the next chapter, enhanced survivability upon planets with different solar intensities and temperatures. The gene changes were the work of the Traders.

Details are beyond the scope of this book, but various degrees of the aforementioned forms of incompetence and avarice were born on all of the nine planets, especially in the early stages. In time, however, those difficulties were overcome and on all of the planets the roving tribes of conquerors evolved into civil societies. Small states merged to become countries and eventually each of the planets was ruled by a one-world government. Since the needs of all the individuals were met, there was relative peace and harmony on all nine planets. In time, the societies of these planets discovered the laws of nature, and each used technology as a way to reduce the burden of work. Each discovered better power sources and machines to increase their explorations and enhance their creativity. (See Note 13.) This was the golden era for this cluster of societies.

Upon one of the planets the scientist perfected vehicles to explore their own moon, the planets of their solar system, and eventually the planets of nearby stars. It was while they were exploring the next solar system they discovered one of the planets flourishing with a great human civilization. News of the encounter electrified both societies. The planet-bound society was in awe of the space travelers, but the space voyagers were somewhat startled by what they saw. This society had progressed along different lines, valued certain habits, used a different technology, and were interested in entirely different things. The voyagers left the planet wondering if other nearby stars harbored planets with similar civilizations. Their search revealed that in all there were nine such societies living in nine different solar systems, and since the cluster diameter was only one light year across, in time everyone would be able to visit everyone else. They observed that the languages were different, the use of technology was different, the habits were different, and most interesting of all, the general appearance of the humans was different.

Epoch of Tears

Once each civilization became aware that it was not isolated, but really part of a cluster of societies, great debates raged on all of the planets. Unfortunately, the primitive hunter instinct reared its ugly head on one planet. Comparing dissimilarities became the central focus there. This was because they had an extremely different sociological structure which caused them to overestimate the unlikenesses. The abnormalities between the societies were greatly exaggerated. The society that fell into the trap of thinking that their idea was the one correct view, began to hate the dissimilarities. This resulted in abandoning the policy of appreciating the differences — the appearance, feelings, interests, and different technologies — for a conquering policy. They did not take into consideration that their own habits, technology, and interests only worked because it was their idea and they, in that particular race, agreed with it. So instead of coexisting, visiting for the sake of conquering and making slaves soon ensued. This was the onset of an "epoch of tears." The conquerors won, aided by the use of powerful machines, and then used the outcome to convince themselves that they were not only better and more powerful, but also the only truly sentient beings.

Having the use of slaves on their own planet made life more pleasant and soon the strong ones thought of exploiting the remaining seven planets. The use of powerful machines did not go unnoticed on the remaining planets and they soon developed weapons of their own. As the conflict engulfed the remaining seven planets, great societies equipped with great machines fought other societies similarly equipped. Those that were superior in weaponry conquered the weak planets, and the conquered were enslaved. For a while, the conflict ceased, but the enslaved soon formulated a plan to learn the secret of technology. Over centuries, they learned how to make their own weapons and when they tried to throw off the oppressors, the race war began again.

Because humans do not have a group mind, they must proceed with their five senses and, as explained, can become their own worst enemy if the golden rule is broken. As far as the Traders were concerned, their belief system was that the war was simply the result of dissimilarities that no one could resolve. So the upset would remain, and the conflict was allowed to continue. While the Traders thought that since a solution might be found by the ones who were involved in the war, and since no extinction event was about to occur, they continued to watch. They observed continual upset and pain. (See Note 15.)

At the time of the great galactic war, humans on planet Earth had evolved only to the Neanderthal stage and, shielded by stellar distances, were not involved. In the other far distant corner of the galaxy, the unfortunate war continued and continued. Even warring Earth humans of today could not conceive of the scope of the original race war. The hundred years war between France and England was nothing by comparison. The war between the planets went on for so long that the original reasons for the war became lost. In those societies, generation after generation grew up only to be taught that there was a war with a powerful and evil race on a far-distant planet.

A society that has learned and mastered the ability to travel up to one light year also has the ability to move planets almost the size of the moon. They can move objects that size and move them in any direction they wished. They could, and they did. So many societies lived in constant fear, knowing that occasionally out of the sky, in the dark of night, great heaps of rock would fall, destroying all of their civilization. Those captured would wake up to find that they were slaves in a strange land, never again to see their home, their friends, or their families.

With that horrible life existing for thousands of years, what started it hardly made a difference. If the intrinsic structure of life is that some far-distant race is an enemy that wants to destroy you entirely, you completely forget why. The truth is, the War of the Worlds raged for **50,000 years!** (See Note 14 and 16.)

To the Traders, watching from a distance, it eventually became apparent that the differences between the societies would not change. The humans would constantly war. (See Note 17.) This was not a war fought over resources, but was a war based on fear and projection. An attempt to simply conquer the dissimilarities by annihilating the other completely was a wasted exercise. It was, in essence, an effort to prove that one's own race had value. At that point, the Traders intervened. They thwarted the warring attacks by using superior technology they had held at bay for the millennia of the war. The aggressors quickly realized that the Traders not only existed, but were in control of the situation completely. Peace was established when all the races were forced to return to their home planets. In one case, however, the original planet was so damaged it was irreparable. Those inhabitants were taken to another solar system.

After that came a period of education when the Traders gave humans an overview of creation and their place within it. The races were different, but possessed the same ability to experience life and create. So the races were equal and should live according to the golden rule. Striving for perfection has become the continuing goal for each of the original races who still live and now thrive on their distant orbs.

At the end of the troubled times, inhabitants of a planet called Lyra of the star Sirius-B, asked for refuge and volunteered to be placed on a different planet, completely out of harm's way, in a galactically-isolated solar system. They had been one of the oppressed races observed by the Traders for millennium. Since they were of basic peaceful intent and were emerging Travelers anyway, the Traders obliged and a large seed group was brought to a safe, distant solar system. The planet had a climate somewhat like Brazil and the Traders helped them make the transition by giving them power, establishing a sustainable food source, and helping them establish social institutions. All was finally well for that peaceful race with blue-green skin and they lived in harmony upon their new planet.

As can be imagined, for these humans, who named the planet Earth, the word conveyed a great emotion. For them it was the answer to 50,000 years of survival against an enemy that was seeking to completely annihilate them. Earth was a word that meant safety, as well as peace, home, rest, anchoring, and a firm reference point. It conveyed the meaning of life itself. (See Note 18.) For millennia the race flourished, but unknown to them there lurked in the solar system a dark secret. Not hostile humans, but this time, nature itself, and one unfortunate day their respite would prove to be quite temporary. (See Note 20.)

NOTES

1. Reference 4 mentions the Brentwood Affair, the story of UFO activity around an US Air Force Base in England. More details about this interesting case will emerge in the future. An acquaintance, Larry Warren, who is co-authoring a book on the case, said he personally witnessed an encounter between government top brass and the aliens for 45 minutes. "The aliens floated and seemed to be in a bubble of some sort." The aliens, of course, were the Traders, and the bubbles were the energy-field protection devices that they used as a shield against any kind of intrusive attempt.

Cloaked in their technology, the Trader view of any military threat is much like a parent's view of an attack by a child. A six-year-old kicking at dad's legs is more of a humorous event than something to worry about. A great deal of money and effort could be saved by discontinuing the Star Wars program, which has the hidden agenda of protecting us from the perceived "intruding aliens." To obtain funding, the government told the people that the space system would protect us from the missiles of unfriendly nations, especially the Soviet Union, but even after the Berlin Wall came down, the funding of Star Wars continued.

2. The book *Roswell Incident* best summarizes what is known about the 1946 episode of crashed saucers. (See Reference 9.) The government actually retrieved one saucer with a damaged bottom and intact interior. At a later date another saucer with a burned-out interior and relatively undamaged exterior was retrieved. The primitive Earth law of salvage rights was applied, and the government decided to keep them. Between the two saucers, all of the parts were available for study, and an intensive program of reverse engineering has been carried out by the U.S. government. (See Reference 51.) Over the years, the government has contracted various companies to try and duplicate the parts and build workable vehicles. They have built 29 versions of the flying saucers in three different locations where they also have been test flown. Area 51, located 75-miles north of Las Vegas within a vast military test facility, is the most famous of the sites. The saucers do fly, although not to the performance envelopes hoped for; they are limited to low altitudes and cannot leave the Earth's atmosphere. The absence of certain metals that cannot be reproduced on Earth has hampered the progress of the research. (See Reference 26.)

3. Recognizing the truth of the God within me, and recognizing the truth of the God within all things, I open my eyes and see them gazing at me as they recognize the truth of the God within them and recognize the truth of the God within all creative species of the Is-Ness. (See Figure 11.3, the Zetas.)

4. The existence of the bodies of Extraterrestrial Biological Entities (EBE) has been a "military secret" kept by the government for many reasons. One might be that presenting news of the existence of powerful alien beings would be an overwhelming shock for society. Perhaps if a period of media conditioning prepared a new generation, the shock could be more easily absorbed.

Since the aliens have a view of creation in which all matter and living forms are manifestations of God, we are immersed within one version of heaven, and everything should be revered. The essence of each individual is that of a forever being and the soul simply reincarnates into different forms within the creation. This contrasts greatly with fundamental Christian thinking in which we are special creatures, favored by God, with dominion over all of the animals and plants of the world. Although original sin hampers our progress in life, through constant vigilance and effort a perfect life can be lived after which the reward for this long struggle is an everlasting heaven. It must be remembered that wars have been fought, not only over border disputes, but over issues such as religion, color of skin, and social behaviors. Could not a confrontation over contrasting religious beliefs polarize Western society into true believers and heretics? Some might decide that the heretics, the aliens and those of like-mind, should die for their heresy. It has happened before, and could happen again.

A contributing factor might be that a certain faction within the government might fear losing their power. This could happen if people followed the powerful ETs and some new dogma that might sweep humanity, hypnotizing humans to behave differently, perhaps refusing to pay taxes, or something that would lead to the break up of the strong central government. Nothing is certain about what the real impact would be and that means it is a sensitive issue for government leaders. As will be summarized in the last chapter, there is no basis for this fear.

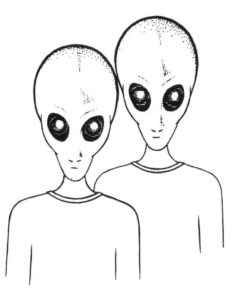

Figure 11.3 Artist vision of the Zetas — large eyed version.

5. The Earth is laced with many bases from which the Travelers conduct their scientific studies and observe Earth humans evolve. The Earth is laced with thousand-mile-long tunnels connecting the far-flung bases. The tunnel transportation vehicles are remarkably swift because there is no contact with rails; they hover like the magnetic propulsion machines our engineers are still perfecting.

6. The universe is full of "secret numbers." As stated before, the value π is one of them. That value is the circumference of a circle divided by the diameter and equals π (pi) 3.14159..., an endless number.

Another secret number is the value of Ø (phi.) In concept, the value of ø is the number by which the length of a string must be added to the length of the new string, so that compared to the original string, it equals the same ratio as the original string compared to the string length, of the original string plus the added new segment. (See Chapter 6 and 7.) That value of ø is unique and is 0.618033..., another endless number. The way to remember the value of ø is to imagine a square with each side equal to exactly one. Travel from any corner one half the length of one side, and turn and travel diagonally straight across to one of the opposite corners and add up the distance traveled. (0.5000 + 1.118033... = 1.618033...) This, of course, is the factor by which any string must be multiplied to yield the original string plus the value of phi. In other words, the value for phi is 0.618033... .

Another secret number is R, the Reality Number. It is an angle by which the least amount of energy is needed to accomplish the most amount of good when rotating from one dimension into the next. A UFO will use this technology to get from third-dimensional reality to the other dimensions. The value is 54.277 degrees and will be mentioned in more detail in Chapter 12 since that secret number is also encoded into the Great Pyramid.

7. Anyone who has read the Billy Meiers accounts, realizes that even the Pleiadians have technology to beam up an individual into the saucer or scout ship. (See Reference 25.) Meiers has surprised many of his friends by materializing before them. Good reading. Meier's literature is based on factual events.

8. The scout ships come in many sizes and types. The scout ships return to a cigar-shaped mother ship after each mission. The cigar-shaped mother ships are of two types. One type has tapered ends and are used when a mission might involve passing into the atmosphere of a planet. The untapered mother ships are for deep-space missions (in a vacuum) and normally do not enter the atmosphere of a planet. With this in mind, review the photographs taken by Adamski. (See Reference 22.) Also see the illustration in this chapter. The Zetas are depicted doing field work for the Traders, visiting humans at the prosimian stage. Other small mother ships or carriers exist in a variety of forms. The forms are deltas, boxes, or even boomerangs. The large carrier that flew over Phoenix, Arizona in March of 1997 was of the boomerang variety. The beings who controlled it were from a race that evolved from a form of bird. They are now very tall and have hollow bones and are extremely intelligent. They descended very rapidly, but flew 35 mph when close to the ground to prevent air-turbulence related damage to the cities. Then they would ascended only to repeat the performance on another city. They did this world wide and over a two week period. They will be back.

9. Many have seen the aftereffects of a visit. Not only are landing-pad prints found, but occasionally it is possible to sense a presence in the air that is not unlike the sense of standing next to the ocean when large waves are breaking. This is actually the exhaust that is left behind, but it is not like exhaust from an automobile. The ship floats near the surface on an ionic cloud. The ship is of the same polarity, and since like-charges

repel, a force exists to hold up the ships. This disturbance to the air leaves ions, it is simply the exhaust, and has nothing to do with marking the presence of Satanic demons, as suggested by some authors frightened by the unknown. Let knowledge fill the void.

10. The Earth-bound humans sometimes fail to understand why some events happen. It is natural for us to be confused, we are limited to five senses and we cannot easily look up into the group mind. For us, that normally occurs at death. Even by observing from this planet, it should be apparent to us that we are **not** actually some special favor to the Is-Ness, expecting It to exist as a good father. Nor should we expect It to exist to glorify us. These concepts come from the time when we were children and rightfully looked up to our parents for shelter and guidance. Now that we are adults, it is time to explore the universe, and the first step is to realize that the Is-Ness simply allows all things. It does so in order to discover what it truly is, and it exists because everything within the Is-Ness is creative. As free-will individuals, we create the Is-Ness with every action that we take. If anything happens within It, it happens because a member of the Is-Ness created it.

A poignant example of the principle is this: If you do not want murder in your society, do not be a murderer. It is as simple as that. Sooner or later, all of us will re-incarnate into the world that we have created, and there is no one to blame for that world except ourselves.

11. As complex as this account is, there exists yet another piece of the story. A Traveler group had a hand in the creation of the primates and that story will be told in Chapter 12.

12. Each human as a small child needs parents for direction and guidance, since education and guidance balances the comparison perception. The child learns to cooperate joyously with others and solve problems in groups. Once he is an adult, he should not need direction and guidance, but those adults who still require it look to others, even the government, for direction and guidance. Our government has even accepted taking on the responsibilities of the family and tries to teach and guide adults. This is the source of many Earth-bound problems, as "father governments" actually hinder our progress.

13. Evolving intelligent beings can discover the laws of nature and build machines to reach other solar objects close by. Using crude rocket power, humans have already reached the moon, and by the same techniques could even travel to some of the close planets. The next quantum jump in space travel is the understanding and use of element 115. Science will discover that when it is bombarded by an energetic proton, the resulting element 116, will quickly decay. That decaying process produces by-products, some of which are somewhat like tiny black holes. They are particles of antimatter that can be harnessed. Vast quantities of electricity can be harvested by properly, designed equipment and, combined with certain advancements in metallurgy, will allow humans to easily travel to about one light year from the solar system. No cooperation with the Traders is needed to achieve that since any evolving race is allowed to travel as much as one light year from its star of origin before the Traders step in. The rest of the universe will not be within the reach of humans until they have overcome their adversarial relationship with nature on Earth, and with themselves.

14. As human beings begin to explore the universe we must be very careful. There are 128 races in the universe that are empowered by souls such as ours, and some of these look almost like large insects. Others look like large fish with gills. Some of these species have four legs, and one has six legs and two heads. The latter is an animal that grazes like a cow and lives a peaceful existence on a planet with no predators.

Just by looks alone there is no clear distinction as to the true sentient nature of these species. We should also note that some of them do not build machines. It must be remembered that because a creature does not build machines to explore at a great distance, does not mean it is not sentient, aware of its position in nature through its senses, and cognizant of its creations. There are examples of this on our own planet: elephants, dolphins, whales, octopuses, and several others.

They are sentient, but they are different. Humans could not share feelings or thoughts with them. That does not mean these creatures are not sentient. The reference point for all of the animals of the universe is different. That is all, simply different.

The original flaw that has occurred in the early exploration of every race that can explore is: disregarding others and assuming that the explorer's view is the only view. The Earth human must not repeat the mistakes of the 50,000-year war. Humans cannot possibly know the existence of something else, but can recognize that there is that existence. At any time that the Earth human does not recognize that existence, hurt and upset will happen.

Consider that the original view the Traders had of humans could have been that because the Earth human did not have a group mind, they were alone and separate and thus very similar to rocks. Fortunately for us, they did not enslave a thing because it is possible to do so. Fortunately for us, by the time the Traders did come to observe us, they were already appreciating the differences. Fortunately they had already adopted the Universal Golden Rule: **Regard everything that is alive to be sentient.**

It is even more preferable for the vivisection-capable Earth human to begin to adopt the policy to regard everything he sees in the Creation as sentient in its own right, in its own reference, and everything means that: **Even the rock is sentient.** Even the rock knows and is aware of itself.

15. One of the great rules of the Is-Ness is that "No thing within the Is-Ness ever gives warning." This is true for all of the splits. Without that rule the Is-Ness could not discover all that it is. Consequently, the Traders rarely intercede and do so only when an extinction event is imminent. In this case, one of the races would have eventually become extinct because of the enslavement.

16. If this information brings an emotional response, it may be a soul remembrance on the part of the reader. It is possible to have been the oppressed or the oppressor, and perhaps both. Could this be the incarnation to make a difference? If so, following the principle means do not be the oppressor.

17. There is a microcosm of this right now on planet Earth. The racial differences look like this: Black people live that way, Mexicans do those things, White people behave that way, and so on. Societies and institutions exaggerate the differences, the oppressed adapt the slave mentality, and the differences become self-perpetuating.

18. Of course the word for Earth is different in each language. The word Earth, or the word Terra, are both interpretations of quality. If one were to translate it into some original language the closest that one could find would be "Itya," which is closer to ancient Sumerian than anything else. Up until ancient Sumerian, this planet was referred to in grunts and whistles, and without an absolute form of agreement. Thus, the word *Earth* is not ancient, it is a comparatively recent invention of the ancient word.

19. There exists another popular version of the Lucifer rebellion that takes the form of misuse of technology. Lucifer, one of God's favorite angels, had the idea to create externally instead of internally. Although this had been attempted unsuccessfully three times before, God allowed it. Essentially, everything technological is faulty. The UFO ships and the beings that have mastered them, especially the Grays (Traders and Zetas) are the example of the Lucifer rebellion in its final stages. This is because what powers the ships is an external merkaba, a sort of synthetic chakra system around the vehicle that rotates and allows movement as well as inter-dimensional travel. Using these devices (creations of the left side of the brain, the male aspect,) eventually leads to the loss of the right side of the brain, the female aspect. The result of this is the loss of love. Without love, one is stuck at the current level of development and cannot evolve to the higher realms. The Grays are stuck and are doing genetic experiments on the loving Earth humans to see if they can regain the lost love aspect. Their uninvited experiments are the evil abductions and associated sexual invasion. This is all nonsense and will be detailed as such in Chapter 14.

20. This simplified version gives the reader a basic understanding of what happened. The situation is far more complex since humans have been seeded upon hundreds of thousands of planets. For a more detailed view, order the tape "The Great Experiment." Call (760) 940-8910. (See reference 21.)

Chapter Twelve

Synopsis — Part One

Nemesis is a 100-mile diameter densified iron-nickel planet core. The sun's gravity captured this wandering orb billions of years ago. Its highly elliptical orbit occasional takes it on a destructive track through the inner planets. The tranquillity of Earth One was shattered 360,000 years ago when the planet was torn apart by a close pass of Nemesis. What remains of that planet is the asteroid belt. The Traders, who monitor all things and especially look for extinction events, saved a sampling of each species, including some of the blue-green race. They were beamed aboard the SMS where they waited for another suitable planet. This planet is Earth Two. The blue-green race was seeded here in two waves. From the point of view of the local inhabitants, the "Lemerians," the newcomers from out there were ETs. These ETs, or Atlantians, had been brought to Earth several times in earlier epochs. The Traders brought the Physical Angels here 225 million years ago as part of a dispersal program for that highly advanced sentient species. These Atlantians had evolved from a bird species, had hollow bones, but no longer flapped their wings because they had learned to float by mentally controlling the Primal Energies. They were one of the ETs that enjoyed DNA research and actually created new life forms. Much to the horror of the Traders, however, the Physical Angels would often create unsuccessful species who would live in agony, be unsuccessful at reproducing, and become extinct. The Traders never do that type of DNA experimentation, but only make small changes that give naturally-evolved species increased adaptability when placed into a new environment. When the Physical Angels discovered the five-fingered Prosimian they recognized a potential for a more creative species, one they might one day incarnate into. It was altered many times until it became what scientists of today have identified as *Australopithecus*, the precursor to man.

It had a fight-or-flight mechanism controlled by the left brain/right brain design with an amazing ability to dream about a future and then take steps to achieve it. *Australopithecus* was placed on many planets by the Traders. The blue-green race was placed on Earth in two waves. The first wave was 130,000 years ago in the Savannas in the middle of Africa. No technology was given to them. It was the intention of the Traders to have them evolve adaptive genes. It took 80,000 years for their descendants, at that point roving bands, to successfully evolve these survival genes. The Traders mixed those genes with the remaining stock aboard the SMS so that their children would easily survive when their turn came. During the 80 millennia of wave one, the Traders were also teaching the nine quarantined races of man. To prove to them that their differences were really superficial, the Traders convinced them to participate and watch an evolution experiment. The races agreed to contribute genetic material, which was mixed with Neanderthals living in Mongolia as well as the Serengeti. The purpose of the stealthy seeding (females impregnated in the middle of the night onboard alien craft) was to slowly improve the brain capacity from the 1,000 cc average of the time, to nearly 1,500 cc. Many forms of Pithecanthropus and Neanderthal man emerged from the seeding. The races on the other planets observed that no matter which seed was used, the offspring were equal in ability, only the appearance varied. In wave two, 10,000 men, women, and children, were set down 52,000 years ago. Their children, born aboard the SMS, already carried the survival genes from wave one. These are the legendary Atlantians who built the Great Pyramid. They were ruled by a triumvirate, Osiris, Thoth, and Isis. The Traders beamed microwave energy to the society which they used to cut stone with laser-like devices and float them with anti-gravity "walking sticks" into final position if they were core blocks. The outer casing blocks, on the other hand, were sprayed with glue and then slammed into final position using rail guides and electrostatics. Besides providing microwave power for the society, the Great Pyramid was a teaching and healing tool, and it was encoded with important knowledge that gave clues about the genius of the society that designed and built it. The power output was enough for the island community because their electrical devices operated at 100 percent efficiency. They controlled their population carefully and took care not to pollute the environment.

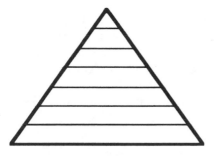

Chapter Twelve

EARTH TWO

The Great Pyramid Society Flourishes

Dark Wandering Orbs

The fiery deaths of meteors are always a delight. The brief trace left by these rare events stir wonder about the universe. More magnificent events are comets that spew enormous tails, visible for weeks as their frozen matter vaporizes during the close pass by the Sun. There is nothing in the design of the universe that limits the size or composition of this space debris. Large meteors do not always completely burn up in the atmosphere, they sometimes hit the Earth, where they are collected, studied, and even put on display in museums. Others exist, so large that a collision with the Earth would cause great destruction at the impact point and fill the atmosphere with dust that could last for months, even years. If the mass and velocity were large enough, a direct hit from a meteor or comet would be a catastrophe.

Unfortunately, all of these large meteors were not neatly swept away in the early formation of this solar system. Several large, well-known and huge meteors from the asteroid belt have elliptical orbits and actually cross the orbit of the Earth. One not so well-known comet is orbiting the Sun and is especially feared because of its highly elliptical orbit and giant size.

This monster comet is not measured in feet, but is measured in miles. Its diameter is 100 miles. On its rare penetrations into the planetary system, this demon body actually disturbs the orbits of the planets. The magnitude of its gravity is such that, even when passing at a great distance, it triggers earthquakes and other upheavals to the surface.

Besides that gravitational disruption, it delivers unexpected and hellish electromagnetic destruction. The reason for the massive effect from such a relatively small body is because it is nearly 100 percent solid iron and nickel in composition. This is not an ice comet that will vaporize as it passes the Sun, but a densely packed metal sphere — an old planetary core. Think of metal so densely packed it has the density of lead. Combine this density with its high velocity, and the deadly projectile has the kinetic energy of a planet 9,000 miles in diameter.

The reason this object is relevant to solving the complete mystery of the Great Pyramid is because the race that was relocated after the War of the Worlds found themselves on a planet between Mars and Jupiter in this solar system. This planet was chosen because all of the inner planets were too warm. (See Note 18.) The inhabitants of Earth One were not told of the existence of any menacing celestial object. Unfortunately the Earth One population, after thousands of years of pleasant life, discovered the dense orb and forever remember it as the "Destroyer."

This metallic comet was first discovered by their scientists, but the effects were eventually felt by all. The agony of the event can only be imagined, but from the contact notes of Eduard "Billy" Meier, the Pleiadian Semjase tells of the reality of the effect on the surface of a planet, even when such a killer comet is millions of miles away. (See Note 1.) Although this account by Semjase describes another planet in another solar system, the events would be similar:

"Now already recognizable as a dark sphere, the evil comet reflected the sunlight while it drew behind it a thin veil of luminous particles. Still some hundred thousands of units of distance from the nearest worlds, it evoked on them hellish storms which destroyed great areas cultivated there by peaceful human beings. In the night of the third day after penetration of the comet into the courses of the planets, the cosmic traveler invaded the elliptical orbit of the sixth planet. Evoking great cosmic storms, it displaced this planet some units out of its course and dangerously near the sun. Immense eruptions and storms rent the flourishing beauty of this planet. Mountains collapsed into themselves and oceans were thrown from their beds as that planet found a new course around the sun. Filled with horror and fright from the vast power of nature, the human beings fled to the large plains scattered over that planet, but the released natural forces overcame them. Two thirds of the inhabitants of that planet were lost in the tempests of nature. Wild water tore away great parts of the solid land, while exploding volcanoes buried huge plains under glowing lava and laid it in ashes and ruin. The rotation of the planet slowed and the day became twice as long and the planet changed direction in its orbit about its sun."

In this account the planet, as well as one third of the population, survives. But the reality of Earth One in this solar system was far worse. The destroyer passed so close that the energy transferred was equivalent to a direct collision. Those who did not die in the storms and quakes that preceded the impact obviously perished when the planet exploded. (See Note 2.) Some pieces decelerated and spiraled into the Sun and some pieces were accelerated into the far reaches of space. Most pieces managed to stay within the solar system, finding highly elliptical or nearly circular orbits depending on their speed and direction after the impact. They can be seen today with telescopes because thousands of these rocks and boulders endlessly drift around the Sun and are known on Earth, not as a splendid planet, but simply as the asteroid belt.

Before the planet was destroyed, some escaped to this planet by their own means.

They had the ability to travel within the solar system and they did. Under the conditions they found on this planet they survived for only one generation. Their inability to quickly adapt to the hotter environment led to reproductive problems. That was not the end of that race, however. The Traders did intercede and a small sampling, enough to insure that the species would survive, was saved. (See Note 3.) The survivors were placed within the enormous SMS in emergency facilities that awaited victims of disasters. To re-seed them, the Traders had to find a suitable planet, but in this solar system none existed. This planet, at the time of these events (360,000... years B.C.), was too hot.

After the close pass-by with the Destroyer, the output of the Sun was reduced and the atmosphere of this planet cooled. After 230,000 years, the atmosphere and the climate were suitable for the new arrivals. As stated in the last chapter, the Traders routinely passed into fourth-dimensional realities where the time frame is scanned. By this fascinating technology, they possess the ability to move between time and place. They emerge into three-dimensional realities in the past or the future, and into any location desired. Amazingly, it was by this "suspended animation" technique that the rescued survivors were brought to this planet. This planet is thus "Earth Two."

250-Million Years Ago

Before proceeding with details of the most recent seeding of this planet, consider seeding events of the remote past. Long before the Destroyer's close encounter with the fifth planet in the distant reaches of time, this planet had one ocean and one continent. This great island continent is referred to by the scientists as the great landmass of "Pangea."

In one form or another, the dinosaurs reigned supreme, prevailed in every evolutionary niche, and roamed almost every square mile of the planet. There was, at that same time, a small creature related to what we think of as a mammal. This small, five-fingered creature was much like the lemur or prosimian of today. They were social creatures and banded together for enjoyment as well as for survival. It can be considered that they had a civilization, although not by the skyscraper standards of today.

These small beings, known as the Lemurians, were satisfied to forage for food and did not alter nature much. They looked for natural places to live, caves within which they constructed their cozy dens. Despite their small size, they had cognizant intelligence. They were aware, sentient, societal, and conscious. In fact, despite their small size, they had social skills that their distant warring cousins, the "giant" human beings of today, might wish they had.

The Traders, even at that time, were bringing species from one place to another to preserve life forms. The Traders were also bringing Travelers from one place to another so that they could study and explore new environments. One group of Travelers was brought to Earth from a planet near the star Betelgeuse, but that planet was not actually their planet of origin. This highly evolved and intelligent group was expanding out into the universe, populating planet after planet.

They looked upon this planet with favor and decided to stay. These were the legendary "Atlantians" who made their original appearance while some of the dinosaurs were still here. Scientists would measure it as 250 million years ago, but in reality it was only 65 million years ago. (See Note 4 .)

The Atlantians had evolved enough to understand a great deal about nature and the atomic structure of all things. They knew about DNA, the double helix that contains the code for all life forms. In fact, for their species, the manipulation of DNA was child's play, no more significant than an Earth child learning how to walk and talk.

When they studied the DNA of Earth's lifeforms, they found a confirmation of what the Traders had already told them, that the Atlantian genetics and the genetics of the creatures upon this planet were very similar. This was because the creation of life forms in this region of the universe originally occurred upon a planet near Sirius. On that planet a cooperative effort at the Double Christus level did the original lifeform creation. (See Reference Figure 10.4 and related text.) It was the Traders who, in their never ending seeding efforts to preserve all life forms, brought those physical life forms to this planet.

The Physical Angels

The physical form of the Atlantians was very different in comparison to the Lemurians. The Atlantians were tall and had hollow bones, like those of birds. They had elongated heads and long wing bones, a carry-over of the bird-like species from which they had evolved. They had abilities that we today would dream of having. Although they had an individual mind, when in close proximity they could project and share completely and accurately each other's thoughts. The communication was always perfect and no mis-understandings ever occurred. They created quickly, they never fought over resources, and they were always cooperative. These Atlantians had the ability to float and needed no forms of transportation. Their long wing bones had evolved to become a means of steering their motion, while the lifting was done by thought alone. They might even be thought of as Physical Angels, although these physical "angels" were quite capable of making mistakes.

The Physical Angels and the Traders use their genetic engineering abilities in different ways. The Traders never attempt gene splicing except to preserve life forms. They help a genetic strain pass through the first stages of adapting to a new environment (horizontal evolution). The Traders will not alter a species by genetic manipulation for the purposes of having it survive in a place that is counter to its own survival to begin with. The Traders consider all life as equal, and with a right to its own opinion of life. All the Traders will do is insure the continuation of that opinion and genetic structure.

The Atlantians, or Physical Angels, consider their opinion of life the only one that counts and that everything would be better if everyone believed in the same way. When on this planet, the Atlantians even decided to create new lifeforms in a direct gene-splicing way (vertical evolution).

Because DNA is the double, helix spiral that transmits the knowledge of life during mitosis of the cell, it can be interpreted as the "tree of knowledge." The Traders forbade the Atlantians to tamper with DNA (eat the apple of the tree), but the temptation was too great, and the Atlantians began to experiment (ate the forbidden fruit).

The story of "Adam and Eve" is not entirely a fable, it is the sad story of the xenophobic Atlantians, trying to create another world based on their limited understanding that considered that nothing could be grand unless it was just like them.

Creations of the Atlantian gene-splicing experiments began to appear on the planet. It was an era of giant species reeking havoc on environmentally-balanced niches and the era of freaks. Trolls, dwarfs, and many forms that did not perform as expected, lived out their distorted existence in agony. Looking back, those new life forms could hardly be classified as successful.

Despite all of the misery, one form survived that we would consider a success, simply because in some regions of the planet we use it to cultivate the soil and we even eat it. That creature is the cow. The other creature that we might consider successful, although the jury is not in from a galactic or even planetary point of view, is the Homo sapiens sapiens of today; that is, the one we admire in the mirror!

Homo erectus equals Neanderthals and the like. Homo sapiens sapiens is the average earthhuman of today. Homo sapiens sapiens Plus are larger-brained human ETs that visit this primitive planet for scientific reasons like the ones that built the Great Pyramid.

The era of experimentation and consequent emergence of humans and other species did not all happen in a day. Long before anything like humans appeared on the scene, when the Lemur species was at its height (and incidentally, had already been injected with genetics of Atlantian design) there was a surprise move from the natural forces of the universe. A very large and fast-moving meteor hit the center of the ancient super-continent, Pangea. (See Note 5.)

The energy of the impact was sufficient to change the motion deep within the planet, in fact, part of the atmosphere was ejected into space, solid debris was thrown off, and some of it hit the Moon. This violent event started the movement that eventually tore Pangea into many fragments, and as it did so, great magma eruptions, volcanoes, and earthquakes roared across the land. Plate tectonics is a fact that scientists have recently documented by observing upwelling magma and stretch marks on the sea floors. Even today the movement continues, several inches per year.

The environment suffered swift, cataclysmic changes. The planet surface cooled as the Sun was blocked by vast quantities of ash and silt. Great volumes of sulfur were released into what remained of the gaseous part of the atmosphere. All of that contributed to a great decline in the animal population.

Warned by their own scientists, the entire Atlantian population escaped to other planets of the solar system before the great collision. They would have to wait eons to return to Earth to continue their experiments, if anything remained.

In all, the turbulent weather continued for 100,000 years. The atmosphere was so poisonous during this long period that all sensitive lifeforms perished. Of all the natural and unnatural species of the planet (since it might be said that the Atlantians "infected" the planet) only the hardy forms, a mere five percent of what once existed, survived. One survivor was the little Lemurs, a hardy species indeed.

What made the Lemurs so hardy was intercession on the part of the Traders who, during such catastrophic events, either move species to other favorable environments, or do genetic alterations to help species cope with extreme conditions. The Lemurians at that point were surviving well due to the efforts of not only the original genetic engineering of the Physical Angels, but also the more recent genetic engineering by the Traders.

The Atlantians were aware of, and were somewhat jealous (although that is not their exact concept of it) of the one-mindedness of the Traders. After all, because of that ability they had the navigational skill to travel between the galaxies, and experienced virtual immortality.

The intent of the Physical Angels was to develop a creature that had great creative abilities and the potential for one-mindedness so that they could travel the universe by incarnating into the new species. Each Lemurian had the herd instinct, the awareness of being a part of a larger thing, and the one-minded awareness that pulls the whole herd to run when one animal runs. That is why the Lemurs were selected by the Atlantians originally, but the Earth changes put a temporary hold on the project.

In time, the Physical Angels returned, and decided to carry on with the experiment. The Earth environment was a challenging place. A species not only had to be adaptable to the environment, but adapt the environment as well. The more a species could learn about how to alter the environment, the more successful and environmentally efficient it became. The Atlantians knew that a balanced omnivore had the potential to be the most creative of all species. A carnivore is too much of a predator. The dog, for example, is an omnivore that doesn't graze. A cat is an omnivore, but it can't get enough protein to maintain health by simply eating plant food. An animal that was totally carrion was not creative, nor was an animal that only grazed. These are examples of unbalanced omnivores. The only true, balanced omnivore on this planet is the human.

The Endocrine Changes

One part of being a balanced omnivore is to cool by perspiration through the skin, which implies a different skin than that of a dog, cat, or furry Lemur. Skin that sweats allows an animal to get rid of toxins and shed heat while enjoying a constant blood temperature as well. Time is lost by sitting around trying to cool off by panting. Having more time to explore and build not only enhances survival, but is part of the creative formula that the Physical Angels were seeking. When the Atlantians returned to continue their experiment, the Lemurians, thanks to the Traders, had lost their fur, had little body hair, and skin that could sweat.

The creature had great potential as it was, but the Atlantians realized that the one-mindedness of the herd animal limited their potential for more creativity. The endocrine system was reworked genetically to give each individual their own flight or fight survival mechanism. This enabled them to learn from past events, develop a greater sense of time, and become more self-aware. With a reduced herd instinct, individuals gained greater creativity and the individual joy that goes with it. Unfortunately, what comes with that territory is individual terror, the pain of defeat, and the imprisonment of the soul into what seems to be an exile or isolation.

For the Physical Angels, an important step in increasing the creativity of the Lemur — the precursor to humans — was changing his experience of time. The adrenal gland allows learning from events and this facilitates survival in extreme conditions, whether an attack by wild animals or extreme conditions imposed by nature. It is the endocrine system that allows humans to remember and have a sense of the past. Even emotional fear is part of the endocrine system. (See Note 19.)

As interesting as the newly-designed Lemurians seemed to be to the Atlantians, their existence triggered the old debate between the Traders and the Physical Angels over what Travelers are allowed to do. The Traders practice horizontal evolution, and vertical evolution disturbs them, although to them that is not the exact emotion.

Eventually the Traders disallowed traveling for the Atlantians, not as a punishment, but as a means of stopping the conscious upset. The Traders rounded up all of the Atlantians and brought them back to the planets they originally inhabited. That meant evolution in the Solar System would be natural, horizontal, and without outside intervention. This rounding up was against the will of the Atlantians and that episode could fill volumes. Tales have filtered down from what is known as the War of the Gods.

What followed were 120 million (actually 30 million) years of natural evolution, during which time many changes occurred on this planet and the planet of the Physical Angels. The Traders, noting a change in the Atlantian's thinking, agreed to allow them once again to travel from star to star. They were quite curious to know what happened to their experiment on Earth and returned as soon as possible.

The Final Touch

They discovered that a great potential existed that needed but one last major genetic change to fulfill their vision. The temptation was too great, and the Atlantians altered the genetics once more. The change led to certain synaptic nervous-system adaptations that evolved into what scientists of today have cataloged as *Australopithecus*. Creative souls such as our own found it to be a beneficial animal to bond with. This is the species that evolved chronologically to become *Homo erectus*, and later still to be Homo sapiens. The specific change of the Physical Angels, the Atlantians, is what we now consider the separation of the brain into left and right hemispheres. This allows dreaming about an outcome, and then the ability to actualize that vision by manipulating the environment. Another change modified the wing bone, which is somewhat bird-like, although very small in our form compared to the bird species or the Atlantians. In addition, there are strange genetic remnants, including *Lupus vulgaris*, characterized by soft brownish skin lesions, which sometimes manifests in the Earth human of today. Finally there is the curse. There are traces of the menace, xenophobia, and the warring problems heightened in our species by the inability to communicate completely. Our verbal and written efforts are only slightly effective when compared to the Atlantian's mind-linkage abilities — they don't fight among themselves.

Although these more recent changes allowed the new species to achieve higher creations, it stirred up the old debate between the Traders and the Atlantians. The creators, the Physical Angels, were once again put on the do-not-invite list, were taken back to their planet, and not allowed to travel to other stars. The Traders are under no obligation to take anyone anywhere, especially if it means an ideological upset on the SMS.

From this brief view of the evolutionary jumps, it can be understood that *Australopithecus* had the left-brain and the right-brain separation as we do today. He was capable of thinking of changing nature to suit himself and then taking action to make that change, much as we do today. *Australopithecus* evolved through many stages and eventually to *Homo erectus*.

At the time of the seeding 130,000 years ago, there were about 600 million *Homo erectus* types living throughout the planet. They were of rational mind, could make dwellings, design and build tools, and survived mostly by eating roots, fruits, nuts, and participating in the great hunt, which meant eating meat when the opportunity was present.

Events of 130,000 Years Ago

Eventually the climate of Earth cooled and the transfer of humans from the fifth planet was possible. On the great SMS the survivors were being divided into two groups. The Traders had been doing this work for a long time and cautiously held a large group in reserve. The advance wave was prepared and the decision to land them was made. They were placed on the land somewhere in the savannas in the middle of Africa.

The Traders provided a certain amount of aid for the transplanted society. A previous very subtle skin change for better solar absorption on the fifth planet, Earth One, altered their skin from the blue-green to a dark olive, but this worked against them on the much warmer Earth Two. The quickest remedy was a genetic manipulation, allowing more sweat release so that people could better adapt to the higher average temperature of the planet.

Another form of aid was the introduction of a few animal and plant species from Earth One so that people would have something familiar among the bewildering spectrum of new plant and animal lifeforms. It would take some time, one generation in fact, to adapt to the new plant and animal species as a food source that the body could assimilate.

The first generation was fed a protein wafer from the SMS called manna. This vital food source has been used more than once during the history of Earth to sustain populations in extreme conditions. The Israelites were given a similar substance and that account has been recorded in the Bible as "manna from heaven."

The manna was slowly withdrawn to encourage the next generation to learn to hunt and farm, but the transition did not go smoothly. The knowledge passed on from the previous generation was useful for a technological society, but quite useless in the new and unfamiliar wild world. All they could really rely on was their wit and an urge to survive. Tensions began to rise as the manna ration became more scarce.

Basic hunger needs soon destroyed all concepts of civilized conduct. People divided into small bands, each adopting a slightly different survival strategy. It was not very long before some bands got the idea to attack a well-off neighbor, and avarice and all of the vices were rediscovered. Learning to conquer to survive soon degenerated into killing for the sake of killing. The new settlers of Earth Two spiraled backwards into chaotic behavior. (See Note 6.)

The Traders, however, were monitoring the events from another level of perception. Since each planet is different and the preservation of the life form is dependent upon its adaptability to the new environment, it was ultimately the survival of the species that counted. The Traders were busy doing genetic manipulation to improve the percentage survival of newborns. In time, the reproductive cycles, the lungs, and the sweat glands improved. The genetic stock was finally demonstrating signs of complete adaptation to the new environment.

It took many millennia, in this case 80,000 years, but step one had finally been accomplished — the species had adapted to nature. Step two was to change nature to fit the species. For that, a complete technological society of sustainable design would be encouraged.

The Great Proof

Before the interesting details of a second wave of people merging with the first wave are divulged, it is paramount to note that two changes were going on concurrently: the saving of the species by placement in a safe zone on this planet and addressing the problem of xenophobia. As described in the 50,000 year War of the Worlds (Chapter 11), there were catastrophic results when the different races discovered one another in their planetary travels.

Because a human's first sense of things comes from its vision, it is susceptible to what it first sees. The physical differences between the people of the different planets was clearly observed, but the difference was interpreted in a way that considered one to be less and one as superior. This came from an underlying fear that said, "If I consider that you are sentient then I must understand that you are equal, and if you are equal then you have what I have."

That "equal place" became a point of argument. One who steps out of a flying disc to observe one who does not have the disc or all the attendant technology, can easily fall into an "I am superior" comparison that supposes that the other cannot be sentient.

The Traders at this time were monitoring a truce between the warring factions. They were trying to teach that the basis for the mutual fear was essentially unfounded, only skin deep and, given the recent demise of Earth One, here was an opportunity for a great experiment. An agreement was made among all the races that they would each contribute genetic material, and each have the opportunity to observe and monitor the experiment.

This experiment would actually be proof that the apparent differences were not quite true. It would show that if each race were stripped of its technology, which provided the illusion of great differences, the races of humans would be seen as simply the races of humans. It would be seen that the superiority complex was founded entirely on the belief of uncertainty. If the technically superior ones did not believe that they truly deserved what they had, or truly understood how they got the machines, they might be tempted to prove their superiority by using their power against a race that did not have the same technology.

The collected genes were used to enhance the two regions of Earth where humans could exist, in Mongolia and the Serengeti. These regions became scientific enclaves for seeding. Quietly, during periods of sleep, females of the *Homo Erectus* species were taken aboard and inseminated with the progressive genes from the far-distant planets. The fact that this could be done at all proved that the different races were really very similar. Even in their dissimilarities the races were similar. Over a long time period, many forms of the Pithecanthropus human and Neanderthal human emerged from the seeding.

The results always appeared to be from natural breeding and no one had the recognition that said, "I must have come from another place." This was because adults were never brought, only the seed. Those who were born knew no other home than this planet, and none had a belief system that thought they were going to be rescued.

At first there were large differences in the genetic structures. Since it was impossible to make the changes everywhere at once, there were places where highly dissimilar groups felt safer living in complete isolation. Eventually, the more advanced men began to mimic the seeding, although they had no idea that the seeding was going on. They often reacted to deformed or retarded newborns by putting them to death, effectively making sure the genes were not carried forward.

Overall, the seeding, the mingling, and humanity's reaction to them led to the success of the progressive genes. Differences between groups disappeared and the creative capacity of humanity increased. With the understanding that the Traders were supervising the seeding experiment with the cooperation of nine Traveler races, the story will now return to the arrival of wave two. (See Note 7.)

The Great Landing of 52,000 Years Ago

Intricate preparations were made on board the great SMS. Then one day in northern Egypt, the routine of the early morning was broken by a convoy of discs floating in the sky, bringing 10,000 Travelers with unusual attire and strange tools. Of this group, some were survivors from the destroyed planet, and some were children born on the mother ships. These children already carried the adaptive gene. This was the beginning of the great merging: wave two would meet the descendants of wave one.

The Society of 52,000 Years Ago

Any group of extraterrestrial origin is given the designation "Atlantian." These new Atlantians were humans this time and were about to create a new civilization, the Great Pyramid Society. They would create the societal structure that would adapt nature to fit humans. Many following generations would enjoy those institutions, and the knowledge of how to live together sustainably in peace and harmony on a new planet with a different environment would endure for thousands of years.

Part of the new strategy of survival was implementing high technology to produce boundless energy, grow food, make clothing, make comfortable shelter, and organize great institutions of knowledge and healing. Everything was planned for, including a penal system to protect society and its institutions from those would not obey the law. Under the new system, the marauding bands began to dissipate and were absorbed into civilized society. (See Note 8.) The time of this second wave was approximately 50,000 years B.C.

Government

The accomplishments of this small group of people cannot be overestimated. In more than one way they have influenced societies on this planet ever since. One artifact leftover and immediately recognizable to all of us is, perhaps, the greatest wonder of the world, the awe inspiring mountain of stone, the subject of this book, the Great Pyramid. More than one form of currency has the Great Pyramid reverently inscribed on it. Why is the Great Pyramid considered sacred? How did a relatively small group of men accomplish this monumental task? For what, and how, did they use it?

The society was initially ruled by a triumvirate, one woman and two men, the legendary Isis, Osiris, and Thoth. They were known through the ages as the powerful and enlightened ones, the ones who administered justice. (See Note 9.) In the millennia that have passed they have been metamorphosed into gods. This is because they not only had the knowledge of the Primal Energies and the enlightenment of the Universal Truths, but they also had the Great Pyramid. This combination appeared to give them unlimited power. They were the first with the physical power and knowledge of a technology so great that in most ways nature itself was virtually under their control. They had the last say in every detail of matters of state. They ruled over scholars, teachers, farmers, builders, police, judges, and virtually everyone in society. In reality, they were as powerful as gods and, happily for all who lived in that society, they ruled with fairness and compassion. The triumvirate helped to design and then rule over the beginning of a golden age that was to last for 3,000 years. Details of that era are absolutely fascinating.

The Construction of the Great Pyramid

Perhaps the most intriguing paragraph ever written about the Great Pyramid was written by Willaim Flinders Petrie, a researcher of the 19th century, who was truly amazed at the finish of the outer casing blocks. It must be remembered that although only two blocks remain today, at that time, there were many blocks still in place. During Petrie's lectures, he often quoted Charles Piazzi Smyth from his work *Our Inheritance in the Great Pyramid*, 1890 Edition, page 20:

"...the mean variation of the cutting of the stone from a straight line and from a true square is, but .01 inch in a length of 75 inches up the face, an amount of accuracy equal to most modern optician's straight edges of such a length. These joints, with an area of some 35 square feet each, were not only worked as finely as this, but were cemented throughout. Though the stones contact, and the mean opening of the joint was 1/50 of an inch, yet the builders managed to fill the joint with cement, despite the great area of it, and the weight of the stone to be moved; some 16 tons. To merely place such stones in exact contact at the sides would be careful work, but to do so with cement in the joints seems almost impossible."

In other words, for anyone who has practical building experience, it is a mystery as to how such large stones could have been carefully positioned, and then, before the glue set, pressed both vertically and horizontally by some unknown means to squeeze out excess cement before it began to cure, achieving these thin joints in every one of the outer casing blocks. A photograph in *National Geographic* magazine, November 1993 issue, clearly shows the struggle of Mexican workmen trying to reposition a toppled five ton block. The repair project of an ancient Mayan ruin shows modern humans with muscle power and some technology at great odds with a block that weights only one fifth that of a casing block.

Cleverly, the five-ton block is suspended at each end using two modern heavy duty chain hoists. These are suspended from a thick beam, which is held eighteen feet over the ground level, using large wooden posts for legs. This wooden framework is heavily lashed together with rope and the whole assembly has many guy wires running off in many directions to prevent it from falling over. Despite this successful attempt to render the block weightless, there were about a dozen people, all closely packed and surrounding the block, trying to swing the stone back on a wall only six feet above the ground. After the block was positioned on two wooden blocks, the rope was untied. The last step was to remove the wooden blocks. In order to accomplish this, metal levers or wedges were used to rock the block down to the final resting position.

The whole process appears to have taken several hours, if not a large part of the day. Because the length of time needed to position a block is longer than mortar-set time, no mortar could be put in those joints, especially the vertical joint, because there is no way to exert the needed pressure manually. Despite these obvious problems, many books have speculated that the Great Pyramid was built with even more primitive techniques. Yet when a Japanese team tried to build a tiny 35-foot pyramid using muscle power, they failed. They resorted to modern technology, including cranes and diamond cutting tools, but even with such aids the desired accuracy could not be achieved.

In the case of the Great Pyramid, exotic equipment was used. The extreme accuracy is found only on the casing blocks. The inner blocks revealed visible gaps. These inner blocks were, for the most part, laser cut and the tolerance needed was only one eighth of an inch. In truth, the inner blocks, except those that line the passageways and chambers, were positioned by hand with the help of a soon to be discussed anti-gravity device.

In contrast, the amazing outer blocks were formed in perfectly smooth molds by a slurry technique. Recent investigators now realize this agglomeration method afforded the economy, the proper piezoelectric formula, and the needed precision. (See Reference 7.) Thus a proper agglomeration, of a quality that exceeds construction-grade Portland-cement concrete of today, was mixed and then poured into inverted molds so that the widest dimension was up. The extremely accurate molds assured that the blocks would be accurate to better than 1/50-inch tolerance. Once the concrete formula dried, the molds were inverted to remove the blocks easily. Blocks within the Great Pyramid that formed the walls of the chambers and passages, or any part that needed great precision, were also agglomerated and sometimes made directly over others.

The placing of the inner and outer blocks followed this sequence of events. One level of core blocks was completed and finished at the outer edge with casing blocks before another layer of core blocks was finished. This sequence was followed because the core blocks were needed to position the casing blocks properly.

The casing blocks were accurately aligned using a special metal fixture called the casing-block-alignment assembly. This was a complex, movable framework that clamped to the completed core blocks on the inner side. On the outer side it had guide rails that directed the casing blocks to the exact position. Attached to the guide rails was a mechanism that held the heavy casing block above its final resting point. The alignment assembly held the smooth blocks with an electrostatic field. Dry casing blocks were highly piezoelectric and could be charged to the point that they could stick to the charged, flat plate element that was part of the alignment assembly.

Each casing block was coated with glue at the contact surfaces while suspended ten inches above and to the side of its final resting place. The buttering knife for the glue was an electrostatic-type spray gun, which applied a thin molecular layer of silica-based adhesive. With the adhesive in place the stone was ready to position. The movement to the final position was not simply vertical, but horizontal as well. The guide rails were designed to allow diagonal travel, down to the lower course of blocks as well as up against the preceding block of the same course

The weight of the stone did not do all the work. It was not simply dropped into position. The drop was not only vertical, but horizontal as well. The field was reversed and the block was shocked by electrostatics onto the vertical and horizontal surface of its final resting position. This technique made the exceedingly fine, water-tight joints that have been the marvel of investigators for thousands of years.

The reason for these water-tight joints was not to prevent rain water seepage into the interior workings of the Great Pyramid. The real reason was to prevent the water and gases that were inside from getting out. The outer casing blocks formed a water tight pressure vessel around the core and its machinery. The core was not meant to be water-tight at all. Examination of the core blocks today reveals the 1/8-inch gap that has always existed.

Picture a typical work gang of only three people, one boss and two workers, carrying and positioning huge 15 to 30 ton inner core blocks. The workmen were natives and wore the dress of the time. The human with the strange headdress and staff was, of course, the "alien" or Atlantian.

The reason for the hat was more than simple recognition. The humidity of the planet's atmosphere at the time was too extreme for direct inhalation, and it greatly disturbed the breathing and sinuses of the new arrivals. Their dwellings were sufficiently sealed and contained equipment that created an indoor atmosphere to their liking. Venturing outdoors for a long time, however, required they use a special apparatus that consisted of a light-weight harness with a small bottle carried on their back. From the bottle, a flexible hose, filter, and injector led to a face mask of clear material similar to acrylic plastic. This lens was fastened to a headdress that kept it properly positioned. The fabric of the headdress fell shoulder length, covering the equipment and protecting the shoulders and neck from the sun. The plastic visor, similar to a welder's mask, held scrubbed natural air already passed through the bottle where it was dried to a tolerable level for the aliens.

After a few generations, their physical form adapted enough that the apparatus was no longer necessary. During the building of the Great Pyramid, however, all of the landing party by necessity wore the headdress. Even as succeeding generations of the sky people were weaned from the breathing apparatus, the headdress — minus the mask and tank — remained a colorful symbol of the ruling class. In fact, even after the cataclysmic events of 45,000 thousand years of history in that region, the headdress continued to be used by the Pharaohs and noblemen of Egypt. In truth, this period around 4,000 B.C., considered "ancient" history in our learning institutions, is actually part of recent history when compared to the roots of the Great Pyramid civilization.

By comparison, the "native" laborers had no need for such breathing apparatus, having long ago abandoned such devices. Of course, by this time the native people had no awareness that they were the successful survivors of a grand experiment, the exalted descendants of wave one and the bearers of a great gift, the survival gene for those who were descending from the sky.

Consider the perception of those descendants, now hunter-gatherers, as they compared themselves to the people stepping from silvery discs wearing strange hats and using tools quite unlike any spear or ax. Imagine them viewing the flying discs, the laser cutting tools, pulverizing tools, drilling tools, and lifting staffs for the first time. Would it be impressive to watch dense stone being cut and carved as if it were soft clay? Could uneducated men possibly understand microwave energy transmitted from an invisible, far distant SMS to keep the magic machines working? Under the conditions it was quite natural for the ones from the sky to ask the local people to work with the promise of shelter, food, and entertainment. Who would not enjoy working for a god from the sky, even if that meant many hours of manual labor in the distant mines?

One piece of equipment especially became legendary. The "star" people, the Atlantians, were often seen with long staffs in one hand. These became known as the great walking sticks. The staffs were more than ornamental or symbolic of leadership. They were actually lifting devices the natives thought of as "miracle" power rods. Actually they contained internal circuitry that received energy from transmitting stations that even today would appear to be magical.

When the rod was activated, the operator could simply touch a large rock or cut stone to render it nearly weightless. At the end of the staff an electromagnetic field literally spread the gravity lines radially outward. Like energy itself, gravity waves cannot be destroyed, but they can be bent. The flux lines of the gravity field could then bend around and "find" the object from the side or, with sufficient power, from the top. The field's intensity was adjusted until the rock's weight could be handled and positioned by one or two men.

Using a power staff required a bit of talent. Applying too much power could result in a floating rock, and if the operator fell off the rock, it would fall too. This dangerous situation was avoided by applying just enough energy so that the rock weighed approximately 1/1000 of its original weight and two men could carry it. The staffs were calibrated to be exactly six Great Pyramid-feet in length, which was handy for the layout and positioning of core blocks. (See Note 10.) This explains why the typical work gang was a three-man team, one man with the headdress and the staff, and two men on each side marching a dressed block to position on the Great Pyramid.

In this manner, the lower two thirds of the Great Pyramid was built. Because of its height, the top third required the use of many flying discs. For several years it was common to see a disc with a block "attached" to the bottom, held by electrostatics, floating up and away to the construction zone near the top of the Pyramid. With these advanced techniques, the people of wave two easily built the Great Pyramid in less than seven years — not 20 or 30 years as some speculate.

The Great Pyramid had to be located on a stable geological formation to insure longevity. The site also had to be a major vortex for power production. The location was chosen with the help of the Traders, whose monitoring abilities were quite impressive. They can monitor the intentions of society, the individuals within the society, and even the health of the planet itself. Planets are entities to the Traders, a fact they learned the hard way. (See Chapter 10.) Monitoring a planet involves measuring the output, the number, and the position of each vortex. Like a doctor measuring the pulse and blood pressure of a human, vortex information gathering provides the data needed to determine the health of the planet and determined the ideal location for the Great Pyramid.

The designers and builders of the Great Pyramid did have flaws, and one great miscalculation is etched in the blocks that line the Ascending Passage where it joins the Descending Passage. Why this point in the passage appears to have been hewn out of blocks already in place is an interesting story. After seventeen block layers had been positioned, an energy reading was taken. This was possible because the sloping outer casing stones were already collecting subatomic energy. The power was not as strong as it should have been and the early test proved a design correction had to be made. One of the results was that the cross-sectional area needed to be enlarged. Thus, existing courses already in place were simply hewn to the needed larger cross-sectional dimension and from then on the construction proceeded without change.

The flaw of the unfinished chamber was not a flaw at all, as this chamber was intentionally unfinished. During construction it was only a functional sump, so the room was a place to get water and flush out equipment used in the agglomeration process. The room contains the rough and irregular dried slurry remains from the original construction, as well as from the "repair" attempt of other ages. The flooding Nile was used to provide water for the project, and a low depression near the site was dammed and then filled with water, thus providing enough water for the next year of construction.

The true base of the Great Pyramid has been the subject of debate by many investigators. Should the perimeter be measured from the top of the pavement, or the top of the bedrock as delineated by the bottom of the depressions found at each corner? These square depressions deliberately carved into the bedrock have been called "sockets" and there is one at each corner. The answer is the top of the pavement. The proof will eventually unfold when the underground source of the water is discovered.

Among its many functions, the Great Pyramid was also a teaching tool. The Great Pyramid represented the Is-Ness, a mythical inverted pyramid above it represented the Is-Not-Ness, and where they touched, apex to apex, was the eternal Now, the present event. The mythical inverted-pyramid, the mirror image, was moved under the Great Pyramid to join base to base. The macro circuit was contained within the mirror image of the Great Pyramid, and the apex within the Earth. The apex is defined by the entry point for the water. (This concept will be expanded in Chapter 13.)

The water entry point is at the exact inversion of the pyramid shape. Thus, that point to the true apex, divided by two will be the top of the pavement, and the much debated true base of the Pyramid. Some argue this is incorrect because the perimeter dimension, defined by the base at the top of the pavement, does not exactly equal two seconds of angular velocity at the equator. The measurement has an error of one half percent. The reason for the error, however, is due to cataclysmic Earth-shifting during the last 52,000-year history of the planet. Originally it was quite precise.

Most human beings of today would hardly place philosophical knowledge into the design of a power plant. What was the perception and purpose of the ancient designers and builders? The actual designer of the Great Pyramid was a human from Lyra, the home planet of the blue-green race of the star Sirius. The technology already enjoyed on that planet was sustainable pyramid power. Not only was the technology different in many ways from the electromechanical technology of today, but the designers also placed more than a single function into their structures. There were at least two, and if possible a full seven functions. The mind of not only the planners, but also the ones who built the Great Pyramid, held a moment of ecstasy for everything executed into three-dimensional reality. They held reverence for the Primal Energies that would lend themselves to the creation, the past that delivered them to their present moment, and the precious opportunity to create something in the now — a monument that would make enormous impact upon the future.

For them, that sweeping thought was awesome and thrilling. Every structure had to be more than functional, it had to be a creation of beauty, an object that reflected the truths of the universe and, therefore, a place of reverence. Each architectural achievement was a teaching tool, and a key to knowing the universe, and no functional thing was created with less than 100 percent efficiency. This careful attention to what and how they created automatically eliminated any pollution that might impact future generations.

It became a joy to incorporate into the Great Pyramid many useful bits of knowledge to be seen by users of the structure. It is therefore the combination of the biggest and best library in the world along with the biggest and best power station, worthy of study for those who would explore and ponder it in the future.

Although our society should take pride in its technology, especially in recent years, these designers and builders of the Great Pyramid were significantly more advanced. Place one of them next to the greatest builder alive today, ask them to build the same thing, and it would be quickly evident that our finest builders are primitive in comparison.

Seven examples of what the designers incorporated into the Great Pyramid:

1. To honor the seven Primal Energies that combine in proportions to form all things, there have been designed into the Great Pyramid seven sources of power production. Anything that can represent the seven Energies and still be functional was included. For example, the walls of the Grand Gallery have been designed with seven corbels. Each was functional and tuned to the appropriate PEP.

2. The understanding of three universal numbers is celebrated by encoding them into the geometry of the structure.

(1) The value Pi, π = 3.14159... (an endless number) is the ratio of the circumference of a circle to the radius x 2. The π value is encoded as the ratio of the base perimeter to the height x 2.

(2) The value Phi, ø = 0.618033989... is another endless number and unique ratio. If an existing line of length AB is added to its length by a segment, BC, there is one unique length of BC such that the ratio of BC/AB = AB/AC; that unique value is 0.61803... This value is encoded by the ratio of the pyramid height divided by the apothem. To precisely get that value using the existing slope angle of 51.853... degrees, a mark must be drawn near the top. This was done by designing the capstone so its base was that mark. Thus the distance along the apothem from the base of the Great Pyramid to the base of the capstone divided into the height of the Pyramid equals 0.618033989...

(3) The Reality Number, R, is the unique angle between two swirling energy vortex systems that yields the maximum transfer of energy. R = 54.277 degrees. This value is encoded into the structure in this way: since the Pyramid has the apothem angle of 51.853... degrees, and since the Ascending and Descending Passages needed a specified angle between them (many angles would work), the value exactly midway between the apothem angle and the R number was chosen. Step one is from 51.853... degrees to 53.065 degrees. Step two is from 53.065 degrees to 54.277 degrees. The two steps honor the three-dimensional reality existing in duality, and the three angles honor the ascension principle.

3. The primary Earth-resonate frequency in cycles per second, cps, is 8 cps, and for the Moon it is 4 cps. Different frequencies add, so the combined frequency is nearly 12 cps. The Great Pyramid was highly efficient because everything about it resonates at 12 cps. The size and thickness of the facets were chosen to resonate at 12 cps. Each casing block had an individual resonance at 12 cps. Each casing block had a volume that was divisible by 12 G.P. ft: 360 cubic feet = 12 x 30. Each foot was divided by twelve segments and this defined the unit of the inch. This inch represents, in the calendar encoded into the monument, one orbit (one year) of the Earth around the Sun.

In the ancient past, the Moon was slowed to a different orbit with the cooperation of the Traders to make nearly twelve orbits per year. (See Chapter 14 for details.) The output frequency was 10 to the 12th power, that is 10^{12}. Thus the value 12 appears over and over again in the analysis of the Great Pyramid's physical dimensions. (See Chapter 5 for other relationships to the value 12.)

4. The designers were taken on journeys into the future to glimpse important events, including transitions. To honor the future, and the transitions that are the creations of Consciousness at the fundamental splits, a calendar of events was encoded into the structure. One inch equals one orbit of the Earth about the Sun. The calendar starts at the beginning of the Descending Passage, and the path, rather than a linear measurement, is a spiral downward and then upward towards the King's Chamber. A point in the King's Chamber represents this particular transition, two precessions of the planet since the Great Pyramid was built. Other events are recorded as marks or as features along the spiral path.

5. The spiral path from the apex, downward along the surface of the Great Pyramid to the base, was always used as a symbolic teaching tool. One aspect of it depends on whether the spiral is viewed as being on the surface of a "π-pyramid", i.e. with an apothem angle of 51.853... degrees, or the equivalent in cone geometry, the π-cone, in which the major angle equals 45 degrees. Of the two, the smooth-sided cone is the closest representation of how Primal Energy dances between the Is-Ness and the Is-Not-Ness, many times each second. (See Chapter 8.) The spiral, represented by either the π-pyramid or the π-cone, points to the value π, 3.14159... in this way: the distance traveled downward divided into the distance traveled along the surface, no matter how tight or loose the spiral, is always a multiple of the value π. The spiral is endless, the numbers of the value π are endless, and our lifetimes and creations are endless.

Energy spirals within the Pyramid until its frequency is raised to 10^{12} cps, at which point it radiates outward. Note that units of time, the definition of the value of the second, are also defined by the base perimeter of the Great Pyramid. Humans near the Pyramid feel the energy because the double-spiral DNA that make up every cell resonate to that value of energy, just as the Primal Energies are also focused by the Great Pyramid. In contrast to the mathematical predictability of the value π and the illusion of what the spiral represents in terms of our endless creativity, our lives do not follow mathematical certainties at all, and that is the fact that makes our lives endlessly creative.

6. The reality of this planet is that it exists in duality. In honor of that duality — the up versus down, left versus right, day versus night, happiness versus sadness — the value *Two* was grandly incorporated into the structure. There are *Two* steps from the apothem angle to the Reality number. There are *Two* main chambers within the Great Pyramid. There are *Two* main passage ways within the Great Pyramid and *Two* access shafts (combination tuning cavities) to each of the *Two* main chambers. There is the base perimeter that defines *Two* seconds of angular rotation at the equator. Because of that definition, and because of the cycles that exist within the universe, it is true that *Two* diagonal lengths, in which one inch equals one year, multiplied by *Two*, equal the precession of the planet. One physical Great Pyramid representing the Is-Ness has its counterpart beneath it representing the Is-Not-Ness. Hence, there are actually *Two* pyramids. The physical Great Pyramid monument was built with a second monument next to it, the Sphinx, thus at this site there were *Two* monuments. The entry to the Sphinx was a portal of *Two* obelisks. Every value that is divisible by twelve is further divisible by *Two*. And there are many more of these symbolic representations, if one only looks.

7. The Great Pyramid Society itself realized that they would not endure forever and that they would be lost in the cataclysmic events to come. There was also the understanding that future intelligent descendants would evolve and in time try to decipher the Great Pyramid. So a clue was left, designed into the geometry of the structure. The clue had to last through all the Earth changes, and so the pyramid was built in the most geologically sound location on Earth. That location was to "shine the brightest" compared to all other possible choices.

The Great Pyramid, being Earth commensurate by design, naturally is symbolic of the planet. In that sense, the Sphinx, the small monument next to the Great Pyramid, is symbolic of the Moon, Earth's companion. The Great Pyramid is, by pyramid standards, the most sophisticated, largest, and "brightest" of them all. The Great Pyramid's symbolic counterpart among the stars is the brightest fixed star, the "leader of the host of heaven," or the "scorching one," a star in the constellation Canis Major. Its name is Sirius.

Sirius, now called Sirius A, was recently discovered to have a tiny companion star, called Sirius B. The small companion of the Great (and bright) Pyramid, the Sphinx, is highly symbolic. It also happens that the advanced Atlantians, who built the two monuments on this planet (a planet with a companion moon) originated from the companion of the brightest star. They came from Sirius B.

When did they build it? It could have been one, two, or three precessions ago. The pyramid could have been built with a perimeter that was one, two, or three seconds long. Two was chosen. They built it *two* precessions ago.

How could they know this information would be decoded on an exact precession? That, and what the proper motion of the stars has to do with this, will be clarified in Chapter 14.

The Farms

The climate in Egypt 52,000 years ago was much different than it is now and it affected the great river system that passes the length of that country. At that time it was not a desert, but a lush and verdant land, filled with thick forests, rich with life. Green valleys glowed in the Sun as the sparkling water of the Nile made its way and eventually emptied into the sea. Then as today, the Nile flooded annually, although the flooding was so great then that whole regions became lakes.

It might seem as though such a flood would be beyond humanity's abilities to control, but walls and levies were built and cultivation was achieved. The levies used to hold back the water were earthen, just as would be constructed today. In addition, however, technology controlled flooding quickly converted certain areas into reservoirs. This was accomplished by simply placing energy pylons at either side of the river so the water would have to reach a certain height before it could cascade over. Cascades of this electromagnetic opposition wall design were placed at strategic locations, and could control surges during the rainy season. Other flooded areas were instantly harnessed into reservoirs by the same instant gate technique so that the water could be used in the dry season.

The gates had a device resembling an obelisk and the Great Pyramid beamed energy to the capstone of the obelisk, converting it to magnetic energy that radiated outward. In the case of a reservoir, water molecules that would migrate close enough to touch the force field would be repelled back into the mass of water and the water would be constantly shimmering. Fish close to the edge, however, could be seen. Everything in the water, including floating debris and even logs, would be repelled by the magnetic opposition walls. The magnetic cascades used to control surges would appear to be typical waterfalls. The gates and cascades, however, were not very high, insuring safety in case the Great Pyramid power was suddenly unavailable.

Imagine the sight of a farm operation near a reservoir with an electromagnetic gate. A disc lifting off with a container, seemingly glued to its bottom, filled with freshly-harvested vegetables and fruits, would disappear over the horizon on its way to Cairo. The growing vegetables, the blooming orchards, and the grazing animals would seem similar to today's, except one might see a raft near the shimmering water gate with several men on it, Neanderthal hunter-gatherers, with spears poised and ready, their attention fixed on catching the fish below them.

The sight was as common as the barbed-wire fence cutting across grazing lands in the farming regions of our society today, and those of that era took it as just another normal day. In all, fifteen percent of the population was involved in the highly-mechanized farming occupation; some were farmers because they wished to be, while others were farmers because that was their method of trade.

The transportation system was the property of the society, and everyone could travel at will. Because of the ever-present disc technology and landing courtyards to accommodate them, there were no wheeled vehicles, neither trucks, tractors, nor cars. There are no artifacts or evidence of these machines to be found because the discs themselves were no more advanced in metallurgy than the automobiles of today. After 50-millennia, they have oxidized, and remain in the soil as thin veins of oxides. Only the device that converted the power for the machines remains, and that of course is the long-lasting limestone crystal, the Great Pyramid itself.

Despite the fact that all transportation was accomplished by hovercraft, there were a few roads. These were used by the Neanderthals, the Lemurians. To these original earthmen, what they observed was pure magic. They quickly learned to overcome their shyness and trade with the city people. The Atlantians lived essentially within enclaves of the much-larger Lemurian population, and there was a certain amount of social exchange between the two extreme cultures.

The Cities

Six out of seven people lived their lives in the cities, which were convenient and efficient. Although our cities would outdo them by their sheer size and quantity, the Great Pyramid Society cities out did ours in quality and in their sustainable sophistication.

Skyscrapers were neither needed nor desired. The beautiful buildings of the Great Pyramid Society were rarely 200 feet tall, and even these contained only seven stories, each with a very tall ceiling. From a distance, such a building would appear to be obelisk-like, a functional shape, since the roof was similar in geometry to the Great Pyramid and not only provided protection from the elements, but collected radiant energy from the Great Pyramid. This roof-antenna combination supplied not only the power, but also the communication for the building. The exteriors were often decorated with columns and other intellectually and visually pleasing designs.

Just as we do, they used what materials were available. They could mine and produce any element or any compound, but only chose substances that would last regardless of what happened to their society. Each part was reverently considered, carefully produced, and inherently strong and difficult to break. When metals, were used, they were uniquely formed and long lasting because the alloys used were almost impervious to corrosion.

Although they could manufacture any alloy, they favored elemental simplicity, and consequently no steel was used for reinforcing their building structures, even in concrete. They favored various long-lasting agglomerated-stone formulas, using perfectly-formed block glued upon perfectly-formed block. Given a little care, these structures were useful for thousands of years. This strategy assured that many generations would inherit systems ready for use. Breakage was rare, but when it was required, the repair work could be accomplished intuitively by anyone within the society.

The interiors of their homes were comfortable, lavish, and convenient to a degree that is only possible by a sophisticated technological society. They used indoor plumbing, sophisticated electronic communication, and mastered countless agglomerated formulas with which to recreate all the beautiful rocks and crystals that exist in nature. They molded any shape, and some elements of pure metals or alloys were used to decorate those forms. The interiors were decorated with splendid designs and objects that appealed to their sense of esthetics and need for convenience.

The design of their environmental control systems was infinitely more sophisticated than our society has yet achieved. Energy from the Great Pyramid was used to convert water into its elements, Hydrogen and Oxygen. Devices were positioned at different levels to control the building's lighting, heating, cooling, and moisture level. Energy was supplied by the burning of Hydrogen. Having a double function was always a design criterion of the devices, so a light bulb also burned Hydrogen in what looked like a porous pink rock producing not only light, but also heat. The heat energy from a light source was used in either the heating or cooling system.

In simplified terms, this is how it worked: If a building was too hot, Hydrogen would be burned near the apex of the roof where there was an escape hole for the hot vapor. The rising and escaping heat caused the interior pressure to drop. Vents at ground level opened to allow air to enter over screens dripping with water. Evaporating water lowered the air temperature and this cool atmosphere was directed into the habitable parts of the building. If the building needed heating, Hydrogen was burned near ground level, and the heat was directed into the habitable rooms. This climate control was done automatically using sensors and thermostats.

In essence their designs were more like living organisms. Using motors to turn axles and then compressors was too inefficient for them to consider. The electromechanical technology that today's Earth scientist naturally uses is a product of our society, not the Atlantian society. Atlantians never burned natural gas or any other hydrocarbon. They never used incandescent light bulbs or even "efficient" neon light bulbs. Long ago, they had gained respect for ecosystems, and learned never to tinker with systems that were less than 100 percent efficient.

With this technology, they lived in peace and harmony with nature. All their needs were met and, in fact, they did everything that we could think of doing. They mined the Earth and had factories. They learned and created. The activities in and around the Great Pyramid consisted of more than what was necessary to produce power. The Great Pyramid was used for many purposes, including scientific and medical research, medical and spiritual healing, supporting an intricate communication system, information storage, as a learning aid, and for initiation ceremonies.

Life Around the Great Pyramid

Workmen used handholds to climb and make internal adjustments to the pyramid by turning valves where the "air vent" portals exited at the outer casing blocks. Since the surface temperature during the day, especially on the south side, reached as high as 270 degrees Fahrenheit, these ascents were normally made at night. At the north face, specially trained and conditioned dwarfs entered the sloping shaft to the King's Chamber to access the inside of the Great Pyramid for maintenance. For other functions, especially when large parts needed moving, they entered through the Descending Passage and even the subterranean passages of the Sphinx, through the macro circuit, and then into the bottom of the Great Pyramid from the "Unfinished" Chamber.

During the day, and even while the Great Pyramid was producing power, they could remain within it and work. The interior of the Great Pyramid, except for the King's Chamber, was not boiling with heat or microwaves, so no one would be cooked while in the passages. This was because the frequency spectrum was dispersed and some of the frequencies tempered any possible damage. The frequencies only coalesced around the output frequency, which was in the terra hertz range, and that was primarily within the King's Chamber. That particular frequency does not hurt the human organism.

Lower frequencies, however, were dangerous to a great percentage of the workmen. Some suffered a radiation damage similar to X-ray or Gamma-ray overdose, that developed into cancer and shortened their lives. Part of this group, however, lived normally, scarcely feeling the effects. They were always aware that, at the very least, they would suffer reproductive damage to their RNA and voluntarily did not reproduce to avoid deformed descendants.

Despite the dangers, there were always enough volunteers for these assignments because the society held them in great respect. They had the personal awareness that they were no longer the same as others. They felt it, knew it, and even experienced out-of-body realities. Living partly in the physical realm and partly in the astral, they still managed to relate to others normally. They were the heroes who made the power possible.

The ultimate sacrifice for one's fellow human is to give up one's own life for society. A mythology was created around these brave men, they were the "eunuchs." This was the origin of the notion about making sacrifices to fulfill one's needs. By pharaonic times, the eunuchs had become defined as the special ones stood halfway between Ra (the Sun god) and humans. They lived partly in the world of the dead and partly in the world of the living, a teaching that was quite accurate.

The Grand Gallery held the Arc device, a sophisticated instrument that had a tuning function as well as a communication function. Through it, the operators could modulate the power beamed from the Great Pyramid. The Arc was the communication source, and by utilizing many frequencies the society could talk to anywhere on Earth. Another communication beam fanned out from the apex of the Great Pyramid and that energy source could reach the distant planets of this solar system.

Another function of the Arc in their society was to provide energy at frequencies useful in their healing technique. A few were trained in this technology and lived their lives as medical practitioners, dedicated to positive changes. It was a fine art, since continued close proximity to the Arc meant exposure to radiation that could cause RNA changes. Monitoring that exposure was also part of their job.

The education of the young always began with understanding the workings of the Great Pyramid and the Arc. These served as teaching aids and in many respects a direct connection to all aspects of their society in both the physical and spiritual realms. Included in the teachings was the idea that happiness in the physical realm resulted when members of society combined their energies, which encouraged participation and joyous involvement in community projects. The Great Pyramid was used as an example of this principle. Because the great power output of the pyramid came not from one source, but from seven sources, it taught that when you join, you are more. It was a celebration of diversity.

Many who chose to be scientists were first educated in advanced learning institutions near the Great Pyramid, and then boarded their hovering discs to fan out across the beautiful water planet in scientific pursuits. With a new and unique ecological balance, everything on the planet was of interest — the rocks and crystals of the mineral kingdom, the diversity of the plant kingdom, and of course, the animal kingdom from the smallest plankton to primates, four-legged beasts, and creatures that lived in the sea.

The *Homo erectus* of the day had spread around the world and were quite often witness to these scientific expeditions. They observed them with great mysticism, because their rational minds had difficulty interpreting what they saw. The flying discs, often with the green electrostatic glow of ionic repulsion on the surface, appeared as hovering platinum pedestals. Tight-fitting, solid stone doors flashed open revealing bright lights and silhouetted long-legged beings who were surely gods from the Sun. These strangely clad beings seemed to float to the ground with the only purpose of collecting things with strange devices. They had absolutely no concern about the presence of the hunting party, even when their numbers were great and they were armed with sharp spears and deadly blow darts. The hunting party stared, awestruck. Imagine the stories they told around the campfires of the glowing ones who could make food appear without the need to hunt or forage, and instantaneously appeared and disappeared without the need of time-consuming journeys over the land. Their rational minds led them to invent many forms of mystical beliefs about the "gods from the sky."

The Great Pyramid Output

The truth was that the Great Pyramid Society was an island community that contrasted greatly with the vast undeveloped regions. One pyramid supplied all the power needed because they were small in numbers and used devices that operated near 100 percent efficiency. The Great Pyramid Society region was especially beautiful because it existed without power lines, telephone poles, advertising billboards, traffic signals, slum areas, or barbed-wire fences.

Try to imagine the tranquil existence of a society that held no fears, and cooperated completely. There was no fear of dying or even of getting sick from their own pollution, because they had developed a sustainable society. Their abilities at mining and industry were directed towards achieving a society that would exist forever. The Atlantians could not conceive of existing as a throw-away society. It was a non-expanding society, and long-lasting. Using well-constructed products resulted in a minimum of drudgery and little maintenance, which dramatically contrasts with the present-day system of planned obsolescence.

The majority of employment consisted of services, education, communication, healing, entertainment, artistic expressions, and science. Imagine living in a society where everything was already created and belonged to the society. Imagine that each human existed as a result of careful planning and not unplanned pregnancies that destabilized society.

Concurrent with the design of a stable and sustainable society is the willingness to keep the population small. They knew from experience that using technology can be inherently dangerous. Each thing produced with technology with less than 100 percent efficiency creates pollution that threatens the very biodiversity that supports the society. The biosystem for this planet, for example, can support only two billion people, because it can only reabsorb the toxins created by that many people. The population is currently at six billion and is growing at the alarming rate of almost 100 million per year!

The individual's only concern, then, was for education and maximum creation. This they did. Throughout the three-thousand-year period that comprised this relatively small, island-like Great Pyramid Society, their population was maintained at only three-million people. This included many other island communities that eventually spread to all the continents.

The Great Pyramid was able to supply unlimited power for all of their creative endeavors, no one was in need, and everyone had their wants fulfilled. In contrast, the rest of the planet was populated by the *Homo erectus* hominid types, whose population swelled to 600 million. This number was periodically reduced, not by education, but by natural forces that often included disasters resulting from poor planning and their general inability to project adequately into the future.

The Traders Depart

The Atlantians had in time achieved stability, and the Traders were able to leave them on their own. They left the new outpost on Earth Two with a working pyramid that provided for all the Atlantian's wants and needs. They had discs for travel, large mechanized farms for food, and great cities of obelisk buildings decorated in a variety of themes, all warmed and cooled with power from the Great Pyramid. They left the Atlantians only after centers for law, communication, healing, education, and the arts had been established.

When the Traders left, a great ceremony was held in the vicinity of the Sphinx. Everyone was there. The Atlantians recounted their long journey, from the hellish torment of 50 millennia on the planet Lyra of the star Sirius B, to what the blue-green race thought was a respite on Earth One, where they sadly discovered that they had to move once again after the encounter with the Destroyer. Now after being rescued once again by the Traders, the Atlantians bid them farewell. The Traders lifted a safe distance into the sky and left them with a brilliant aerial display. The ships were ionized, causing them to appear as if they were on fire, and the spectacle was awesome. In this way they rode away, as only God could do, as only Ra could do. They rode away on their chariots of fire. They carried the Sun with them — thus another legend was born.

Even the *Homo erectus* population witnessed the departure. To them, however, the Atlantians were God. To the Atlantians, their purpose was to survive doing what they did naturally, using technology. Next on their agenda was to christen their sparkling new city, Cairo. Could anyone not understand why they named it Cairo, which literally meant, "end of journey"?

Chapter Twelve - Part Two

Synopsis

The Sphinx was built at the same time as the Great Pyramid. The Sphinx is part of the encoded genius of the Atlantians. It represented many things, including the celebration of existence. It subtly points to the genetic structuring aspects that resulted in mankind, and to the ones with that structuring ability. The serpentine form of a cobra on the headdress represents the twisted form of DNA, the basis for life. This headdress itself was worn by the Atlantians. The first generation had to wear a plastic mask and canister on their backs (never sculpted into the monument) to prevent them from drowning in the high humidity of the new planet. The headdress came to represent the Atlantian boss who got the local Lemurians to join in the fun of constructing the Great Pyramid, the Sphinx, and the city of the Atlantians. The Sphinx is made of a concrete-like agglomeration and was mixed and poured over a two-year period. Within it remain passages and three chambers. The three chambers represent the ascension principle. The passages also lead to the maze of tunnels under the Great Pyramid. Buried to the head for many millennia, the sand turned to sandstone, which was recarved by a later civilization to suit their remembrance of the monument. The head has been recarved nine times. The recumbent feline body was added about 15,000 years ago. To those who modified it, the monument represented man-animal/man-god. The original monument, however, had a slightly different form and different meaning. Part of this remains buried beneath the soft sandstone. It has human arms in a relaxed, folded position. The folded arms represented the infinity symbol and points to endless creation. During teaching ceremonies, the students walked to the Sphinx and passed between two obelisks. These represented the Is-Ness and the Is-Not-Ness. The Sphinx and the Great Pyramid were built on a stable geologic strata designed to last for many millennia. They were intended to be time capsules using a highly symbolic language that pointed to many mystical principals, including the Primal Energies, the combination of which created all things of the three-dimensional reality. After 3,000 years, a large meteor hit Earth Two. The global weather pattern changed, dust filled the sky, and the magnetic poles shifted so much that the Great Pyramid output was greatly weakened. The Nile River flooded unchecked and the society had to abandon the region. They survived in caves and mixed with the Lemurians. Their descendants and the continuing seeding produced a new breed of human, the current people of Earth. Many civilizations have come and gone in the last 49,000 years. About 12,000 years ago a technological society existed that learned to use the weak power output of the Great Pyramid to hydrolyze water into Hydrogen and Oxygen. This was their favorite fuel and it was used for lighting and heating. The tranquillity of that time, however, was disrupted when the Nemesis made another close pass.

This time, the planet wobbled, and water surged from the oceans over the land. This was the Great Flood. Although the scientists saw it coming, they couldn't decide what to do. One group decided to abandon technology and teach how to survive by living a simple agrarian lifestyle. Another faction sought to use technology to brace for the coming catastrophe. The argument over what to do led to a battle. The warring caught both sides off guard and most perished during the Great Flood. Those who survived settled in the land of Sumer. Eventually the flooded Nile valley was resettled, but it was a simple agrarian existence. Some remembered the power of the Great Pyramid and tried to restore it. They altered the internal design and built other pyramids around it. The largest pyramids at Giza and at Dashur are the result of those efforts of about 10,000 years ago. They didn't realize the Earth vortex had shifted, so their efforts were partial successes producing only a little local power. About 5,000 years ago a king named Zoser had united most of the people along the Nile River. Imhotep came from Sumer with some of the secret building techniques he learned in the libraries in Sumer. Imhotep and Zoser eventually formed a great partnership and the new building techniques transformed Egypt. The long-forgotten agglomerated stones were used to build huge mastaba burial monuments which evolved into small step pyramids. This revolutionized the economy of the country. The step pyramids actually increased the resonance of the Primal Energies near them and a healing center was built there. Zoser was soon healing the sick and began to be seen as more than a king. He became the pharaoh, a god-king. After Zoser, other kings attempted to keep the king/healer tradition going, because it had become the cohesive element that held the country together. Ever-larger step pyramids were attempted. Eventually they built smooth-sided pyramids similar to the Great Pyramid and the other smooth-sided pyramids in existence. Now, the pharaohs were as good as the ancient ones, the god-builders of the past. Then the pharaohs began to claim the smooth-sided pyramids built in ancient times as their own. Khufu built several small pyramids and a monument next to the Great Pyramid, claimed it as his own, and was even buried in it. After that, no large pyramids were constructed, but small pyramids were used as decorative elements in more economical-style burial compounds. By that time the religious practices had become very complex and required a large priesthood. There were many lesser gods and many priests were required to tend to the various ceremonies required to bring good weather for a good harvest, to prevent the Nile from over-flooding, and the like. When Akhenaten and Nefertiti were visiting from Lyra, a planet of Sirius B, their ship malfunctioned and they were stranded on Earth. Their intelligence soon gained them the throne, and they were proclaimed King and Queen of Egypt. They then tried to change the polytheism by reintroducing the knowledge and awareness of the Primal Energies. They were successful only during their reign. When they died the priesthood reverted to the old-style polytheism. Through all the changes of Egypt, two monuments stood in mute testimony to the ancient god-builders the original monuments, the Sphinx and the Great Pyramid.

Earth Two — Part Two

About the Sphinx

The Sphinx appears to us now as a recumbent feline body with a Pharaonic head adorned with a headdress and a serene gaze. What is seen today is a rework of the original. Construction started concurrent with the Great Pyramid, and the Sphinx was finished within two years, much earlier than the Great Pyramid itself. The Sphinx is the oldest monument on Earth built by the Atlantian human beings. Why and how was it built? What did it represent? What secrets, if any, are still held within the Sphinx?

The Sphinx represented living form, and was a celebration of existence. It rested on the planet to extol all aspects of three-dimensional, physical life-forms here, to the ones who need a planet to exist. It subtly points to the genetic structuring aspects that resulted in humanity, and to the ones with that structuring ability. The Traders, in contrast, do not need a planet to exist.

An important ornament at the very top of the headdress, the cobra and its serpentine form, symbolized the origin of life. Science has come to understand that there is the smallest of all serpentine forms residing at the molecular level and existing within each cell. That microscopic serpentine gives the knowledge for all forms of life. It is the DNA or double helix that divides during mitosis. DNA passes on the information necessary to create a new cell and, ultimately, the completed living form.

The serpentine shape has always reverently represented the understanding of the role of DNA in the life process. Of all the snakes, the cobra was chosen, because it fans out and appears larger than it is. This also represents the creative aspects of humans that are maximized when he becomes involved in the community. The creation that occurs when two or more join is much larger than any individual creation. Humans are an animal form powered and driven by a soul, so humans are part animal and part god. The Sphinx in its current form obviously represents the half-human, half-animal concept. The Sphinx also represents the spiritual half-god, half-human aspect as well.

How the Sphinx Was Built

Since the Sphinx represented important truths of the universe, it was conceived and built with great consideration and reverence. The Sphinx was not carved from living bedrock, it only appears so. It was actually made of the same material as the limestone casing blocks.

The pad for the Sphinx was leveled from the dense, stable bedrock. Once the base was prepared, a giant mold with a complex designed was built. After the pour there remained cavities the size of rooms within the finished monument complete with connecting passageways. The finest bonding elements were combined with the finest and purest ground limestone to form the long-lasting agglomeration that left the monument's surface extremely smooth. An around-the-clock effort of mixing, slowly pouring thin layers, and carefully removing the excess heat of curing, assured that one singular, solid block, without cracks or defects, would be formed. The Sphinx was completed in two years, but the result has lasted for over 50 millennia.

Geologic Mystery of the Sphinx

Today the strata lines of the body of the lion appear to match exactly the strata lines of the surrounding bedrock, so how could it be a poured structure? The answer lies in the fact that the original poured Sphinx is at the heart of what is now visible. There was a period of time when the region was abandoned, and during that time sediment built up. For many millennia, only the head projected from the surrounding land. That epoch was long enough for the sediment to congeal into a soft, sandstone-type rock, much softer than the interior blocks of the Great Pyramid and the true bedrock, but hard enough to carve. This fact alone gives a sense of the great age of the monument.

The fact is that, except for the head, the original monument is underneath the feline body of the Sphinx. If the Sphinx were studied in relationship to the surrounding Earth, it would be obvious that it is a recarved structure, since it's mostly in a pit and the strata layers of the monument and the surrounding pit line up. Workmen today are constantly working to remove the sand that naturally blows in.

When it was first recovered by digging into the soft sandstone about 12,000 years ago, it was decided to change its shape. The form of a lion was chosen and it represented the currently-held idea of god-human, human-animal.

Secrets of the Sphinx

There are three cavities or rooms within the Sphinx. One is in the middle of the body and the other two are carved partially into the bedrock. One of these is in the front of the Sphinx and the other is towards the rear. The triangular orientation points to a pyramid that represents the Primal Energies and all of the creations that derive from the combination of them.

In front of the Sphinx is an opening leading downward to the room at the bottom. From this room, passageways lead to the other chambers as well as to the Mega Circuit under the Great Pyramid. The alignment and shapes of the rooms are both symbolic and functional.

The arrangement of the rooms represents the ascension principle, in which the soul of humans can ascend to reincarnate into 128 different living forms. It can do so endlessly or, if desired, it can ascend to form a unity with another soul. When it does so, it reaches the Christus level, and the creations of these entities are different, not necessarily better, but equally endless. Eventually two entities at the Christus level can merge and form the Double Christus. Christ was from the Double Christus level and in some teachings this is known as the ascended master level. Those entities are again capable of different types of creations, not necessarily better, simply different. It is not appropriate to contemplate much about these levels other than to understand they exist, because it takes from us time well spent in joyous creation here. Those realms will be reached in time and without any effort by humans at this level.

From the vantage point of the Double Christus there are another three levels that can be grasped as future possibilities for future ascension. This is because built within the universe is the capacity for endless change, forever creation on 666 levels. When the "final" level is reached, there is the realization that the inside of the outside is really the outside of the inside, the top is really the bottom. This linkage is much like an endless belt, hence the infinity symbol. It represents the realization that energy and creation are always flowing and new creations are forever replacing old ones. The Was-Ness constantly makes way for the Is-Ness, lest one good creation should spoil all. The Sphinx was a monument in honor of that understanding.

The lower two rooms were ceremonial and educational centers, and the upper room was a communication center. The crystalline wall structure and the size of the upper room formed an emotional resonance such that a human being could confront his own issues. If he was of the proper resonance, he could ask the Traders for access to the intergalactic elevator, the SMS. This was best done in the evening hours when the Sun did not interfere with thought transmission, and if the human was of the proper frequency, the Trader ship would simply appear. More on this later but, for now, the point is that the Atlantians always had a link to the stars.

There was only one Sphinx, but in another sense there were many. The reason is that from the time of antiquity, the Sphinx has been reworked into nine different configurations. There were periods when the surrounding society collapsed and the area was abandoned, but the region would always be rediscovered and remembered. The leaders who put society back on track became the favored model for the Sphinx's head, either at their own hand or by popular demand. The result is that the original size of the head, which was comparatively quite large, diminished in size with each recarving. The head's style eventually resembled that of royalty. Observations from the ground looking up at the Sphinx with the Great Pyramid in the backdrop, instill the impression of a colossus, with the head in proportion to the body. This is a distortion of perspective, since the observer is near the head. From an airplane, the head appears to be disproportionately small when compared to the body.

The original design did not have the recumbent feline. The face was similar to the face of the Pharaoh Akhenaten, a being from Lyra, a representative of the olive-skinned race who journeyed through incredible episodes of space and time to arrive at yet another location, and grateful for the opportunity. (See the section, "The Fallen Angel, Akhenaten," at the end of this chapter.) The body was in the meditative lotus position with folded arms. Under the paws of the feline body will be found what remain of the crossed legs of the original design. Before it got covered with sand, the original suffered some destruction and pieces were carried away. The crossed arms with the hands under the armpits were selected for two reasons. It is common for humans to relax in this position and, with a stretch of the imagination, this becomes a slightly bent, symbolic form of the infinity symbol. The figure eight lying on its side represents endless creation. One end of the symbol represents the Is-Ness, what has been created; the crossing over point represents the present-now of creation; and the other end represents the Is-Not-Ness, what will be created.

In the original design, the head was visible through a portal suggested by *Two* obelisks positioned in front of the Sphinx. The obelisks were symbolic of the duality of the three-dimensional plane of demonstration. The *Two* represented up and down, Ying and Yang, sad verses happy, and the *Two* seconds of time of angular rotation measured at the equator and equaling precisely the perimeter of the Great Pyramid at the base. Other coding in the Great Pyramid is based on the *Two* relationship. One of these obelisks has been moved to England and the other to France, and although they still exist, they, like the Sphinx, were recarved with symbolic forms by contemporary leaders during the intervening millennia. They are no longer precisely what they were.

The site of the Sphinx and the Great Pyramid is one of the most geologically sound places in the region, if not the entire world. Chosen for that reason, the Sphinx and the

Great Pyramid, were designed to be time capsules using a highly symbolic language. The Great Pyramid Society was grateful for the special teachings and help given. This came from not only the Traders, but also by higher consciousness channeled from the level of the Primal Energies, and especially the great intermediary, the Primal Energy and Consciousness of Love, Yahweh. So in gratitude of many things, the Great Sphinx was designed and constructed. It is at once a memorial to the understanding of the Primal Energies with which the universe is constructed, it is a sacred commemoration to honor the Travelers and Traders, and also a monument to honor the connection to spiritual realms and the 666 levels of creation.

The End of the Golden Era

After 3,000 years of idyllic life, scientists realized that the regular passing of the Destroyer would bring it extremely close to the Earth. Although Earth was not impacted physically by the great demon, its great mass, speed, and close passing produced a movement within the molten, ferrous core of the planet. Like a swarm of killer bees, many small and large meteors travel with the mother demon, some ahead and some behind. One of these did impact Earth, so the combined effect enlarged the small wobble that already existed between the magnetic pole axis and the rotation axis.

The resulting wandering of the magnetic pole meant that all of the electromagnetic vortex centers shifted. Unfortunately for the Atlantians, the Great Pyramid, lost its primary source of power, the up-welling electromagnetic vortex. In addition, there were great earthquakes and many dormant volcanoes began to vent. Dust from the impact and fine particles from the volcanic activity combined to darken the sky on a global scale. The weather became violent and crops could not be grown. Once again the people of that society were forced to learn to adapt to a changed environment.

The Dark Age

Because there was little time to prepare, 98 percent perished at the onset. For the survivors, circumstances were drastically different. Their clothes and shoes wore out, and food soon became scarce, but they desperately tried to retain some semblance of the civilization they once knew. Unfortunately, their familiar world deteriorated to the point that their traditional life-strategy didn't work at all. Although most of the dust settled after a few years, the Earth had received such a shift that the climate was unstable for 400 years, and life became a daily struggle against great torrents of rain. The planet cooled and the rain turned to ice and snow. The winds and storms were constant, the wet alternating with periods of drought.

Under these extreme conditions survivors huddled in caves, wrapped in animal skins when cold, and shielded from the sun's intense rays when hot. There was the constant search for food. Any scrap of food, no matter how meager, was used. Only those capable of adapting to this rugged lifestyle survived, and it was the naturalists, the *Homo erectus* Lemurians, who were better able to adapt to this rugged lifestyle. Many of the Homo sapiens sapiens Plus species, the Atlantians, also found themselves sharing the same caves and food supplies.

Rarely did Atlantian males mix with the Lemurian females. The Lemurian males, however, quite often found an Atlantian female entering the safety of their cave and mixing occurred because the females didn't have a lot of choice. It was instinctual for the females to raise the descendants from these encounters and Earth humans now had a genetic code with a common female ancestor, that is, essentially Atlantian.

Also in the human genome, there are a lot of genetics that appear to be switched off. They are the instincts of the Lemurians, the genetic remembrances of how to pick berries, which berries to eat, and so on. They also included the ability to stand almost as soon as they came from the womb, and the knowledge of what was a predator and what was not.

With the Nile now flooding unchecked, the great cities, including Cairo, became unsafe to live in. The Atlantian culture was in utter ruin. After 400 years of extreme conditions, the metal structures rusted and lost their strength. Even stone buildings collapsed during the violent earthquakes and the rubble was then buried in the blowing dust. The great city of Cairo was abandoned and some of the outposts in remote regions suffered even greater destruction, either victims of up-welling magma or moving sheets of ice that mowed down entire communities. Today, even if one knew where to excavate, large cities would appear to be nothing more than ore deposits.

In time, the extremes of climate settled into a predictable and favorable pattern that eventually nurtured a new civilization. After a hundred years, mankind began to consolidate enough knowledge from legend and on-site inspection to partly understand the power of the Great Pyramid. Hope grew as a plan developed to re-establish the Great Pyramid as a viable power source for the people. Evidence of that effort remains carved within the pyramid and tells of the effort of those people.

Entry was made via the "air vent," in reality the main control shaft leading from the north facet to the King's Chamber. An inspection shaft was first carved at the top end of the Grand Gallery up high to provide access to the cavities above the King's Chamber. Another shaft was dug from the bottom of the Grand Gallery downward, eventually emerging after a twisting path into the Descending Passage. This passage has become known to researchers as the Grotto Passage.

It was concluded that the Great Pyramid had suffered a grounding disconnect during the period of earthquakes. An effort was made to "re-ground" the Great Pyramid with water. Another twelve inch diameter pipe was placed within the passage to the Queen's Chamber which led to the lower end of the Grand Gallery and then downward to the junction of the Ascending and Descending Passages. The pipe, along its way downward, fanned out into 21 smaller pipes to increase the back pressure and slow down the water. The idea was that with the heating action of the Great Pyramid on the water, thermo-siphoning would, once again, naturally raise the water up to the Queen's Chamber and then return to the depths via the pipe system. The cycle would continue endlessly, with the water becoming electrically charged along the rise by the action of the piezoelectric crystals on the surface of the passageways.

Electrical energy from the thermo-siphoning operated electrolyzers within the Queen's Chamber. Hydrogen and Oxygen were released upward to be recombined in the combustion process in the King's Chamber. (Details of the process have been discussed in Chapter 9.) The heat produced increased the efficiency of the battery in the King's Chamber, and the Great Pyramid thus produced weak amounts of power, enough for cooking, heating, and cooling for communities of the immediate vicinity. The new scientists failed to realize that it was the vital electromagnetic vortex, now in a new location, that produced the vast quantities of power that legend held. The new Great Pyramid Society limped on, but never again was there a society with hovercraft, nor a Nile River harnessed by great magnetic walls.

The Great Experiment

The Neanderthals, designated here as Lemurians, were of several varieties and had an average brain capacity of 1,000 cc. Hominids, with a brain capacity of 1000 cc, predominately operate by remembering instinctual behaviors that they are born with. For the most part, their lifestyle consisted of repeating patterns and habits that were more than adequate for survival. These natives generally existed on a vegetarian diet, although meat was eaten opportunistically. While these original earthlings were quick witted and had rational minds with the ability to think and change nature, learning new ways and discarding the old was not their favored survival strategy.

One might say they were mostly traditionalists who enjoyed living on their instincts. In regions where *Homo erectus*/Lemurians met Homo sapiens sapiens Plus of the first wave, the *Homo erectus* generally retreated into remote regions where their lifestyle would work. That movement continues even today. Of the many varieties of *Homo erectus* that existed 130,000 years ago, only one type survives today. Sightings of this survivor are even more rare than sightings of the great ape. He is called by many names, and one descriptive name is based on the large footprint he leaves behind. He is Big Foot to some, or Yeti, and even the Abdominal Snowman to others. (See Note 11.)

As stated earlier, besides helping the Great Pyramid Society get started, the Traders were simultaneously overseeing the great seeding operation. The descendants of the rival races on distant planets were contributing genetic material, so in various places around the globe there were populations of *Homo erectus* that were going through the process of "rapid evolution." The experiment went on literally for thousands of years with two results. First, the brain capacity expanded from 1,000 cc to 1,500 cc. Second, the egg and sperm began to closely match that of the Great Pyramid communities of the Atlantians. Any breeding at the time of the first arrival would have been a sterile mixture, but by 47,000 B.C., breeding between the two groups was possible. Thus the Lemurians gained more ability to project into the future, became more long-legged, and physically more attractive. Although the quote, "the gods saw the daughters of humans as fair," is not completely accurate, surely during the pressures of this Dark Age, more and more of the daughters born were becoming fair.

Many societies came and went during the long millennia of 47,000 B.C. to 8,000 B.C. The task for modern researchers is to understand that there were many "endings" to many post-Great Pyramid Society civilizations, and what happened could fill volumes. Underlying that period of history was that the persistent seeding accomplished not only by stealthy technology, but by voluntary involvement. The result is that any trace in the present population of the pure Atlantian (*Homo sapiens sapiens Plus*) or the pure Lemurian (*Homo erectus*) does not exist. Instead, the population with an average brain capacity of 1,500 cc exists, and the people of 10,000 years ago and the population of today are essentially the same. We are as different from the Atlantians as we are from the Lemurians. We are *Homo sapiens sapiens*, the Earth humans.

Now that the story of the Great Experiment has more fully unfolded, its purpose should be restated. The effort of the Great Experiment focused on finding a place of cooperation, to demonstrate that physical differences were not something to be judged harshly.

On a distant planet in the remote past a landing by a technologically advanced race, the visitors, resulted in an erroneous thought process. Because the planet-bound race looked different, the visitors believed erroneously that they not only were obviously technologically superior, but were superior in intelligence as well.

There still remains on planet Earth an echo of the same forms of recognizable differences, and in isolated places there still exists obvious racial tension and at times, warring. The tension is fostered by societal structures that exaggerate small differences, and economic and educational inequities serve to stratify the perception.

The Travelers have observed from their distant vantage point that different-looking people, with a given average brain capacity of 1,500 cc, have very similar abilities and only slight differences in capabilities. All have the ability to feel the same intensity of love or hate, pleasure or pain, feast or famine, and dream of surviving and creating in comfort. The aliens see that on a global scale there is relative cooperation among the races and that the small differences in capabilities are all but equal in regions where the races mingle voluntarily and have similar opportunities.

This planet is a microcosm of what happened to the Travelers on their distant planets. The conclusion was drawn thousands of years ago that the differences are skin deep and are of appearance only. The experiment is essentially over. The races of humans are simply the races of humans, and given equal opportunities, the "winner" of the "race" can never be predicted. Millions have been born, lived their lives, and have died in this grand experiment, but the effort has been worth it, because it has helped foster cooperative strategies and peace upon planets in far-distant reaches of the galaxy. Only one planet is left with vestiges of the warring state.

The Great Flood

In the last 100 million years the destructive Nemesis has plunged through the inner planets 200,000 times. Because of the vast distances between the planets, there has been only one catastrophic pass. That pass was relatively recent, and a once splendid planet, now the asteroid belt, is the evidence of that distant event. More numerous, however, are close passings that cause great shifting in the planets, and Earth has felt many of these. One such close pass caused an event that is recorded in ancient texts around the globe. In our culture it is known as the Great Flood. There was a gravity lock for a short period of time of enough intensity that anything not attached to the mantle kept moving of its own momentum. All great bodies of water surged over their banks, smashing everything they encountered. Even though the Earth quickly resumed its original rotational cycle, the displaced water was already on its way to delivering its kinetic energy and would do great global damage.

Since the Traders understood that the event would not cause mass extinction, simply a great upset, they took no part. Travelers from the races represented on the planet were allowed to bring information, and there was an upsurge of UFO sightings and eventually humanity once again became aware of the existence of the Travelers. The information was spread among the people, but there was hardly a consensus about what to do.

In our culture we have an understanding of what Noah did as protection from the Deluge. He built the "Ark," a large floating barge into which he and his family placed a sampling of the animal kingdom; mostly farm animals for his own use. Although that part of the legend is true, the other story that is not known is about the great debate of the time.

What was at first predicted by the Travelers was eventually observed by the Earth astronomers, and then society perceived it as certain cataclysmic death. During that phase of constant interaction, there emerged differences of thinking, and a polarity of opinion developed. The approaching object could not be stopped and the Traders refused a rescue, so humanity realized it must quickly do what would insure survival. That was the only point everyone could agree upon.

One side thought that increasing technology would insure survival. They thought that the shutdown would be very brief, perhaps three days at the most, and then things would get back to normal. The other side thought that technology would be wiped out and never return to normal, so humans had better learn how to survive without great amounts of technology. This polarity of opinion created a dilemma. The ones who wished to find ways to survive without technology needed control of the entire technology to teach the fearful society how to survive in the aftermath. The opposition needed the force and will of the society to build a sort of shield to protect the technology so it would function afterwards, and there was precious little time left for that.

The argument became so disturbing that the factions began to battle. One faction destroyed part of the energy-producing equipment. They thought that since the technology was partly gone, then society would surely have to resort to living without it, which would be for the betterment of all. However, the act of destruction motivated the opposition to seek out the saboteurs to stop and punish them. The attempt to squelch the destruction angered the opposition and their reaction was to commit more terror. Each side escalated, until continuous war broke out.

With their focus on battling, the Destroyer was no longer considered, but it continued to accelerate towards the Sun. Even before the flood waters flowed, the effects of the enormous electromagnetic wave that was coming could be felt. This was anticipated by a group that was trying to protect the Great Pyramid, so they shut it down by blocking the Ascending Passage. They were the ones who installed the granite plugs.

The plugs were not dressed stone dragged through passageways and then carefully slid into place, as many have speculated. Nor were these blocks quarried from the Grotto. The dense stones were formed by the agglomeration process and poured into place. There were several blocks poured as part of the plug assembly. A wood partition was placed across the bottom of the Ascending Passage and this formed the bottom of the first plug. After the agglomeration was poured into place, a wood cover was placed over the fresh concrete. Then a heavy block was lowered to force the air out of the mixture and to better seal it against the walls of the passage.

Once dried, the top block was removed, and the process was repeated two more times. Since the wood has decayed over the years, there is a gap between the stones. Also, since the blocks were formed of a different stone than the walls, there has been enough oxidization over the years to form a small gap between the two differing stones. The idea of some researchers, that "tight fitting stones were slid into place by the pharaoh's loyal priests to protect the king's mummy and burial treasure from the grave robbers," is not accurate. One of the stones used for the pressure at the top is the mysterious stone now located in the "resting room" of the Grotto Passage. Others were destroyed by Al Mamun's workmen as they chiseled their way upward around the dense granite plugs.

Eventually, the destructive flood did arrive and the surging water flowed for three days and three nights. It was this quickly-flowing water, and not glacial action, that caused the detectable water erosion of the sandstone body of the Sphinx.

The war left everyone unprepared for the onslaught of the water. The once-ordered society was decimated. Most of those not destroyed in the fighting were consumed by the ravaging waters. After the waters receded into the deep basins there were still hardy survivors on each side of the argument who blamed each other for their lack of preparedness. Fueled by anger, warring between them continued for another nine months. Eventually, the anger was spent and the battling ended as each side simply withdrew.

Who really won the war? Those who understood technology retreated with their knowledge of technology, but also with the realization that the destruction was so great that it would be impossible to restore its use on a grand scale. Obviously they were losers. On the other hand, those opposed to technology won the battle, but lost the war. Without the technology, their original goal of informing the people and preventing chaos was hardly achieved. They lost as well. Both sides lost, and thus ended another great civilization of planet Earth.

Because the soil remained contaminated for almost one year, and some effects lasted for five years, many abandoned the Nile River in favor of the land of Sumer. As survivors in isolated pockets began to rebuild, the debate about the Flood continued, and became the favorite campfire conversation. The physical battle was reduced to arguing, and the disturbance, the lack of agreement, and the belief in the necessity of having absolute agreement in which someone is right and someone is wrong, continued until shortly after the time of Christ.

The great debate surfaces even today. The original event that formed the polarized positions is hardly remembered, but it manifests as the high priests of technology, with all solutions based on science, battling the herbalists, with all solutions based on natural techniques. Each is the enemy, and each side is determined to be absolute right.

Besides the flooding waters, there were earthquakes, deep plate shifting, and some volcanic eruptions. Deep within the Earth the molten core shifted slightly with respect to the crust, causing the vortex points to wander even further. Any power that the Great Pyramid could generate on the already-shifted and weakened vortex began to wane more and more, about 4,000 years ago there was no significant radiation that could be used to electrolyze Hydrogen. Thus, no useful heating or cooking could be done even when in close proximity to the Great Pyramid. The energy that still emanated was from the focusing of PEP, basic combinations like neutrinos, and the variable gravitational energy, especially from the cyclical movement of the Moon and Sun. This energy is real and can be felt. The effect is a subatomic-resonance phenomena that continues even today, and for those in the proximity of the Great Pyramid, it yields the pleasant sensation of being home.

After the loss of energy and technology, humans adjusted to living with simple technology. The population at large forgot that the Great Pyramid was ever a source of power and did not rely on it at all. They "sinned" ecologically speaking and began using wood for fires and burned animal fat for lights, but in a small, elite class of intellectuals, there were the stories of the grandeur of the society that once flourished along the Nile. Some of the elite continued to make simple batteries from Carbon and Zinc to hydrolyze water into Hydrogen, to store it in animal bladders, and to use it for heating, cooking, and even ventilation-type cooling.

The possibility of doing this on a large scale required a working Great Pyramid, and since it was not realized that the true cause for the loss of power was the loss of the vortex, those interested in restoring the power concluded that the Great Pyramid had a faulty foundation. Their solution was to build a new pyramid and choose a new foundation without fractures. Another pyramid was actually constructed, and the result of that effort is the pyramid now known as Khephren's Pyramid, the second pyramid at Giza, adjacent to the Great Pyramid. Although large, it was simple in design and execution. It also increased local power, but again it was only useful for those in the immediate vicinity. (See Note 12.)

The power received was disappointing and no further attempts were made for many years. Eventually, it was thought that some inner complexity was the secret to the power. In time, resources were available to build a small pyramid to test the hypothesis, so another pyramid at the Giza site, the third pyramid, now known as Mycerin's Pyramid, was built. This one had a complex portcullis fashioned after the clues still remaining in the Great Pyramid. Even though many styles of doors were attempted, that pyramid yielded similar disappointment. There was no radiation at a distance.

It was concluded that the site was the problem, and although this was correct, they didn't really know where the proper site was. The hope for the return of pyramid power drove them to build another large pyramid, and at a new site many miles south of the Giza plateau. That pyramid, at Dahshur, is known as the North Pyramid, or the Red Pyramid. It had an incline of only 43° 36', a shallow angle compared to the 52° for the Great Pyramid. It was quite large, and the design and construction of its chambers and passages were complex. Sadly, it too did not radiate power at any great distance. Only those people living near the pyramid reaped any benefit.

Critics of this last effort reasoned that the shallow sloping sides did not allow the energy to resonate properly. Another pyramid was built nearby with a steep incline, 54° 31'. It is now known as the Bent Pyramid, because about half the distance to the apex, the angle changes abruptly to 43° 21'. (See Reference 3.) The originators of the steep-sided pyramid abandoned the project because it seemed to radiate very little even with the redesigned facets, so it was concluded that the energy did not exist at that location either. The story of who and why that abandoned Bent Pyramid was finished is told later in this chapter.

Leaders of that area had little to show for their labors, and to make matters worse, a new difficulty was soon to be upon them. By experimenting with different sizes and angles, the builders eventually struck a note of great discord. Everything vibrates at a natural frequency, and each pyramid being slightly different had a slightly different natural frequency. Although the pyramids were radiating feeble amounts of energy, it was strong enough to reach out and cause what would later be called the "wrath of the gods." Technically, all of the radiation of these Great Pyramids combined into what is known as beat frequencies, the sum and the difference of the frequencies.

Unfortunately, one of those was a frequency which equaled a mating call found in nature. A catastrophe resulted by introducing the frequency into the environment, because it reached out far enough to call the locusts. They responded to the calling lover in thick waves, but eventually, as hunger over-drove the mating instinct, they began to devour what remained of the verdant forests of the area. No one was aware of what caused the plague, which was actually designed and built by the hand of humans. It continued for so long that the region slowly turned into a desert. When there was no more to eat, the locusts died off. The scar of that event is the fact that the region has remained a desert ever since.

A lot of time passed and a new agrarian society emerged along the banks of the Nile. They had adapted to the changed weather pattern and had learned to cultivate and thrive in the desert. Always near the desert-enveloped pyramids was an elite group that had a remembrance of the society that had the legendary power. The hope to build yet another grand Great Pyramid Society remained a dream. As the centuries passed, the vortex wandered farther and farther from the Giza plateau, and what little power remained continued to weaken. Perhaps the great power available then was nothing more than a myth.

Their reality, between 3,000 and 6,000 B.C., was that only weak energy existed, enough to heighten their ceremonies. As far as relieving the agrarian drudgery, no solution was available. They simply learned to cope with the seasonal floods of the Nile, now much less intense, and would till the fertile soil aided by manual irrigation.

Then history took an interesting turn. The different groups that lived along the Nile were united under a charismatic King who's name was Zoser. There is much speculation about this period of history. What great thing did Zoser and his court accomplish?

The Egyptian Pharaoh Zoser

The change began with the arrival of one man to the fertile Nile Valley. That man came by ship, and he was the great historical figure, Imhotep. Some have speculated that Imhotep had come via space ship, because his life's achievements were so extraordinary, but he actually came in a ship with sails. The sailing vessel made its way from the land of Sumer, across the Mediterranean Sea, and then up the Nile River.

Many of the original inhabitants of the Great Pyramid region had fled to the fertile crescent region of Sumer after the devastating effects of the Flood. The scholars among them had recorded all they could of the technology of the day. The information was kept in libraries, one of them in Ashurbanipal, and it was in this library that Imhotep obtained the knowledge of his ancestors. (See Note 13.)

After years of study, he realized his knowledge would be incomplete without a first-hand inspection of the Great Pyramid itself, but in those days it was dangerous to make such a journey. In the face of possible harassment and even physical danger at the hands of the strange and primitive society that was rumored to exist in Egypt, Imhotep made his way there.

In Egypt at that time, the true history of Earth Two, the true understanding of the power of the Great Pyramid and the application of technology had become distorted by the disturbing events of the Great Flood, the great debate, the war, and finally the dispersal. By then, Isis, Thoth, and Osiris, the original leaders of the ancient Great Pyramid Society, had metamorphosed in the minds of the local Egyptians to the status of "gods." Even the concept of the soul and the next dimension became distorted into the belief that the physical body had to be preserved or the spiritual part of a humans could not enter the realm of the afterlife. Hence, shallow grave burials, in which the low moisture content of the desert preserved a buried body, had become the standard practice of the day.

One religious distortion was that the mysterious presence of huge pyramids in their land was the understandable remnant of Creation itself. The hieroglyphic record suggests that the Egyptians believed that Benben, the most sacred object in a temple, probably represented by a conical or pyramidal stone itself, symbolized the mound that emerged from the primeval waters in the beginning of Creation. Upon the Benben, the Sun-god revealed himself in the form of the Phoenix. The Sun-god, Re-Atum, generated himself out of the primeval waters, Nun. The Sun-god created Shu, the god of air and

Tefnut, the god of moisture. These three comprised a basic trinity. Shu and Tefnut pro-created Geb the Earth-god and Nut the Sky-goddess. Geb and Nut procreated other deities, Osiris, Isis, Thoth, Seth, and Nephthys. With this composite belief system sup-ported by the priests of the time, people could be harmoniously merged into one nation with a central authority.

One can easily see how this cosmology evolved even before the Egyptians of Pharaonic times built any pyramids of their own. It was simply an embellishment of their own basic ancient history. After 40,000 years of existence, the Great Pyramid, and then later the smaller pyramids, five in all, were imposing monuments visible on the horizon from miles away. They had become the Benben, so in effect, these primordial mounds had always been there. It only takes a simple shift to imagine that they created the ancient astronauts — Osiris, Isis, and Thoth — and not the other way around. The Sun-god was not a single entity, but could manifest himself in many different forms, or as lessor gods, hence all of the nomes of Egypt (like states in America) could have their own favorite god-form with a particular ability, thus uniting the diverse clans that existed along the Nile River.

Some intellectuals in the court of the rulers, however, always knew the pyramids were human-made. They thought a lot about the ancient ones who could build stonework to mountainous proportions, and wondered if they ever could. This was the setting in the early days of the reign of King Zoser and, at that moment in history, Imhotep made his entry.

When Imhotep arrived in Egypt, he discovered that another society was flourish-ing, but by his standards it was quite primitive and uncivilized. Although his intentions were scholarly, the Egyptians upon seeing this unusual looking foreigner, perceived him as being a possible threat, perhaps a spy, and so he was brought before Zoser. Imhotep told Zoser that he was from the land of Sumer, and that he was a descendent of the builders of the Great Pyramid. To a great extent, the technical knowledge of those ancient pyramid builders was understood by him and his quest was to examine and review the Great Pyramid firsthand. His passion was to see the great power crystal in all of its minute detail. It would be the culmination of his education.

Zoser listened to Imhotep's stories and to the knowledge that he taught and saw a great opportunity. Zoser asked Imhotep to do more than just teach the knowledge. Imhotep was invited to put the knowledge to use, to actually build a power-producing pyramid for Zoser and restore to Egypt the power and glory that was once hers. Imhotep actually was in no position to deny the request, for he was for all practical purposes under house arrest. He decided to cooperate and take the opportunity to show the Egyptians the marking glory of his civilization and his genetic understanding of his ancestors.

His first step was to complete his studies, which meant that he needed to explore the Great Pyramid in detail and observe its many subterranean passages. During that study he realized that the magnetic poles had to relocate before any hope of restoring the pyramid power, because the vortex and the Great Pyramid simply did not line up. After Imhotep gained all the information he desired, he filled most of the subterranean passages with sand as a protection against the unruly ones who would not cherish it. He then told the truth of what he had discovered, except for the weakened vortex.

A trust was formed between Zoser and the high priests. Imhotep fell in love with Egypt, and decided to stay forever. During that stay he changed the country by teaching them how to use new equipment and techniques. Under his guidance an Egyptian renaissance began.

First Imhotep reintroduced the lost skill of making agglomerated stone. Egyptians were taught how to pulverize quarry stones by making them hot with huge fires and then dowsing them with vinegar. The resulting aggregate was then easily moved to the building site where it was blended with water and a strong binder. Like cement, the slurry could then be poured into molds of any size or shape. The binders were many times the quality of the Portland cement used in standard construction projects of our society, and the new geopolymer stone increased by a hundred-fold the efficiency of making dressed blocks by hand.

Stone products by this technique were not only durable and hard, but could be made to look like any polished limestone, granite, diorite, or marble found in nature. The Egyptians became greatly skilled in using this revolutionary technology crafting vases, bowls, jewelry, tiny beads with holes the diameter of hair, and even megalithic blocks for their monuments.

Imhotep next functioned as the chief architect directing the building of the huge Step Pyramid. At over 200-feet in height, this Great Pyramid was over 100 times the volume of any mastaba of the time and it was built in just over nineteen years. Egyptians now had a new image of themselves. No longer in awe of the ancient Great Pyramid builders, they too could build mountains. Even though the project had revolutionized the society, had taken almost two decades of effort, and totaled millions of man-hours, there was one glaring detail that was hard to overlook, where was the radiant power?

For his failure to produce the expected power, Imhotep was not beheaded or even expelled from the royal court. How he pacified Zoser and the court when the obvious became apparent is one of the more interesting accounts in history.

Imhotep taught many things besides how to build monuments with agglomerated stone. He also expanded their knowledge and understanding of medicine, the ten dimensions, and even Primal Energy and Consciousness. He taught that all things — stone, plant life, all animal life, and even the very soul of Pharaoh Zoser— was a complicated construct of Primal Energy and Consciousness. Imhotep enhanced their awareness of the spiritual body that surrounds the physical body. He taught that when a physical illness manifests, there is a corresponding change in the spiritual body. Healing can occur with proper nutrition, rest, exercise, the use of herbs, and when facilitated, healing can occur by a direct change to the spiritual body in cooperation with the Primal Energies.

Healers can be the source of this extra Energy. When the healer prays over an ill individual and touches the forehead or certain parts of the body, a short circuit occurs that allows additional "healing" Energy to flow from the healer. The result of combining two spiritual bodies is an expansion, because by joining we are always more.

A properly-designed pyramid focuses and resonates to the Primal Energies and, in the case of the Step Pyramid, there was increased resonance to the lower frequencies, especially Will and Power, Allegiance, and most of all, to Allowance. In the vicinity of the pyramid the healer was able to gather more energy and healing was enhanced many times. The pyramids are natural healing temples, and those who experience the Energy of the pyramids, even today in their weakened state, describe it as a pleasant experience.

Zoser made full use of this feature. A great wall was built around his pyramid and within the huge courtyard, chapels were constructed. Great crowds were attracted to the healing services, and on that special day when the doors were opened, the line of people moved first through an impressive portal in the wall, then a colonnade and eventually, a series of chapels. The process allowed time for personal prayer, which served to increase one's frequency and receptivity. The ceremony culminated by walking up to Zoser posed in front of the Step Pyramid immersed in the giant swirling vortex, where he invoked Primal Energy and Consciousness and touched the person either on the head or shoulders, which completing the short circuit and transferred the Energy.

Thousands of people came to be healed, receive spiritual education, and be initiated. All felt the power and were awed by the ceremonies, which continued for many years, especially during the time of Zoser and Imhotep in the special courtyard at Saqqara. Zoser gained fame as the Healing Pharaoh, and Imhotep was remembered as a great medical practitioner.

Imhotep clarified what was known about the closest dimension to this physical realm, the Astral. In that and this plane of demonstration, atoms are made of the eight Primal Energies in combination, but the molecules vibrate at three times the frequency. Time does not exist as a linearly-shared feature in the Astral dimension, but instead each entity is creating time at his own rate and it is not necessarily a common experience.

Imhotep had a grand way of demonstrating the existence of the Astral plane. A mixture of the proper proportions of a chemical from the puffer fish with calcium carbonate and other chemicals ingested in the proper dosage will induce a form of paralysis that causes consciousness to temporarily leave the body. In just such a manner, Zoser experienced the Astral plane for a few minutes, after which his etheric body merged with the physical and consciousness returned to his body. The experience taught him that life does continue, and that knowledge was included during Zoser's Great Pyramid initiations.

Within the Great Pyramid was a chamber designed and constructed in such a way that it amplified the Primal Energies, and caused a resonance in a gland in the brain. A person in meditation might have great dreams, actually depart the physical and use the etheric body to communicate to entities of other realms and even other planets. Useful information could be exchanged, so the dream chamber was also a communication chamber, but the benefits of the room were reserved for a precious few, and they were usually those in the priesthood. (See Note 14.)

The construction project was a great boon to the economy. It helped to stabilize the society and centralized power. The very size of the project demonstrated the new strength of the political system that was able to pull together a large part of the society to work diligently on a new, promising technology. Zoser not only helped create a stable society that fed, clothed, and sheltered people, but with the building of the first skyscraper in centuries, a new camaraderie was stimulated. The king, the pharaoh, more than ever before took on the characteristics of a god. For his part in these great accomplishments, Imhotep became a deified official and was known as patron of the scribes, healer, sage, and magician. Egyptians were taught to worship him. Imhotep was honored in Egypt for almost 2,000 years, because to them he was as important an historical figure as Christ is to our own Christian society.

The "god" connection, or belief that the pharaoh was the representative of God upon the planet, became the power that bonded the Egyptian society. Zoser sincerely had lived his life with impeccable intentions, to serve the physical and spiritual needs of his people and return glory and power to the land of Egypt. Pharaoh Zoser had presented himself as God (capital G) to the people, and since God can do all things, God had to deliver. In this case god could not move the vortex 500 miles. The criticism mounted, and the populace was tired of being pacified with only the benefits of medicine and healing. They wanted the power first promised to reduce the drudgery of their daily work, and the credibility gap had to be addressed. In order to deal with this growing dilemma, Zoser resorted to much prayer and meditation in his communication chamber. He was told by helpful beings on the SMS that the inevitable solution was to leave the physical body — a pharaoh cannot be wrong, and a dead pharaoh hears no criticism.

What was to transpire would be unheard of for us, with our belief system, but for them with their limited understanding of the technology, it fit. The belief developed that if the body of the Pharaoh were buried inside the pyramid, the soul, composed of the Primal Energies, would be released to activate the pyramid. In one final, unselfish act, Zoser saw an opportunity to deliver to Egypt the promised power. The ironic twist was that it was Imhotep preparing the poison for Zoser, his long-time friend and ruler of the land, and not the other way around.

Imhotep's final teaching to Zoser and his court was the correct blend of herbs for an effortless, painless, transition for the Healing Pharaoh, and so, with the greatest ceremony and reverence, the dose was administered to Zoser. The King was reverently buried within his great Step Pyramid. What greater love has any human than to give his/her life for another, in this case for a whole country? What act could follow that?

Zoser took full responsibility for the failure. With no one to blame, Imhotep and the priesthood managed to quell the rage by explaining that Zoser had failed to use certain precious metals in key locations of the pyramid. It was too late to tear it apart and fix it, and besides, the healing center was operational and the country was better integrated than anyone could have ever imagined. The next pyramid would be a complete success.

Zoser's revolutionary rule and great accomplishments became the standard for the rulers that followed. Trained from birth by the royal priesthood, each succeeding ruler was indoctrinated with his preordained purpose in life, and was taught what Zoser had been taught by Imhotep. Each Pharaoh became enlightened through the use of herbs and prided himself greatly in his role. Each Pharaoh was determined to heal and serve the economic needs of the country, and each attempted to leave a Great Pyramid edifice, temples of healing and learning, as proof of the "god power" of the Pharaoh. So each Pharaoh took his role as the representative of god on Earth seriously, and most could not be accused as being slave driving megalomaniacs because, during that period of time, the building of pyramids was the entrenched formula of success for the Egyptian economy.

The Egyptian Pharaoh Snofru

The first few pyramids after Zoser's Step Pyramid were also step pyramids, with plans to build them to ever-increasing heights. Several large ones were started, but never finished. One of these was built by the King-Pharaoh Huni. This one, located at Maidum, was eventually finished as a seven-step pyramid.

The following ruler, Snofru, decided to reach greater heights by simply building another step onto it. After completing that project, the largest step pyramid in the world, the builders decided to transform it into a smooth-sided pyramid. Working the mines feverishly, Snofru's builders had enough material to mold thousands of beveled casing blocks. They were successfully hoisted into position by crude technology, resulting in the first smooth-sided pyramid in thousands of years.

Compared to Zoser's Step Pyramid, the Maidum pyramid yielded a manifold increase of power in the local region. It was taller than the ancient pyramid of Menkaure' at the Giza complex and, because it had recently-polished facets, reflected the sunlight more brightly than any other pyramid. It was a quantum leap for Egypt, another milestone of achievement and, for the moment, the Egyptians literally out-shined the ancient pyramid builders. (See Note 15.)

Even this great achievement, however, did not radiate power at any great distance. Snofru, still young enough, decided to try one more time. At Dahshur there already existed two pyramids, one complete and one unfinished. Snofru and his men examined them both and wondered about the apothem angles. The most northerly pyramid, the North or Red pyramid, had the unusually shallow angle of only 43° 36'. By comparison the unfinished pyramid to the south had the unusually steep angle of 54° 31'.

The hypothesis developed that the steep angle would better reflect the magnetic spectrum of energies and the shallow angle would better reflect the electric spectrum of the energies. The idea was extrapolated to predict that a pyramid with a combination of the two angles would behave as if it were much larger, and since large pyramids radiate large amounts of power, the new design would produce the large amounts of energy desired.

The geometry of a pyramid with two angles, one steep and one shallow, was not only conceived, but finished. A bent-looking structure was produced, hence the name the Bent Pyramid. The attempt, however, was a wasted effort. The concept was erroneous, and there was no more radiation at a distance than around the pyramid at Maidum. In fact, there was less. Although the power produced is small, even today these two pyramids at Dashur, the Bent and the Red, produce PEP-induced power. It is rare to be able to visit them because they have been protected by the government. It is wise to keep people away because there have been instances of people being harmed in ways not fully understood. Additionally, the off-limit policy protects the pyramids from unscrupulous archeologists and looters.

To the south and only a few feet from the Bent Pyramid was a relatively small subsidiary pyramid. Subsidiary pyramids, in general, were step pyramids or smooth-sided pyramids. The purpose of these small pyramids was to test the building skill of the new team of builders. In the case of the Bent Pyramid, the small subsidiary pyramid was not intended for the Queen as some speculate, but was simply a test to see if they could master the smooth-sided technique. This particular pyramid was built before the top of the Bent Pyramid was even started.

Snofru is credited with the creation of a new architectural style which was repeated at each succeeding complex. He finished all of his pyramids with the usual protective wall, but added a "causeway" to the Nile River where a "valley building" was built. The causeway led to the "mortuary" or "funerary temple" that touched the east side of the pyramid. Thus the developed pyramid complex, the causeway, and the valley building, all were designed with wall protection for complete privacy. The royal burial ceremony could proceed along the river to the valley building up the causeway and to the mortuary and be protected from view, and the walls provided further protection from thieves.

The Egyptian Pharaoh Khufu

Eventually the great builder Snofru died, and his son, Khufu, inherited the throne. Khufu continued the large pyramid complex tradition and claimed the Great Pyramid as the center piece for his effort. He had three smooth-sided, subsidiary pyramids built on the east side of the Great Pyramid to prove his abilities. Enclosed within the walls of this massive complex were not only the Great Pyramid and its three subsidiary pyramids, but also a mortuary building connected to the valley building via a long causeway. Each of these were carefully decorated with statues and hieroglyphs to honor the life and deeds of Pharaoh Khufu and his court. One making the ascent from the valley building along the causeway to the mortuary building would be visually bombarded with this sculpted message of the Egyptian royal court.

In stark contrast, the major element within the splendid complex, the Great Pyramid itself, remained absolutely untouched. There are no royal hieroglyphs of any sort in any of the rooms or passageways. The reason for that is their ancient treasure, the Great Pyramid, was in reality the accomplishment of the gods. In respect for the ancient builders, only their buildings, the subsidiary pyramids, the valley building, the causeway, the funerary building and the enclosure walls were adorned, because these truly belonged to them and celebrated their accomplishments, the works of men.

Eventually Khufu died a natural death, and his body was ceremoniously carried down the Nile in the largest boat of a long flotilla, with the valley building as the destination. There his body was brought ashore and after a short ceremony, serenely carried up the long causeway and placed into the mortuary building, where the priests mummified the body. Now ready for its last journey, the body was brought to the Descending Passage of the Pyramid and lowered all the way to the start of the Grotto Passage. The bearers continued up the Grotto Passage, past the Grotto Room, on up to the top of the Grotto Passage to emerge at the bottom of the Grand Gallery. From there it was an easy ascent to the King's Chamber where the mummy was lowered into the sarcophagus. The massive stone lid was positioned over the coffer and the ceremony concluded. The priests retreated, blocking the entry to the King's Chamber. For a time the room actually was a King's Chamber, and the king was King Khufu.

It might appear that for a pharaoh to actually use a revered national treasure, the ancient Great Pyramid, as a personal burial crypt would be the ultimate act of self-glorification. The economy of the country, however, depended on the building of these large complexes. From childhood, the pharaoh was taught that it was his duty to his country to build such a complex, and he was specially selected to have the honor to include the Great Pyramid. The belief that the spirit of the pharaoh could actually restore the power was still taught, and why it had not yet yielded results was considered the fault of the priesthood, whose job it was to perform the correct burial rites. So it was actually an unselfish act for the pharaoh to agree to a life in service to the people of Egypt and to be buried in the Great Pyramid. After all, any act that might reactivate the radiant power of the Great Pyramid was not too great a sacrifice to make. It would mean restoring Egypt's glory and power.

Yet far more than Khufu's mummy was interred into the Great Pyramid. In Khufu's case, the priesthood actually interred his essence. The story starts with the understanding of the lid of the sarcophagus. The lid was destined to be part of the effort to restore the power to Egypt and could not be an ordinary lid. Consequently, it was not chiseled from the living rock of a common quarry. Instead the finest craftsmen of the art of agglomeration were given the contract to build a lid according to the priest's specifications. The dimensions, including the type of stone, minerals, metal dust, and a specific rare and sturdy binder, were all detailed by them. By trial and error they eventually fashioned a lid that met the approval of the priests, who desired a particularly dense rock with the texture and beauty of marble.

They already knew the lid was too large to fit the narrow entry to the room, but they hadn't planned to carry it there anyway. They planned to use an alternate method that not only placed the lid where it belonged, but demonstrated the power of the priesthood. Their effort would clarify the teaching that the sum of group-thought was more powerful than the individual mind. This was to be demonstrated by building the lid by hand, dematerializing it where it lay at the factory site, and then rematerialize it near the sarcophagus, in the King's Chamber.

Can one human, by him or her self, manifest something solely by thought? The potential is there, but most men can accomplish tasks more quickly by building with their hands. The project can be accomplished by thought if a group with a unified mind and good planning does it. The formula for success that the priesthood used is this:

1. The object to be dematerialized must already exist in three-dimensional reality.

2. The physical aspects of it must be well-known: the basic shape, size, composition, where it exists, and so on, which help form the unified picture of it.

3. The location or position in which it will be materialized must be known in detail to form a clear picture of the materialized block.

4. To amplify the weakness of one mind, there must be a complete and clear resonance of eighteen to twenty unified human minds.

Primal Energy and Consciousness will simply cooperate with the single, strong purpose and intention of the group. Manifesting by thought is an ability that humans have, and the priesthood understood that truth. In a ritual that included chanting, to blend the minds into a unity, they imagined the lid glowing white hot, disappearing, and reappearing into position, first white hot, and then cooling into its shape.

The high priests performed another ritual that was to inter, almost forever, the essence of Khufu within the Great Pyramid. From childhood, Khufu was taught that he would one day be part of a great experiment, the purpose of which was to return the power and glory to Egypt. He came to accept the grandiose task, routinely meditated and prayed throughout his life, and upon his death bed, cooperated by focusing his consciousness upon the ritual chant of the eighteen priests surrounding him.

That effort looked essentially like this: The ships used to transport royalty upon the Nile had a spiritual counterpart thought of as solar boats, or sky chariots, that could transport royalty from the court of humans to the court of the Gods, the court of Ra, which was believed to exist within the Sun. (Reread The Traders Depart, Chapter 12 — part 1.) To accomplish this, the group mind of the priests imagined that the essence of Khufu was placed into such a ship. Sailing away, the rising solar boat was pictured turning into a chariot. The last view of the chariot and the strong charioteer had them merging into the

Sun, into the entity known as Ra. At that point Khufu would have become part of the court of Ra.

This strong picture of the ritual, reinforced by a life of meditation and selfless training, trapped Khufu upon the Astral plane. He expected that he, with every effort for the glory of Egypt, faithful from birth to death to the instructions of the priesthood, would merit entry into the court of Ra. He expected the brilliant light of the Sun itself, but instead, saw mostly darkness. The expected picture did not materialize. Occasionally, over his shoulder, his Oversoul glowed, but to Khufu, the faint light could not be the Sun God, Ra, so it was ignored. Through the ages the presence that many felt was Khufu, as his spirit hovered about the Great Pyramid. At last he has been set free. (See Note 16 for details of how Khufu has been freed.)

The Pharaohs Khephren and Menkaure´

The building of the colossal pyramid complexes continued for many years after Khufu. The second largest pyramid at Giza was claimed by another son of Snofru, named Khephren. His son, Menkaure´, eventually claimed the third pyramid at the Giza plateau. Despite their efforts, the radiated power never returned to Egypt.

Once the largest pyramids at Dashur and Giza had been converted into pyramid complexes, the building of large pyramids of that scale was never again attempted. There were pyramid monuments built, but they were modest by comparison, and the emphasis slowly changed to different styles of expression.

The Great Decline

The use of many columns, the sculpting of large statues, and the building of richly-decorated courtyards became the norm in this post elaborate and massive, pyramid-building period. The use of the pyramid geometry as the primary element lessened, and eventually it was used only as an architectural accent.

During this time, several great obelisks were built and moved into place hundreds of miles from the quarry. The Eypgtians, by then master craftsmen, chiseled these obelisks out of living rock and moved them to the waters edge using stone rollers on stone tracks. These several-thousand-ton stones were then placed on the decks of huge wooden boats. These boats, planked with wood from Cypress, were sealed with animal skins. The obelisks were eventually stood upright by excavating under the base and easing the obelisk over the pivot point using long ropes manned by hundreds of men. The obelisks still stand, and are mute testimony to the determination and craftsmanship of the men of that time.

During this period of Egyptian history, the tradition of initiating new priests was considered important and the standard training evolved into a routine of learning advanced knowledge, which included years of prayer, meditation, and spiritual work. Finally, when the new priests were considered ready, they made the journey between the paws of the Sphinx, the "Keeper of Secrets," and would then be guided into the subterranean corridors. They passed around and over doors with strange hinges that appeared to be traps to catch the impure of heart. In reality they were the old valves and tuning chambers of the macro circuit. Eventually they emerged into the passageways and chambers of the Great Pyramid. Since any passage or chamber with parallel walls within the Pyramid served as an amplifier of the Primal Energies, they resonated to the cells and very DNA of initiates. It was the perfect place for out-of-body experiences, and the notion that the sole function of the Great Pyramid was to serve as an altar was firmly entrenched.

Nothing they tried restored the ancient, radiated power. Debates and speculation resulted in several misconceptions, one of which was that it was the metal alloy used on the top-third exterior of the Great Pyramid that was the true source of the power. Another point of misunderstanding was that there was a connection between the radiated power and the physical and intellectual strength of the ruler and his aides. The Kings who came to this belief perceived that to place gold on top of their palaces would insure success. They initiated efforts to steal this metal, and it became a primary undertaking.

The Great Pyramid was mined for every ounce of its gold, whether it was attached to the exterior or part of the machinery within the passageways or chambers. Anything that looked like gold was taken, and for this reason the floor to the Queen's Chamber was torn up. The floor was not actually gold, but the rock that it was composed of sparkled somewhat like gold. All of the gold from the pyramid was taken, melted down, and reshaped into other things. This was the origin of gold temples, gold spires, and gold Byzantine toppings.

In time it became obvious that the gold itself was not the source of the power either, but the damage had been done. The Great Pyramid was stripped of its exterior and interior gold and no longer glistened in the Sun. Today the Great Pyramid has little reflectivity since the white casing-blocks were all used to rebuild the temples of Cairo after devastating earthquakes hit 1,500 years ago.

The Fallen Angel, Akhenaten

During the decline period the priesthood was teaching a distorted version of the seven Primal Energies. They taught that each Primal Energy was a separate god with multiple subservient gods. This system resulted in over eighty gods to honor and the complexity required a large priesthood to administer.

This state of affairs was studied with great interest by certain Travelers whose society had contributed DNA here years ago. From the planet Lyra, third planet of the small star Sirius B, Akhenaten came to study the primitive Earth culture. He made regular visits, stepping out of his scout disc and physically communicating to the leaders at that time.

Because of their advanced mode of transportation and high intelligence, Travelers are often thought of and revered as gods or angels. This particular angel had difficulty flying away. To make the leap to a Traveler's home star, the scout ship and its occupants had to attain the frequency of the Traders' mother ship. This was accomplished by machinery on the scout disc that was activated first in the sequence of operations to get back to the SMS. Rarely did the equipment malfunction, but one day Akhenaten found that his ship could not attain the proper frequency. He and his wife were stuck on Earth.

It was not the first time in history that Travelers were forced to live out their existence on Earth. These "fallen angels" — not by morals, but simple equipment failure — usually have no trouble mixing with Earthlings. The Travelers quite often became part of the ruling elite. Such was the case for Akhenaten and his wife Nefertiti. They were soon raised to the position of Pharaoh and Queen of Egypt.

They found the standard culture of Egypt to be quite oppressive, however, and soon began to make changes more fitting to the lifestyle they were accustomed to. They built a new palace from which to rule Egypt. Except for public ceremonies, they and their court practiced nudity. The purpose of nudity was to teach truth and honesty among the officials. They began to introduce the truth of the seven Primal Energies and the true position of humans as fine paintbrushes on the 34th split. They taught that purpose and intention was everything.

They assumed the changes would be good for everyone and be accepted as the best course for harmony in the land. Their vision to revolutionize Egypt and reform the polytheism, however, began to be misunderstood even among the priesthood intelligentsia, especially when it meant fewer priests would be needed. Upset was brewing.

By clever leadership, Akhenaten lived out his natural life. After he died, one of his two daughters married a young man who became the Pharaoh Tutankhamen. The marriage meant the Akhenaten teachings and revolution would continue. The angry priesthood, anxious to revert to their traditional ways and end the influence of Ahkenaten, put an end to the dynasty — the young couple "mysteriously" died in their teens. Ahkenaten's revolutionary ideas died with them. Every building and monument built by Ahkenaten was destroyed.

Akhenaten and Nefertiti's strange facial appearance and large head shape have been attributed to many things. They are actually quite representative of the people living on Lyra, a planet of the sun Sirius B. Many statues and paintings survive. (See Reference 1 and 5.) Notice profile of the head, the unusual torso and legs of this alien family.

The One True Pyramid

Despite the aforementioned denuding of the Great Pyramid, it maintains the secrets for those who look and consider all of the facts. It allows one to have a new vantage point to see the true order of the pyramids. Because anyone can put his name on a house built by someone else, it is erroneous to assume that the pyramids were built in a sequence corresponding solely to the pharaoh who inscribed his name on a pyramid or buildings near it. Once that is understood, the true order of the pyramids can be seen as attempts throughout history to produce power. (See Note 17 for the true order of the pyramids.) The pyramid that produced the radiated power was the first one, and that was and will always be, the Great Pyramid.

NOTES

1. See Reference 25. Semjase, Traveler from the Pleiades, told Billy Meier, the contactee from Switzerland, about a comet that was also called the Destroyer, but that account is of a planet within the Pleiades cluster, and not this solar system. From the vantage point of entities living on the surface of a planet in the path of such a returning dense comet, the appropriate name is understandably Nemesis, Destroyer, or any similar designation.

Semjase's account states that the Destroyer wanders among the stars, but this book states that the Destroyer is in an orbit around this binary sun system. Both are accurate when it is understood that she described the Mother Body, the giant Destroyer, that makes its rounds through various star systems in this corner of the galaxy. That Mother Body is so large and dense, and is on such a large, looping orbit, that it sweeps planets into its wake and deposits them in other star systems. Our solar system is afflicted by one of these pieces. It was attracted out of the wake of the Mother Body and into the gravity field of this binary system long ago. It alone is enough for us to contemplate. It is our Destroyer.

2. The Traders monitor all things and knew of the impending disaster, so why didn't they move the Destroyer to a less cruel orbit? It must be recalled that in all of the universe, for fear that creations cease, **"No thing gives warning."** (See Note 15, Chapter 11.)

3. There is a percentage of people living on Earth today who have an apparent inexplicable recollection of a cataclysmic event. The terror is remembered, but it cannot be associated to any particular event in this lifetime. The puzzle cannot be linked to any childhood traumas, but continues to surface even into adulthood. It is actually a soul remembrance of either death on Earth One as it exploded, or being saved at the last instant, and then witnessing the destruction of the whole planet from the safety of a mother ship. Some afflicted with these feelings even remember the curved window of the SMS and the aliens standing by — all witnessing the awful specter.

4. Science has many methods to date materials from ancient strata. Some are based on radioactive decay rates, Carbon-14 dating being the most commonly known technique. Science has not yet accounted for the regular occurrence of "transitions," which by definition are the changes to the proportion or ratio of Primal Energy Packets that make up subatomic particles. (Transitions, including the one we are experiencing now, are discussed in detail in Chapter 13.) For example, during a "shift" or transition, a particle might gain more Wisdom in exchange for less Allowance, and this slight difference would affect all atoms and molecules of the mineral, plant, and animal kingdoms. These are normal occurrences and are the creations of Entities of other splits.

How these changing proportions affect the radioactive decay dating methods and even the magnetic resonance techniques will become more self evident as this Transition draws to a close. Gravity and time changes will become measurable to the scientists, so obviously, this means that the Earth itself is not a good reference point for accurate dating.

The break up of Pangea, for example, is given in scientific text at 225 or 250 million years ago, but the actual event in terms of the number of orbits of Earth around the Sun is closer to 65 million years ago. Another example: if the materials of today were measured by current methods 2,000 years into the future, it would look like 8,000 years had passed. Because of this inherent error factor of four, ancient dates in this work will sometimes be presented as: 250 million (actually 65 million) years ago.

5. Pangea is dated in J.E. Pfeiffer's *The Emergence of Man* (See Reference 29) as 225 million years ago. "At that time the world was literally one world. No separate continents existed, only a great, single land mass or island in the midst of a great, single ocean, a super continent known as Pangea."

6. It might be thought that they would simply reproduce what they had achieved on the other planet and, although they remembered it, there was unfortunately not enough time. They realized that they would have to give it up almost entirely, and adopt survival strategies in the new world. Only the necessities to survive were stressed: how to talk, how to communicate, how to hunt, and how to forage for food, and cooperate for existence within a small tribal unit. For each generation, the teaching of the other world grew more faint and distorted, and what was taught about the other world eventually became nothing more than a dream reality, a fantasy. After 40 generations, all details of the life upon Earth One had vanished. Today after over 100 millennia, however, there is a basic remembrance. In some tribes in various parts of the world, included in part of their legend of origin is the knowledge that "our ancestors came from the stars."

7. Fossil evidence will eventually reveal that the Traders have been involved with other seeding programs on this planet. This is what they do, and other seeding events date back to 160 million (actually 40 million) years ago. During the time our precursors of millions of years ago lived, there were other animal types that had the chance to live and evolve here too, and there was genetic manipulation to help them adapt. They were seeded to speed evolution, and some were of a conscious, reasoning species. So there existed, other than humans and their precursors, other sentient, tool-using species. While they no longer exist here, their fossil records and tool artifacts may soon be discovered.

8. The strategy for survival of marauding bands would shock a civilized society, but would appear to be a great success story to the Traders, whose gene manipulation and seeding efforts were aimed at producing a physical form that could adapt completely to nature. The results you measure depend on where you stand. Until the physical form had adapted to nature, the next step, the civilization of the species, could not be taken.

9. The names of Isis, Osiris, and Thoth exist in the cuneiform and the hiero-glyphics of ancient artifacts. Texts on ancient Egypt such as Reference 1, 3, and 31, and even the mystery schools of ancient Egypt such as Reference 10, present these three names as some of the gods revered at the time of the pharaohs.

10. Details of anti-gravity circuitry have been purposely withheld from the author because the state of the Earth human at this time is such that he would quickly use anti-gravity technology as a weapon.

11. In all, there are less than 10,000 Yeti type *Homo erectus* still alive today in remote regions of the planet, and their numbers continue to dwindle as global pollution continues to take its toll. Besides being affected by chemical pollution, their reproductive genes are especially susceptible to radio frequencies and microwave radiation. The Big Foot type will likely be extinct on this planet in the near future.

12. From the time of the Flood there was a period of approximately 5,000 years when the vortex was close enough to partially activate the pyramids. In the last 5,000 years, however, the vortex position has moved so far from the Egyptian pyramids that practically no power has been produced. The reality of them producing any power is now considered a myth. The predominante notion in the last several thousand years is that the

pyramids were actually altars and tombs for the pharaohs.

13. The ancient Sumerians have recorded with great accuracy the orbital periods of all the planets, including Uranus and Neptune, which are not visible without the use of telescopes. The Sumerians are considered the inventors of the 24-hour day with 60 minutes per hour and 60 seconds per minute. The number 195,955,200,000,000, reverently recorded in a library within a palace in Ashurbanipal, was discovered during an excavation in 1875. The information is thought to have been recorded by the same ancient Sumerians. This value is a remembered fact about the Primal Energies, as the frequency of Allowance is 195,955,200,000,000 times per second. (See Chapter 14 and Reference 32.)

14. Recently released videos continue to report paranormal events within and around the pyramids. The Saqqara site has many unusual and interesting temples besides Zoser's Step Pyramid complex. One underground chamber exists that is carved from the living rock and accessible only by a long narrow passage. In this chamber is a sort of sarcophagus hewn out of the same rock. Above it is a suspended stone lid. The lid is too large to have been brought down the passage and is even of a different material than the rock sarcophagus. Those who venture to lay in the sarcophagus report eerie sensations and feel they are about to pass into another dimension. What is this all about?

The lid, built by the Egyptians and made up of gravel, sand, and a fine binder, was simply agglomerated into position. By the nature of the rock and the parallel walls, there is a certain PEP-enhanced resonance in the chamber. Add to that the strangeness of such a room. It has no apparent function as a real tomb. The only idea of the designers seems to have been to get you to try laying in the sarcophagus for a while. You are then left to examine your own emotions. It has been suggested that it is a portal to another dimension. It is not. If anything, it is a portal to one's own emotions. It is quite successful in this, and many wild stories have been told relating to those experiences.

15. The Maidum pyramid today is a great ring of debris, but within the center of the pile of sand and ruble rises a very steep, smooth-sided "skyscraper" almost to its original height. It is quite impressive against the sky, but looks nothing like the smooth-sided pyramid that it once was. The pyramid produced power when it was first constructed, but it did so unchecked, and the ones who built it did not understand the design or functional purpose of the arc within a pyramid.

To properly keep a pyramid under control the arc needs to be lowered or raised depending upon the position of the Sun, Moon, and other factors. The arc functions like the control rods of a nuclear reactor. Without the proper controls the Maidum pyramid ran "hot" several times a year. After many years of this, and long after the life of Snofru and his sons, the subatomic formula began to change, and the once-sturdy limestone turned to a relatively soft chalk-like substance that could not support the enormous weight. Especially since this pyramid used the 75-degree method for the inner core, the outer walls simply slid down into its collapsed state of today. (See Reference 1, page 132.)

16. The story of how Khufu has become freed from a fixed Astral picture helps us know what to do about it. He was instructed strongly from birth that a Pharaoh who practiced a life of good deeds and effort for the betterment of the people of his nation would obtain rightful entry to the court of the Sun God Ra, the most desired place to go

after death. (Notice that this picture is a lot like the gates of heaven story.) This strong fixed picture, amplified by the chanting of priests surrounding Khufu's death bed, created a thought form almost impossible to release when he actually entered the Astral plane. The solar boat that would usher him to the Sun was not there — where was the blazing Sun? Unable to shake this thought form, he patiently waited. Occasionally he noticed over his shoulder a small moon of light, (the tunnel to his Oversoul) but it was far too dim to meet his expectations.

In all, this trapped soul waited 5,000 years for the golden chariot to carry him to the Sun — not a very creative thing to do! Of all the priests in Khufu's death ceremony, one of them at his own death and entry into the Astral plane gained a more expansive understanding of the universe. He realized also that false teaching given to Khufu could be corrected. This priest, after reincarnating on Earth, simply chanted and made contact with the Astral essence of Khufu and suggested that he look over his shoulder at the dim light, the moon he refused to look at before. The priest suggested that Khufu would find what he desired on the other side of that light.

Once Khufu's focus had shifted to that light, he drifted towards it and it grew in size, even larger than any of his dreams of the realm of the Sun. As it enveloped him he, like all of us will eventually do, experienced the transcendence to and the bonding with the majestic Oversoul. With that completion a new creation begins somewhere else in the universe.

17. The information in this book gives some idea of the important features necessary for a pyramid to produce radiant energy, and the features that can be easily viewed firsthand or from recorded measurements of researchers are:

(1) Power-generating pyramids are large. The volume ratio assumes that the power output is directly proportional to the volume. For the volume ratio, divide the volume of the small pyramid by the volume of the Great Pyramid (G.P.).

(2) For the power to be kept under control and to be consistent, internal machinery is needed and a means to adjust that machinery must be designed into the pyramid. That means at least one internal corridor for the tuning, with access shafts like the G.P. air vents for tuning and for maintenance. Set the control factor for the G.P. = 100, since it is the most complicated internally and sets the standard. For a solid pyramid the control factor = 0.

(3) Piezoelectric covering on the outside. For the piezoelectric factor, let high grade limestone = 100, low grade limestone = 50, and mud or plaster = 0.

(4) Focusing lens at the base. For the base lens factor = 100 for the G.P., uncertain because no data is available = 50, definite flat base = 0.

(5) Methods to reflect long-wave frequencies back into the pyramid for further mixing. For the reflecting factor: The existence of an internal room near the focus point = 50, the existence of one or more stone ceiling blocks = 50. Since all gold coverings have long been scavenged this will not be considered.

(6) Correct alignment over a vortex, correct alignment with the magnetic N-S magnetic

flux lines, and an apothem angle near 52 degrees. For the alignment factor, a zero deviation from N-S = 50 and a 45 degree deviation = 0. Pyramids with an apothem angle of 52
degrees = 50, but deviant from the 52 degrees by 5 or more degrees = 0. Since humans can
still not measure the position of the vortex, this third part of the factor will be ignored.
(7) Gap between the casing and the inner core to allow movement of the casing facet and
to trap microwaves and cosmic particle energy. For the movement factor, recessed cores
or bulging casing facets = 100, casing blocks attached to the core or for flat facets = 0.

With these easily-attainable factors, a rough attempt will be made to compare the
first 33 pyramids. Every pyramid in Egypt is awe inspiring silhouetted against the setting
sun, but there exist great differences between them. After the 5th Dynasty another 50
pyramids were built, but they are not considered here. Because of their poor quality and
small size, they would rate zero against the above standard.

The pyramids that merit comparison are given in Table 12.1 through 12.4, listed
according to the scientific chronological order of construction, as well as the location of
the pyramid, the name of the King normally associated with the pyramid, and the name
of the pyramid itself.

What these tables list are the values that will plug into the Energy Equation. This
is the ultimate aim, to calculate how much energy each of these pyramids radiate, compared to the Great Pyramid. This Energy Equation, hypothesized here for the first time is:
Volume Ratio times Sum of Factors:

Energy = Volume small pyramid / Volume G.P. x (F1+F2+F3+F4+F5+F6)

The all important volume ratio is given in Table 12.1 for each of the 33 pyramids.

In Table 12.2, three more power producing factors, F1+F2+F3, for each of the
pyramids are listed. F1 = the piezo factor, F2 = the base factor, and F3 = the lens factor.

In Table 12.3, the last three power producing factors, F4+F5+F6, for each of the
pyramids are listed. F4 = the reflecting factor, F5 = the alignment factor, and F6 = the
movement factor.

All of the factors are summarized by simple addition in Table 12.4. The equation
is then calculated for each pyramid and the relative ability to radiate energy is listed in
the last column of Table 12.4.

These results are plotted against the order of construction in several ways for easy
and effective comparison. Graph 12.1 is the scientific order of construction based on the
chronological order of the Kings. This bar graph shows that many pyramids do not rate
high enough to be seen on the scale of the graph. These pyramids include the unfinished
pyramids, many of the subsidiary pyramids, and other pyramids with very small
volumes.

Graph 12.1 falsely suggests that as the Egyptians first experimented with step
pyramids, and then, based on knowledge gained from those projects, changed their building style. Throwing away the 75-degree core method in favor of parallel courses and
smooth sides allowed them to dramatically increase the volumes of this very difficult

building method by a factor of a hundred or more. But then mysteriously, what follows is the inexplicable decline back to a simple building technology. This is what the standard theory implies, but this book suggests there is a more plausible explanation.

Graph 12.2 removes the Great Pyramid, the Second Pyramid, the Third Pyramid, the Red Pyramid, and one half of the Bent Pyramid from the bar graph because the assumption is made that they were built thousands of years before the time of the pharaohs. What is seen here is the true chronological order of the pharaonic pyramids. These pyramids reflect pyramid volumes that could be realistically achieved in the lifetime of one king. Note that the tallest bars are attributed to projects built during the life spans of at least two Pharaohs.

In other words, in this span of over 200 years the pyramids built by the pharaohs are on the same relative order of magnitude. This is as expected, because while they all used the agglomeration technique to some extent, the moving and placement was all accomplished by hand.

Graph 12.3 depicts a span of time of 50,000 years and lists what is proposed by this text to be the correct pyramid sequence. The first pyramid is the Great Pyramid, built about 50,000 years before Christ, and ends with the small pyramids built by the pharaohs, about 2,000 years before Christ. The graph includes two relevant, cataclysmic events discussed in this book that have altered the course of pyramid construction.

Superimposed on the order of the pyramids is an approximate attempt to show how the movement of the vortex caused the theoretical output to drop off until about the time of Christ, when the power became almost nonexistent. (Not to scale.) The chart shows that humans recovered from the first cataclysm enough to renew pyramid technology, however, the movement of the vortex overcame his attempts to restore power by building more pyramids. The Great Pyramid, the first pyramid, was the inspiration for all the others.

18. The planet was not as cold and desolate as might be expected at that distance from the Sun. This is because at that time there was a greater amount of solar output and the atmosphere of that planet was more dense than this planet, helping to trap the radiant energy. That planet had a large metal core which was heated by its orbital motion around the Sun, and this internal source of heat actually warmed the surface.

19. There is one source of information that teaches that humans were the result of an experiment gone bad. In this account, the original intent was to create a slave that would follow orders and mine ore deposits. Although the names are different, it can be seen that the story is somewhat plausible as handed down generation after generation. (The contact was actually several thousand years ago.) The slave is one who takes orders from the master. In actuality, however, the master was the natural environment, and the Traders simply added genes to allow the new species to survive the harsh conditions. In a sense this was taking orders from the environment.

The rest of the story has to do with the Children of the Feather placing within the species the ability to disobey the orders, and to be rebels. In a sense that is also true. The endocrine system allows individuals to fear for survival, react, and search the events for a means to survive. Interestingly enough, the Children of the Feather are the Atlantians, the physical angels, known as the species that evolved from a feathered bird, although by that time, they did not have feathers.

Scientific Order	Location	Pharaoh	Name	Volume Ratio = $V_{small\ pyramid} / V^{G.P.}$
1	Saqqara	Zoser	Step	0.1288
2	Saqqara	Sekemket	Buried	(0.1320)*
3	Z. E. Aryan	Khaba	Layer	(0.0449)*
4	Seila	Unknown	Unknown	0.0016
5	Z. E. Maiytin	Unknown	Unknown	0.0005
6	El-Kula	Unknown	Unknown	0.0005
8	Maidum	Huni	First True (F.T.)	0.2604
9	Maidum	Huni	F.T. sub	0.0073
10	Dahshur	Snofru	Bent	0.522
11	Dahshur	Snofru	Bent sub	0.0110
12	Dahshur	Snofru	Red	0.651
13	Giza	Khufu	Great (G.P.)	1.00
14	Giza	Khufu	G.P. sub	0.0081
15	Giza	Khufu	G.P. sub	0.0081
16	Giza	Khufu	G.P. sub	0.0081
17	Abu Rawash	Djedefre	S. Star	(0.148)*
18	Abu Rawash	Djedefre	Star sub	(0.0041)*
19	Giza	Khephren	Second	0.855
20	Giza	Khephren	Second sub	0.0068
21	Z.E. Aryian	Unknown	Unfinished	(0.700)*
22	Giza	Menkaure´	Third	0.0932
23	Giza	Menkaure´	Third sub	0.0050
24	Giza	Menkaure´	Third sub	0.0050
25	Giza	Menkaure´	Third sub	0.0050
26	Saqqara	Userkaf	E. Haram (E.H.)	0.05
27	Saqqara	Userkaf	E.H. sub	0.001
28	Abu Sir	Sahure	Ba Rises (B.R.)	0.05
29	Abu Sir	Sahure	B.R. sub	0.001
30	Abu Sir	Neuserre	Established (E.)	0.02
31	Abu Sir	Neuserre	E. sub	0.001
32	Abu Sir	Neferirkare	Ba Spirit	0.12
33	Abu Sir	Ra Neferef	Divine Ba	(0.044)*

( )* indicates never finished, for the most part only one or several layers finished.

Table 12.1 Comparison of pyramids by Volume Ratio.

Scientific Order	Name Control	Piezo Factor	Base Factor	Lens Factor
1	Step	34.	100.	0.
2	Buried	24.	0.	0.
3	Layer	4.	0.	0.
4	Unknown	0.	0.	0.
5	Unknown	0.	0.	0.
6	Unknown	0.	0.	0.
7	Unknown	0.	0.	0.
8	First True (F.T.)	46.	100.	0.
9	F.T. sub	20.	50.	0.
10	Bent	66.	100.	0.
11	Bent sub	10.	50.	0.
12	Red	66.	100.	0.
13	Great (G.P.)	100.	100.	100.
14	G.P. sub	10.	50.	0.
15	G.P. sub	10.	50.	0.
16	G.P. sub	10.	50.	0.
17	S. Star	0.	0.	0.
18	Star sub	0.	0.	0.
19	Second	50.	100.	0.
20	Second sub	10.	50.	0.
21	Unfinished	0.	0.	0.
22	Third	52.	100.	0.
23	Third sub	10.	50.	0.
24	Third sub	10.	50.	0.
25	Third sub	10.	50.	0.
26	E. Haram (E.H.)	12.	100.	0.
27	E.H. sub	10.	100.	0.
28	Ba Rises (B.R.)	36.	100.	0.
29	B.R. sub	10.	100.	0.
30	Established (E.)	12.	100.	0.
31	E. sub	6.	100.	0.
32	Ba Spirit	6.	100.	0.
33	Divine Ba	0.	0.	0.

Table 12.2 Comparison of pyramids by piezo factor, base factor, and lens factor.

Scientific Order	Name	Reflecting Factor	Alignment Factor	Movement Factor
1	Step	0.	69.	0.
2	Buried	0.	76.	0.
3	Layer	0.	76.	0.
4	Unknown	0.	45.	0.
5	Unknown	0.	45.	0.
6	Unknown	0.	45.	0.
7	Unknown	0.	5.	0.
8	First True	0.	99.5	0.
9	F.T. sub	0.	99.5	0.
10	Bent	35.	99.8	0.
11	Bent sub	0.	99.5	0.
12	Red	45.	99.5	0.
13	Great	100.	100.	100.
14	G.P. sub	0.	99.7	0.
15	G.P. sub	0.	99.7	0.
16	G.P. sub	0.	99.7	0.
17	S. Star	0.	49.	0.
18	Star sub	0.	49.	0.
19	Second	20.	94.9	0
20	Second sub	0.	94.6	0.
21	Unfinished	0.	89.	0.
22	Third	0.	99.7	0.
23	Third sub	0.	99.5	0.
24	Third sub	0.	99.5	0.
25	Third sub	0.	99.5	0.
26	E. Haram	0.	98.	0.
27	E.H. sub	0.	98.	0.
28	Ba Rises	0.	96.	0.
29	B.R. sub	0.	96.	0.
30	Established	0.	98.	0.
31	E. sub	0.	98.	0.
32	Ba Spirit	0.	98.	0.
33	Divine Ba	0.	98.	0.

Table 12.3 Comparison of pyramids by reflecting factor, alignment factor, and movement factor.

Scientific Order	Name	SUM = (F1+F2+F3+ F4+F5+F6) (600 Max)	ENERGY FACTOR = Volume Ratio X (F1+F2+F3+ F4+F5+F6) (600 Max)
1	Step	203.	26.1
2	Buried	100.	(13.2)*
3	Layer	80.	(3.6)*
4	Unknown	45.	.07
5	Unknown	45.	.02
6	Unknown	45.	.02
7	Unknown	5.	.003
8	First True	245.5	64.
9	F.T. sub	169.5	1.2
10	Bent	300.8	157.
11	Bent sub	159.5	1.76
12	Red	310.5	202.
13	Great (G.P.)	600.0	600.
14	G.P. sub	159.7	1.3
15	G.P. sub	159.7	1.3
16	G.P. sub	159.7	1.3
17	S. Star	49.	(7.3)*
18	Star sub	49.	(.2)*
19	Second	264.9	226.
20	Second sub	154.6	1.1
21	Unfinished	89.	(62.)*
22	Third	251.7	23.
23	Third sub	159.5	.8
24	Third sub	159.5	.8
25	Third sub	159.5	.8
26	E. Haram	210.	10.5
27	E.H. sub	208.	.2
28	Ba Rises	232.	11.6
29	B.R. sub	206.	.2
30	Established	210.	10.5
31	E. sub	204.	.2
32	Ba Spirit	204.	24.
33	Divine Ba	98.	(3.9)*

(   )* indicates never finished, for the most part only one or several layers finished.

Table 12.4 Comparison of the pyramids using the energy factor.

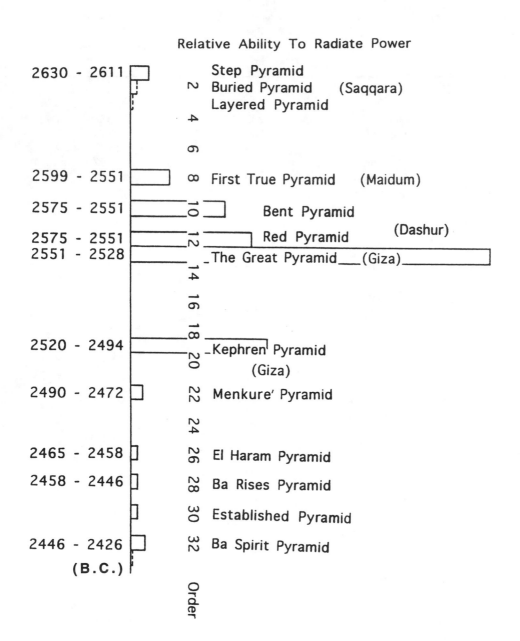

Relative Ability To Radiate Power

2630 - 2611	Step Pyramid
	Buried Pyramid (Saqqara)
	Layered Pyramid
2599 - 2551	First True Pyramid (Maidum)
2575 - 2551	Bent Pyramid
2575 - 2551	Red Pyramid (Dashur)
2551 - 2528	The Great Pyramid (Giza)
2520 - 2494	Kephren Pyramid (Giza)
2490 - 2472	Menkure' Pyramid
2465 - 2458	El Haram Pyramid
2458 - 2446	Ba Rises Pyramid
	Established Pyramid
2446 - 2426	Ba Spirit Pyramid
(B.C.)	

Order

Graph 12.1 The traditionally accepted order of the pyramids matches the King's List, however, quite often this sequence is based on sketchy evidence such as inscriptions on vases, statues, or buildings found near or within that pyramid.

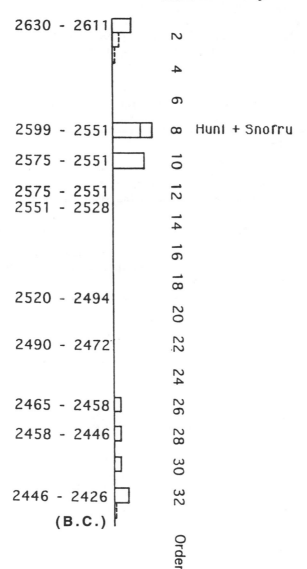

Graph 12.2 The order of the pyramids without the five large pyramids (hypothesized to have been built by more ancient civilizations). The pyramids listed here are monuments of the size and proportion that could have been constructed by pharaohs if their workmen used manual labor and the agglomeration methods of that time.

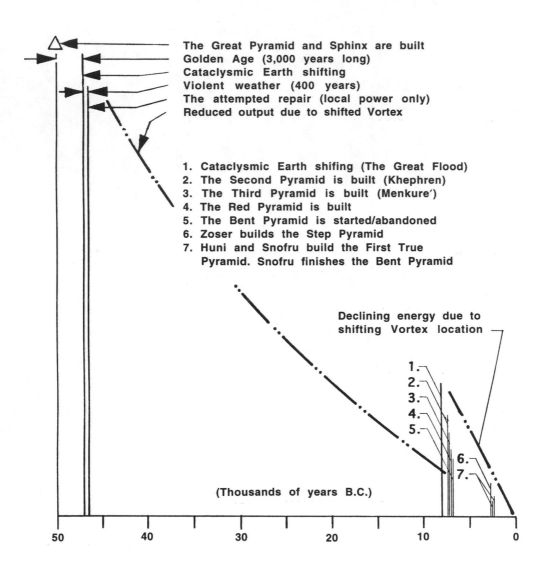

The Great Pyramid and Sphinx are built
Golden Age (3,000 years long)
Cataclysmic Earth shifting
Violent weather (400 years)
The attempted repair (local power only)
Reduced output due to shifted Vortex

1. Cataclysmic Earth shifing (The Great Flood)
2. The Second Pyramid is built (Khephren)
3. The Third Pyramid is built (Menkure')
4. The Red Pyramid is built
5. The Bent Pyramid is started/abandoned
6. Zoser builds the Step Pyramid
7. Huni and Snofru build the First True
   Pyramid. Snofru finishes the Bent Pyramid

Declining energy due to
shifting Vortex location

1.
2.
3.
4.
5.

6.
7.

(Thousands of years B.C.)

50   40   30   20   10   0

Graph 12.3 Depicted is the true order of the Egyptian pyramids. An energy output curve is suggested which, although not to scale, demonstrates that power output has diminished as the vortex position shifted. The reduced output was the driving force for the second, third, fourth, and fifth pyramids, and the memory of the power inspired the pharaonic pyramids.

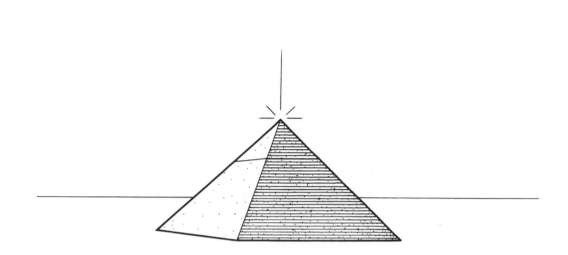

Figure 12.1 Shown is the Giza plateau at 50,000 B.C., and the only pyramid is the Great Pyramid. (Compare with the drawing Int.1 on page v.) The Great Pyramid was built by a long, vanished civilization that used the radiated power from the Great Pyramid to heat and cool their buildings, to help grow the crops, to travel around the planet, to communicate, to heal, and much, much more.

THE PRESENT

Chapter Thirteen

Synopsis

The planet and everything on it is passing through a Transition, a three-dimensional shift at the Primal Energy level. At the end of it, the year 2012 A.D., there will be less WP and more L. Transitions affect us physically and emotionally. Society changes as well. After this change there will be less control needed from leadership since everyone will learn to control themselves and will cooperate to a degree not known before. The Great Pyramid Society taught their children how to pass through Transitions. The teaching started with an overview of creation, the story of the Primal Energies. The endless cycles of the Primal Energies flowing between the Is-Ness and the Is-Not-Ness is represented by the infinity symbol. One loop represents the Is-Ness while the other loop represents the Is-Not-Ness. The crossover point represents the eternal now. A short version of the infinity symbol is two lines crossing, or two triangles apex to apex. The solid geometric representations are cones or pyramids joined at the apex or the base. A balanced life is represented by two overlapping triangles, cones, or pyramids. The overlapping triangles form the Star of David six-pointed star. It symbolizes the god-man cusp, the balance place where one does not dwell entirely in the physical nor in the astral. Another symbol of a balanced life is a line with a circle at each end. One circle is need, the other is desire. The line is want, the balance place between need and desire. During a Transition, stay in the want region. Keep the body in peak performance. Study what is proper to eat. Keep fit by proper exercise. Healing is often accomplished by the power of the mind. When two or more join, the power of the mind increases dramatically, at which point Primal Energy responds. During this Transition, shamans and doctors could improve healing by learning from each other. Meditation is another key to maintaining a healthy mind and body. Use the breath during meditation. Breath means spirit in the ancient languages. Of the many types of meditations, the cleansing meditation, fire breath meditation, and the problem-solving meditation will control the stress of life. The remote-viewing meditation will add extra spice to life.

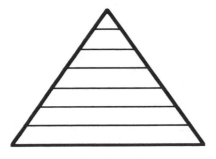

Chapter Thirteen

THE TRANSITION

Living a Dimension Shift in Balance

The Transition Defined

There are many names for the turbulent times we are in today: "The End Times," "The Harmonic Convergence," "The New Age," "The End of the World," and "Armageddon." All are apt descriptions depending upon where one stands. Technically it is the "Transition," a dimension shift, or a phenomena of the universe. In our method of measuring time, transitions occur at regular intervals of about 2,000 years. Another cycle occurs every 26,000 years, and yet another cycle every 69,000 years. Sometimes the cycles overlap, and an extra-strong, double-cusp transition occurs. That is what we are experiencing now.

What happens during a dimension shift? The formula that makes up each atom changes. During this Transition the Will and Power (WP) portion of everything is reducing and the Love (L) portion is increasing. This shift is something that we can feel and it causes great changes in our behavior.

Refer to Figure 10.3, cut and paste it into a three-dimensional cone as indicated, and it will graphically show how dimensions and Primal Energies interrelate. First find the three-dimension column on the cone and notice that it is made up of all eight Primal Energies. Notice that some dimensions have less than eight Primal Energies. Observe also that the three dimensions are very dense with Allowance and very lean with Wisdom. At the end of the Transition we will be in the fourth-dimension column with more L in ratio to WP. This affects everything. Although the ratio is what is changing, this transition is often called a shift from Will and Power to Love.

Where you stand always becomes the place from which to define everything, so as soon as the transition to the fourth-dimensional reality is made, the whole cone must be clocked over one notch. The fourth-dimensional reality will suddenly envelop the world and everything will change. This will eventually become the status quo and be seen as normal three-dimensional reality. If one desires to measure the density of everything, it will be noted that just as before, most things are primarily made up of Allowance, combined with varying amounts of the other Energies, with Wisdom being the least dense. What is not readily apparent is that after the Transition, the new version of Allowance and the new version of Wisdom are of a finer frequency. Life on the planet will be more expansive. Since gravity is a combination of WP and L, gravity is changing. The Earth will expand slightly. If a pound of Earth matter could be quickly taken to another part of the galaxy it would weigh more in that location. If a pound of matter could be quickly taken from out there and brought here, it would weigh less.

This change from Will and Power to Love, which is the decision and creation of entities on the Primal level, will take approximately 50 years to complete. The ratio of L/WP will be higher in every sub-atomic particle, atom, and molecule of the Earth. Everything will be affected, the minerals and elements, the plant kingdom, the animal kingdom, and every human being. No one has the power to change it. Humanity as a whole gets to perceive the Transition and is along for the ride. Already the physical sensations are occasionally apparent. On some days people feel extreme fatigue and on other days a sensation of butterflies, excitement with a little confusion, a strong heart-pulsation, or sometimes a body-ripple.

Love is the Energy that glues all things together and at the same time slightly separates and gives definition to each creation This will be a time when each individual finds he is getting a clear picture of what he is. That clarity allows a feeling that is lighter, a little quicker, and less burdened by the weight of events as they would be. It's a feeling that is more expansive in the way interrelations get to be.

There will be greater and greater difficulty conforming to the social model, especially models of behavior defined by strict conformity and by dictatorial governments. From watching the news the last few years it is apparent that the world no longer accepts that leaders can demand absolute understanding, absolute belief, or absolute paths of social behavior.

Rulers who use corporal punishment to uphold such strict decrees are being exposed and dethroned. Religious leaders will increasingly be found to be untruthful.

There will be no need for harsh rule, since individuals will naturally want to control themselves and society will function with far fewer bosses and rules. Individuals will follow the code of ethics that makes sense to them. Personal ethics will guide everyone, but this changeover will not occur without turmoil. Some of what is to come is changing governments and changing economies.

What worked in the past may no longer work in the future. This will result in a great deal of physical and emotional discomfort for some. Many may choose death. Others will hang on, deciding to experience the entirety. For others it will be the most joyful ride of their lives, because they see and understand that the differences that will become more and more evident are the spark of the movement of creativity.

The excitement of this time will be felt by those who relish differences. The great polarities will not be judged by them to be either right or wrong, but simply different.

That understanding allows living with the least amount of pain.

The Transition of the Great Pyramid Society

The Great Pyramid Society was well aware of the dramatic changes that can occur during dimensional shifts. Since it was one of these shifts they came to that caused the upheaval that brought them to this planet, they taught their children well. This teaching could serve us well now.

The young were taught that the plane of demonstration upon Earth was a dimension of duality, and the emotional realm on this particular planet was extreme. (There exists only one other planet where life for humans is more extreme.) Ethics were vital while under these shifting conditions, but the ethics were not founded on the principle that good and evil exist in the universe. Their society was not taught to be good for fear of going to hell or some other punishment. Fear was never used. Instead, enlightenment was used.

The first step was to teach the overview of the creation. It is the same overview given in an earlier chapter, that the Is-Ness discovers what It is by the splitting of Consciousness and Energy, a process activated by thought. The simple thought of wondering what It is starts the flow that defines the distinction between the Is-Ness and the Is-Not-Ness. Each of these distinctions receives a piece of the original Consciousness and it is that imparted Consciousness that wonders again, "What am I," and that in turn results in another movement and the discovery of the second split. The process continues. At the third split there were four Primal Energies and Consciousness making up the Is-Ness and four Primal Energies and Consciousness making up the Is-Not-Ness. (Sacred geometry was the teaching tool, Note 1.)

Primal Consciousness then decides to create by combinations. At first, the simplest combinations of Energy and Consciousness are created and these are followed by increasingly complex formulations. Three of the Primal Energies, Wisdom (W) Knowledge (K), and Harmony (H) exist in the Is-Not-Ness, however, they wink into the Is-Ness and then back to the Is-Not-Ness. This cycle repeats at such an incomprehensible frequency that they are available for creations in the Is-Ness. Allowance (AL) Allegiance (AG) and Will and Power (WP) exist primarily in the Is-Ness although they also wink back and forth from the Is-Ness to the Is-Not-Ness and are available for creations in the Is-Not-Ness. The winking in and out is similar for Chaos and Love, but they are oriented closer to, and actually straddle, the junction between the Is-Ness and the Is-Not-Ness.

Chaos, the longest wavelength of the Primal Energies, is the carrier for all the Energies. Unimaginable numbers of Chaos particles expand outward to uniformly fill all of the universe and this provides a place for all other Energies to attach to and to ride upon. Chaos is the slow-vibrating base string, while the actual creations are the Energies vibrating on the string at higher frequencies. Love functions as the definer, giving definition to the patterns created, holding them together, but separating them enough for definition at the same time. On a sliding scale, each of the Energies occupies part of a bandwidth with Chaos at one end and Wisdom at the other end. Wisdom is the shortest wavelength of all the Energies and is thus the fastest in vibration.

Creation then decides to discover what it is by combining different Energies in different ways. As explained earlier, these can be simple combinations of two, three, or more Primal Energies. Different combinations form different dimensions. Creations with all eight Primal Energies fill up the three-dimensional reality, the one we see and are familiar with. With each split of consciousness the combinations created become more complex, moving from subatomic particles, atoms, and then molecules. Suns form at the 24th split, planets are formed knowingly at the 30th. By the 33rd split, souls are formed and are entering physical forms on the 34th. (See Note 2.)

Rules of the Discovery

These are some of the rules of creation.

1. Forces of Attraction arise from the basic urge to return to the rest state before the original split. This urge is not an emotional longing as humans would imagine, but the impulse is as real and obvious as the attraction of negative and positive electrical particles, including mysterious gravitational forces and all nuclear forces.

2. For anything to be visible in the three-dimensional reality, all eight Primal Energies must be part of the formula. When a formulation is missing one or more of the Primal Energies, it will be recognizable only from the vantage point of another dimension.

3. Creations can be observed from the first split downward, meaning towards increasingly complex splits, but not the other way around. The reason for this one way mirror effect is that without it, motivation for further creation would cease.

4. The waste of one creation is the food for another creation. This is true for the simplest formula to the most complicated formula. Thus, for the human being, at the end of the physical body's life, the creations of life, the consciousness of that existence flows upward at least one split and gets recorded into the Oversoul. What gets recorded at the Oversoul, the Akashic Record region, are the latest delicacies of the three-dimensional realm, the exciting new experiences of all human beings.

5. The Is-Ness allows all things, however, what does not create will disperse. The Is-Ness is self-cleansing.

The teaching has always been given using symbols of one design or another, some of which are depicted in Notes 1 and 2. Sacred geometry, for instance, used overlapping circles. Although these symbols were originally used to teach ethics from the point of view of enlightenment, they have been distorted through the ages and some have interpreted them to mean ethics based on good and evil. This leads to the opposite of cooperation — polarities and war. Other symbols have lost their original meanings. It is worth looking at the basic ones.

The Infinity Symbol

This endless cycle of the Primal Energies, flowing between the Is-Ness and the Is-Not-Ness, the endless cycle of changing creation, is represented by the infinity symbol:

∞

Why this is the perfect symbol for the Primal Energies is best explained by a review of figure 8.7. In this model, Chaos is shown to be an expanding toroid that spirals to its maximum, after which it decays back to the crossover point, only to repeat the cycle in the reverse realm. When considered in relation to time, the ebb and flow of that cyclic activity looks like a sine wave with the positive side representing the Is-Ness and the negative side representing the Is-Not-Ness. (See Figure 13.1.) Since the cycles from A to B are exactly like the cycle from B to C, C to D, etc., picturing the shorthand version of such a graph would mean placing a hinge at point B and then flipping point C back to point A. That resulting path yields a graph very much like the figure eight on its side, the infinity symbol. In other words, the infinity symbol is a folded, shorthand, version of Figure 13.1.

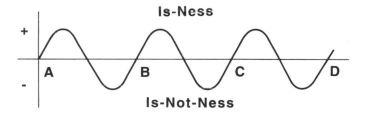

Figure 13.1 All PEP and all creations cycle between the Is-Ness and the Is-Not-Ness. This is the long form of the infinity symbol.

Another way of conceptualizing it is to imagine the path of one of the PEP upon Chaos, as represented in figure 8.7. The path would spiral to a maximum, then decay to a minimum and then cross over to repeat in the anti-realm. (See Figure 13.2.) The hint of the infinity symbol is clearly evident in such a pattern. Thus for the infinity symbol, one loop always represents the Is-Ness and the other loop represents the Is-Not-Ness. The crossover point represents the junction between the two realms and defines the "now" of events.

The Is-Not-Ness is the future from which an event is about to be born, and the Is-Ness is the actualized history of the event. The crossover point is the birth of the event, the "eternal now" of all creations. The loop has no starting or ending point, and each of the Primal Energies continuously move from the Is-Ness to the Is-Not-Ness. The waste from one cycle becomes the food for the next cycle, the end of one loop begins the next loop, and the creations and cycles continue forever.

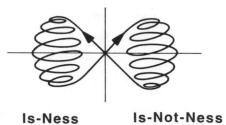

Figure 13.2 The path of a single PEP is to spiral to a maximum value and then to spiral to a minimum value where it crosses over into the anti-realm and the process moves as a mirror image. The infinity symbol is clearly present.

Infinity Symbol — Short Versions

There is even a shorter version of the infinity symbol that is two straight lines forming a stretched out "X." (See Figure 13.3.)

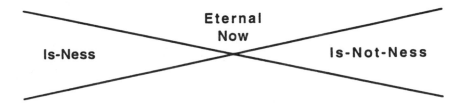

Figure 13.3 The shorthand version of the infinity symbol.

The crossover point represent the eternal now, the open region to the left represents the Is-Ness, and the open region to the right represents the Is-Not-Ness. This easy-to-draw symbol is like viewing a portion of the infinity symbol, zooming in on the crossover point, and imagining that the lines reach out to infinity where they eventually meet, completing the loop.

Another stick version for the infinity symbol is made by closing the open regions with a straight line. The result looks like two cones or triangles joined at the tips. (See Figure 13.4.) It was always included in the teaching that by standing on your head the reverse would be true, and the symbol is equally applicable.

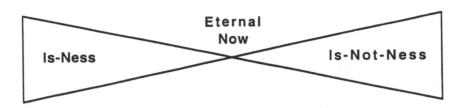

Figure 13.4 The shorthand version of the infinity symbol with closed ends.

Since it is necessary to have all eight Primal Energies participating to create in the three-dimensional reality, each Primal Energy is equally important. It is appropriate to remember this by representing each side of the triangles with equal lengths. Although there are endless possibilities of triangles, there is only one, the isosceles triangle, with all three sides of equal length. With two of these triangles touching point-to-point, the apparent cross over is the Now of the creation, with one triangle representing the past or the actualization of the event, and the other triangle representing the future, from which the Energy for the event was extracted. (See Figure 13.5.)

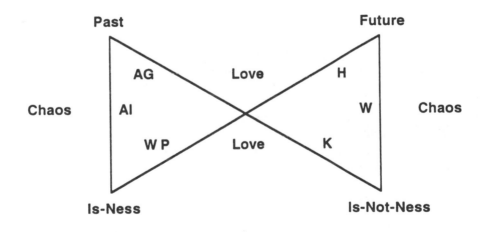

Figure 13.5 Shorthand version of the infinity symbol with equal lengths representing equal importance to each PEP.

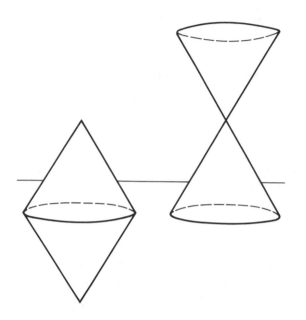

Figure 13.6 The three-dimensional form of the isosceles triangles is two cones tip-to-tip. Since this is impossible to construct, the next best representation is base-to-base.

The three-dimensional representation of isosceles triangles arranged point-to-point, is two cones point-to-point, as shown in Figure 13.6.

This symbol was grandly designed into the Great Pyramid. Since the cone shape is highly complex to build, it was reduced to a four-sided pyramid. The practical method of building pyramids point-to-point was to shift the concept, and to consider it base-to-base, which still achieves the symbolic mirror image. (See Figure 13.7.)

The Great Pyramid has a conceptual pyramid beneath it. This reversed pyramid is defined by the entry point of the water which is at the apex of the inverted form and the macro circuit is entirely within its boundaries. Exactly one-half the distance between that entry point and the visible apex is the base of the Great Pyramid, which is at the much-disputed top of the pavement. (See Note 3.)

Misinterpretations of the Infinity Symbol

The knowledge symbolized by the infinity symbol is so basic and timeless that versions of it have passed down through the ages, however, the original meaning has been lost and the stylizing of it has been highly exaggerated. (See Note 4.)
sical body eventually passes, all new creations and emotions experienced by the Is-Ness

Isolation Fears

The Soul of an individual physical form essentially straddles the 33rd split and 34th split, while the physical form exists entirely upon the 34th split. The emotional creatures that

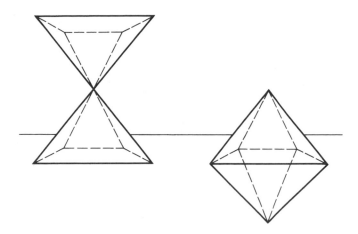

Figure 13.7 A physical monument with curved sides like the cone of Figure 13.6 is very difficult to build. The practical three-dimensional cone is the four-sided pyramid as shown.

are created by the soul-body combination exist upon the 35th split. Even though the physical body eventually passes, all new creations and emotions experienced by the Is-Ness via the physical body get recorded into the Oversoul, which is somewhat like a giant corporation compared to an individual Soul's sole-proprietorship.

It is true now, and was true at the time of the Great Pyramid Society, that of all the emotions there is one that is especially difficult for humans on the Earth. That dreaded emotion has to do with being isolated, one of the greatest fears associated with the five-sense limitation of three-dimensional physical existence. The paralysis felt when consumed by this fear makes each Earthly step almost impossible because motivation is almost non-existent. The master teachers reminded their students how to live in balance without getting stuck in fear. They taught that the Soul focuses onto, and attaches to, a physical form at the cost of great limitation, but at the gain of perceiving its own creations.

Three-dimensional reality, with its associated duality, is not a mistake, nor a situation to be wished away. It is a special gift, a corner of the universe where one creative event follows another, potentially, in harmony with other creators. On Earth, duality has extremes, but this incarnation is considered the ideal choice for adventure. To minimize chaotic events on the adventure planet, which could result from the improper actions of the free-will creators, certain concepts were ingrained. The blueprint for an impeccable life for the children of the Great Pyramid Society was very much like that given in Table 10.1. Since "thou shalt" and "thou shalt not" were never a part of the teaching, every student was encouraged to meditate and exercise great patience to properly obtain the correct interpretation of the blueprint for their life as it would apply to them.

A meditation was given so that students could get in touch with Primal Energy, using the technique for solving problems and interpreting the great blueprint. They were taught that proper interpretation results in a life that is balanced between the selfish and the selfless. This balance relieves the fear of isolation. Polarities were best avoided. A proper selfing lifestyle is characterized by an absence of judgment, little comparison with others, and no projections on others of how they should behave. Each person is on his own pathway through the universe and no two pathways are identical.

Simple Relationships

The meditation helped the students understand that simple relationships most often and appropriately reside within the "want region" of the "relationship creature." That relationship creature can be diagrammed by a straight line connecting two circles. One circle represents desires, the other circle represents needs. The line between represents the spectrum of possible wants. (See Figure 13.8.)

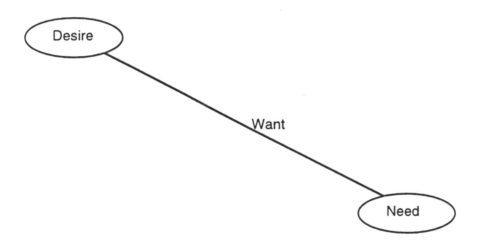

Figure 13.8 The balance diagram for any relationship.

People "need" to eat something, some minimum amount, to stay alive. They "want" to eat a variety of food that is plentiful and nourishing, while they "desire" to eat a variety of gourmet foods that are plentiful, nourishing, extremely tasteful, expensive, and look delightful. With respect to these definitions, students were encouraged to seek balanced relationships that were in the want region. Demanding to have relationships in the desire region quite often results in failure, which puts one in the need category and increases fear of isolation and the inward spiral of defeat.

Group Relationships

It was taught that students would eventually find themselves in groups, and to avoid chaos in groups, it is necessary to find a balance point between dominating a group and being a non-contributor. A group works much like any event, with all the Energies actively engaged. With the absence of Love in a group, there is not enough definition of the individuals and the group will disband. Without Allowance in the group there may not be a goal to keep them together. With no Wisdom in the group the many possibilities that could be accomplished will be absent and the group may fall apart for lack of interest. Chaos functions as the arbiter and its discernments settle squabbles that could lead to dysfunction.

Members within the group should find which function, in terms of a Primal Energy, they can best serve and that will help keep the group functioning. For example, business groups were always formed with eight members on the board and the function of each was to represent one of the Energies.

A Balanced Society

With that model, the society was made up of many small groups. The best way for groups to join with other groups was for each group to recognize the other as equal. Domination and chaos were thus avoided.

Star Of David — A Symbol Of Balance

The master teachers concluded each lecture with the reminder that the ten-dimensional PEP cones, representing the Is-Ness/Is-Not-Ness mirror image (See Figure 10.3.), can be joined in many ways other than apex-to-apex. They can be joined base-to-base. (See Figure 13.9 a and b.), or they can be joined at the conjunctive portions of the cones, intermeshing.

When that balance is found between the higher and the lower in frequency, that desired unity and concept that is called "god-human," was represented by two triangles overlapping symmetrically to form a six-pointed star. That is the Star of David and what it represents. (See Figure 13.9 c.

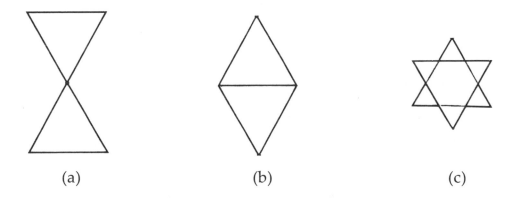

(a)   (b)   (c)

Figure 13.9 The symbolic isosceles triangle can be joined three ways.

The grandest three-dimensional monument ever constructed to honor the Star of David god-human cusp was the Sphinx, which represented the grandest unity of self. As far as human beings are concerned, that god-human unity takes place within the three-dimensional realm. It occurs when the individual is in balance with the world around him/her. That is the place where no one is unconnected and everyone is a participant in harmonious keeping. What counts is involved, joyous creations. This basic teaching has been taught repeatedly to human beings on this planet for more than 52,000 years — and elsewhere, far longer than that.

Astral/Physical Cycles

When joyous creations flow, day in and day out, there exist peace, happiness, and youthful vigor within the individual. Since the Astral is part of the plane of demonstration, life is not to be one long drudgery upon the Physical plane, followed by an endless ride through the Astral. Instead, life's flow will consist of moment to moment cycles. This will manifest as a dip into the Astral, to feel the joy of the good works and to gain inspiration for another creation on the Physical followed by the cycle back into the physical for more good works and more involved joyous creations. (See Figure 13.10.)

Astral joy and inspiration

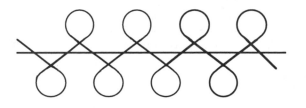

Physical good works and joyous creation

Figure 13.10 The balance point between the Astral and the Physical.

The balance between the two should be discovered, and that is found easily by listening to the body. If it feels wrong, do not participate. If it feels right, then join in, bringing joy to each day while keeping the body from degenerating.

Initiation at the Great Pyramid

Eventually the students were ready for the much-anticipated initiation. With the Great Pyramid visible in the far distance, the teachers would gather the students and repeat that the soul knows it is not actually isolated, but for those living a three-dimensional existence, the reality of the ten-dimensional existence is at best an intellectual concept. In fact, an intellectual understanding of five-dimensional reality is all that is possible once incarnated into a human physical form.

So the master teachers would point to the Great Pyramid and remind the students of the 2π spiral from the apex that wrapped over 200 times to reach the base. (Introduced in Chapter 12.) Countless points were connected to make the line that formed the spiral.

The top point represented their first moment of consciousness in their present incarnation. Each point thereafter represented events of their life. The Base represented the moment of creation, the eternal now. The spiral on the pyramid represented their past, and the spiral stretching outward from the base, their future. That outward stretching spiral expanding over the visible expanse of land was only a small part of what existed over the horizon. Imagine how many points, all future events, would be needed to form a spiral that covered the enormous area of the planet.

One of the reasons a calendar was built into the Descending and Ascending Passageways was to represent that each individual was not only what they had already been, but also already what they were yet to be. The realization that they were much more than the reflection in the mirror — their five-sense physical body — and much more than the positive and negative events already experienced in their current incarnation, allowed them to realize that whatever they thought they were was only one third of what they actually were. Two thirds was still to be experienced and part of the expansive future. When that was experienced, they would essentially remain at the base of the Pyramid and view, once again, another two thirds of the future events stretching out over the horizon.

Instantly, the students were transported by floating discs to the base of the normally off-limits Great Pyramid. Being that close meant they would experience a grand electromagnetic shift, a physical effect of the great power generator. At that close range their hair stood on end. Those who had no knowledge of what it was experienced fear and terror at close range. Even those who understood the principles were awestruck.

The master teachers explained that the Great Pyramid extracted power from everything: the power released by the planet's core moving within the mantle, the movement of the Moon and all other celestial bodies, the solar wind, atmospheric changes due to the seasons, the wind, distant lightening, and even the crashing of ocean waves against the shore. The Great Pyramid picked up the resonance of all things because it was sensitive to the ten-dimensional nature of all things. All things within the ten dimensions have a resonance.

In the ten-dimensional wrap around universe, each person is truly a ten-dimensional being stretching across all existence. Bathing in the intense focus of Energy at the base of the Great Pyramid, the students experienced a complete out-of-body unity with the Astral plane, which included the intense feeling and remembrance of the true home — the pleasing ripples of knowing one is connected forever, and the knowing that no matter what happens hereafter, this Earth plane is only a drop in a much larger reality. Forever afterwards, a contemplation would achieve a remembrance of the event. No student feared death after that. (See Note 5.)

The purpose of the initiation, to eliminate fear and replace it with intense living, was always a success. The experience fostered the balanced lifestyle as well as the realization that it was not appropriate to fixate on the goal of getting to the Astral. The real goal was achieving the balance place between the two realms. Good works and involved, joyous creations resulted in an appropriate daily cycle. Now that students knew of the great mystery of this realm as it relates to the rest of the universe, they took personal responsibility — the key to life — for their experiences. Never did they consider themselves to be the victims of an uncaring universe.

The Body Is the Temple

For a five-sense experience, the body is the vehicle. It is the fine paint brush of the Is-Ness and is the form to which the soul attaches. Truly a precious creation, this temple is to be held in reverence. Appreciation, love, and respect for the body means that each individual will guard against degenerative conditions of the body, and strive to maintain health at the highest level possible.

Since this wonderful, adventure-filled reality is one of extreme duality, it potentially includes not only the passions and experiences of youthful vigor, but also the potential for body degeneration and associated negative experiences. One way to become a victim of the latter is to believe that Western medicine, based on science alone, can solve all problems that afflict the body.

The list of successes by scientific medicine is long and includes the ability to accomplish incredibly sophisticated diagnoses to treat successfully many dreaded diseases and infections, and to surgically repair a wide range of body injuries and birth defects. Another effect on the populace has been the acceptance that there is nothing for the individual to do except to keep the medical insurance premiums paid and see the doctor when a problem arises. This grave mistake has been aptly called by some the "passive patient syndrome." This belief is undesirable, because many are lured into not being responsible for the maintenance of their own bodies. They have transferred the responsibility to the quick-fix medical professionals. In our "pay as you go" society, these medical professionals actually benefit when a great part of the populace is less than healthy. The simple truth is that there is much that the individual can do to maintain youthful performance. The saying, "An ounce of prevention is worth a pound of cure," is quite appropriate.

To become more responsible and jump on the expanding spiral of health success, simply recognize that it is time to take personal action. Action is the key formula for life. That action is never too late. The body always wants to repair itself, and even "terminally ill" patients can and often do make the turn-around.

The reader is urged to read several books to get a feel for what personal action he can take. Start with References 41, 42, 43, 45, 46, or 48 at the end of the book. This will reveal the power of the mind and start you on a new road to discovering health. (See Note 6.)

Power of the Mind

The power of the mind cannot be over stressed. The Great Pyramid Society understood the spirit/mind/body connection and taught their descendants that a spiritual body surrounds the physical body. (See Figure 13.11.) When a physical illness manifests, there is a corresponding change in the spiritual body. The situation can change through proper nutrition, rest, exercise, meditation, and the use of herbs, but many times the process can be speeded up by a direct change to the spiritual body. A rearrangement of the Primal Energies can be facilitated by Energy practitioners, who are a source of this extra Energy.

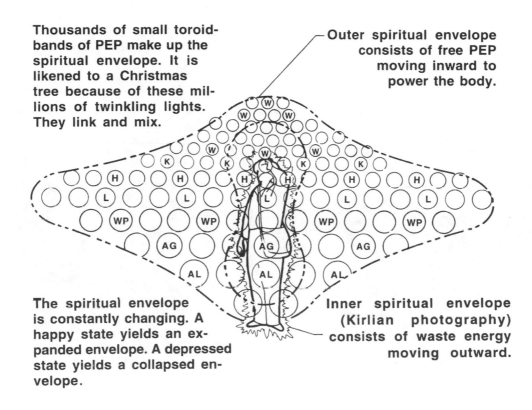

Thousands of small toroid-bands of PEP make up the spiritual envelope. It is likened to a Christmas tree because of these millions of twinkling lights. They link and mix.

Outer spiritual envelope consists of free PEP moving inward to power the body.

The spiritual envelope is constantly changing. A happy state yields an expanded envelope. A depressed state yields a collapsed envelope.

Inner spiritual envelope (Kirlian photography) consists of waste energy moving outward.

Figure 13.11 Details of the spiritual envelopes that surround the physical form.

An interesting example of this combining of two or more spiritual bodies and a demonstration of the principle, "by joining you are more," has been captured on photographic film in the courtyard of the temple of Dendara in Egypt. An impromptu Energy session attracted those waiting to board the tour bus and the resulting photograph (See Figure 10.2.) has resulted in much speculation. Since it was analyzed by NASA and found to have no overlays or evidence of trick photography, the apparent beam entering the woman's body at the throat chakra, considered by some the healing chakra, has led to speculation that the beam was a healing ray from a benevolent UFO. The fact that everyone is looking up at some object seems to reaffirm the notion.

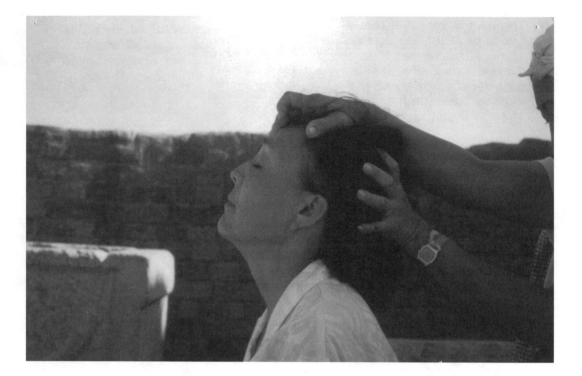

Figure 13.12 The Energy Practitioner is looking down here, but up in Figure 10.2.

Figure 13.12, however, shows the event from another angle and this helps clarify what actually was going on. In this photograph, the Energy Practitioner is looking down and has her hands in a different position, indicating that both her hands and her head were moving. Refering back to Figure 10.2, the three in the photograph were working together, consciously combining their Energy fields in an attempt to create a positive change in the woman suffering with a migraine headache. Because of their position on the planet, the history of the temple, and the effort of the three, a dense swirl of their chakric energy formed to such an intensity that it exposed the photographic film.

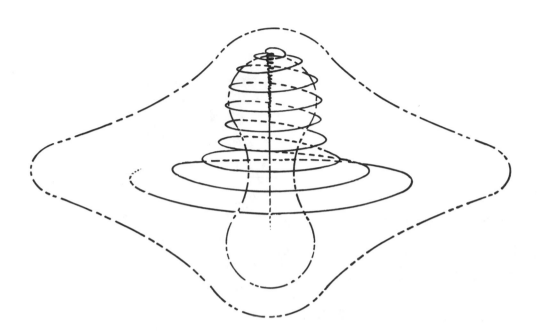

Figure 13.13 Within the complex spiritual envelope, W PEP can often form an inner spiral, a beam that shoots down to communicate with the other PEP.

The standing woman manipulated the scalp, causing a short circuit between the two of them, and this allowed the combined chakric energies to flow into the seated one. Primal Energy answers the command of human beings and, in this case, positive change occurred.

Figure 13.13 and 13.14 show details of the swirling vortex. The Allowance, Allegiance, Will and Power, Love, Harmony, and Knowledge toroids flow together upwards into Wisdom. The flow is cyclical, first up, then down. The Energy of Wisdom mushrooms out and flows downward, communicating with the other Energies on the way. The mysterious beam from above is actually the core of the intense vortex of Wisdom's downward spiral.

Notice that the light around the man is the extra light of his spiritual Energies joining the vortex. (See this in Figure 10.2.) Why the man is looking up is a function of the flow of Energy along his spinal column. In response to an intense energy flow, it is natural to hold your head in that position and then hold up one hand to reduce the intensity of the flow.

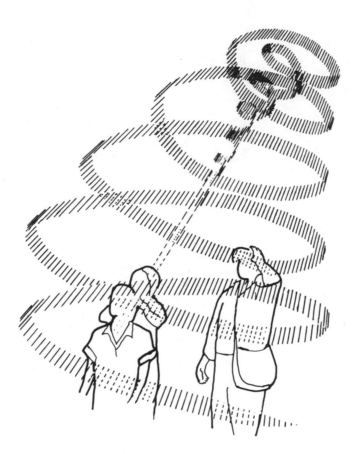

Figure 13.14 The beam from above is the core of the intense vortex of Wisdom's downward spiral.

What are the specific steps that occur during an Energy Session? Is reducing stress the basic function of the procedure? The physical body is dense, low-frequency Primal Energy and even the brain and the mind's thoughts are a dense formulation of Primal Energy and Consciousness. The body gets its hope to be a body from the Earth, and the energy to be a body from the Primal Energy realm. Its form comes from the low-frequency realm and its power, the Soul and Oversoul, from the high-frequency realm.

It is, of course, not like opening a bucket of molecules and one by one building a body and spirit. The process is complicated and beyond technical understanding because it involves the ten-dimensional realm impacting the three-dimensional physical plane. This is precisely the source of all psychic phenomena, the source of all placebo effects, and the source of all spontaneous remissions.

In a setting where two people align in the ten-dimensional realm and act with common purpose, an energy flow and sense of **faith** occurs. Essentially, the one that needs positive change has given up the purpose for the disease, and in one brief instant this celebration of life changes the body's response. What can be measured at the physical level is less constriction of the muscles, arteries, and capillaries. The endorphins flow the moment the change occurs in the neurological system. Soon the pain leaves and the person moves on.

A shaman can resolve many afflictions in this manner and coerce the one needing change by any number of methods to have pure and undeniable **faith** in the shaman's abilities. They all are valid, if they work. It is not that much different than the **faith** we in modern society give to a doctor. Everyone starts with that **faith**, and the doctors do set bones and administer antibacterial pills and other medication, but approximately 70 percent of what is achieved is because of our original **faith** that the doctor knows the healing process. We have **faith** that the doctor knows the right thing to do, and thus the harmony within our system does not fight against the positive change.

So too, the shaman begins by chanting and performing rituals that form a clarity of purpose and increases his **faith** in himself, as well as the patient's **faith** in him. In the process the shaman begins to get in touch with the Primal Energies. Perhaps he calls them by another name, but essentially he makes contact with the spiritual realm, at once realizing a mental out-of-body experience, and touching that membrane between the three-dimensional and the ten-dimensional realms. Then, with the patient willing, healing occurs. Like a dimension shift, a healing is always a two-step process. Step one is suspending the belief that it can't be done. Step two is to taking the first step towards it.

Does it always work? The shaman can not directly treat bones that cannot be properly lined up, nor directly treat huge bacterial infections. But, by relieving stress and calming the patient, the Shaman can speed the positive changes that will eventually come to the patient.

Sometimes investigators discover that strange sounds, movements, and appearances or disappearances that occur during the rituals are fabricated by an assistant. The shamanistic practices are thus branded as the work of charlatans and without value. This is a strange conclusion to the shaman and those cured, because the increase in **faith** quite often yields a cure. Statistical analysis of the claims is difficult. Medical doctors themselves will administer sugar pills and tell the patient there is nothing wrong when they encounter symptoms with no apparent physical cause. In effect they are relying on the same placebo affect that they accuse shamans of using.

Doctors do have a point with regard to certain forms of fast-growing cancers and virulent diseases that require quick attention. It is better to get an accurate diagnosis first. If a doctor's remedies fail, then at least alternative medical practices might yield a cure through the natural methods used by the shaman.

Now both the doctors and the shamans are claiming to be absolutely right. This is a clear example of the polarity that often occurs during a Transition. What needs to occur is for each side to see the benefit of the other, the wonder of diversity, and to work together to discover a balance point.

Any time there is a synergistic energy flow between two or more people who are allied with a common purpose, miraculous things can happen. This is because the ten-dimensional being that each human truly is, is almost unlimited. Releasing the true power of a human being is truly formidable.

The Energy Practitioner, however, must be of an evolved DNA makeup. The patient must be allowing and ready to receive energy to form positive change. The Energy

Practitioner's function is to help energy move from the low-frequency realm to the high-frequency realm. The physical act of touching forms a jumper circuit that connects with the high-frequency act of forming the purpose and intention of a change for the positive. That agreement is what forms a Chaos point. Once a Chaos point of a single piece of Chaos, or a complicated formulation of Chaos, exists, Primal Energy rushes in to fill it.

These Energy sessions are a balancing act between the three-dimensional reality of setting the purpose and intention, and the ten-dimensional reality that fulfills the creation. Cells will alter, endorphins will flow, and blood vessels will dilate. By whatever means, that gift of the ten-dimensional universe will always appear to be magic to humans. (See Note 6 for other sources, including Energy Practitioners.)

Clearing Meditation

By meditating, a person reaches a state where the Primal Energies can be perceived, and the world is very lovely. The techniques for reducing stress used by the Great Pyramid Society included the use of the breath during meditation. They understood that the human being is a relationship of light spiritual energy, or the soul, with dense energy, or the physical form.

Breath was the vital tool to reconnect with spirit. In the language of the Great Pyramid Society, the word for *breath* was the same as the word for *spirit*. Even today the word used for *breath* means *spirit* in several languages, including Greek, Hebrew, and Sanskrit. The breath is used in two types of meditation, the clearing meditation and the problem-solving meditation.

The clearing meditation is used to relax, blow away the chaos of the day, enrich the blood supply with Oxygen, and reconnect to spirit. The clearing meditation gets one in touch with the energies and should be done at least once a day to reduce stress. It should always be done before the problem-solving meditation is attempted, because it is important to be in touch with the Primal Energies before asking questions.

Each of the Primal Energies swirls toroid fashion around the human body and then spirals into and concentrates in the body at different locations. The center of that is the Energy Center or, in the ancient terminology, a chakra. The chakra for Allowance is at the base of the spine. The chakra for Allegiance is the sacral area, which is near the belly button. The chakra for Will and Power is the solar plexus. The chakra for Love is the heart. The chakra for Harmony is the throat. The chakra for Knowledge is the middle of the forehead. The chakra for Wisdom is the top of the head. These chakras are explained in much detail in a book called *The Tool*. (See Resources at the end of Chapter 13.)

The specific method for the clearing meditation has evolved from techniques others have found useful. Here is part of one method. Begin by finding a comfortable position that will allow your back to be straight. The two positions are lying down on your back with the knees bent or in a lotus-type position; both will help to keep the spine straight.

Breathe inward to Energy Allowance. Ask for Allowance to come to you in full strength.

Breathe inward deeply. While breathing out, release your small fears, angers and tensions, and relax yourself into contemplation.

Breathe inward to Energy Allegiance, that it may strengthen all of the sexual organs and endocrine organs within you, and blow away the chaos.

Breathe inward to Energy Will and Power to strengthen the muscles, bones, and connective tissue. Breathe away from you the chaos in those areas.

Breathe inward to Energy Love to strengthen the heart, lungs, veins and capillaries within you. Blow away from you all disturbances to them.

Breathe inward to Energy Harmony to form the most perfect balance to your immune system. Blow away from you all diseases.

Breathe inward to Energy Knowledge to strengthen you to know all, to remember all without fear. Blow away from you all disturbances.

Breathe inward to Energy Wisdom that your mind may be clear in imagining and visualizations. Blow away from you any disturbances and chaos.

Breathe at least seven breaths to each of these Energy Center. Or breathe until the body tells you to wait, hold a breath, then wait, and feel the Primal Energy come to you. By the time all seven centers have been addressed a relaxed state is normally achieved. Occasionally it is necessary to repeat the steps, but eventually a subtle connection to the Energies is felt within and all around the body. The clearing meditation is so invigorating that emotional states can be changed dramatically in as little as five or ten minutes. Do it at least once a day.

Fire Breath Meditation

If there is no time for a complete clearing meditation, a much shorter version can be used to get centered between events. This is called the fire breath. Breath out very fast and forcefully seven times. Then pause for a moment. When ready, repeat the seven breaths. If time permits, try to finish a sequence of seven. It is best to start another event with a pleasant sensation within the body, which this allows. Remember, the quickest way to change your emotional state is to blow out forcefully (develop this as a silent technique if facing an angry person), and let the breath fall in. Do it with connected breaths.

Problem Solving Meditation

Once relaxed, with the Energies pulsing in body and spirit, a little more time can be taken to solve the problems that cause stress. For problem solving, another element added to the meditation is a question and answer period. Primal Consciousness looks down through the many splits and experiences this emotional realm through the eyes of human consciousness. Primal Consciousness and Energy always observe positive and negative emotional creations equally without judgment.

Human beings need not be burdened with a continuous path of chaos and can take steps to move to a joyous, harmonious path. The transition can be made by using the problem solving meditation in which a particular facet of a fear, an anger, or any imaginable problem is addressed to Primal Consciousness in a particular order. First, Wisdom is asked to show the fear or anger. It is presented to Allowance to show that fear in clarity, without judgment of you or others. Remove the right or wrong and you have released the fear, and it can be changed if desired.

The process continues and uses all the Energy centers in order. The answer from one is presented to the next Energy for correction, clarification, or for an entirely new focus. The process is described in great detail by an excellent manual, *The Tool*, written by Larry Hawes. The process is clearly and simply presented and there is even a work section in the back of the manual. The author and several students of the process assure those trying it for the first time that it is well worth the effort, because the internal dialogue that is a constant menace may finally be resolved. As the manual suggests: "there is no right way to do it. While it is possible not to do it, it is not possible to do it wrong. Just do it." (See Resources at the end of this chapter.)

Recreational Remote Viewing Meditation

Not all meditation is used for stress reduction or problem solving. Remote viewing, if done with intent to enhance the common bond and good will of humanity, can be an added joy to the thrill of incarnation. In as little as two heart beats one can travel to a distant planet and bring back enough information to write a book. For the tools to remote view contact Balance Productions. (See Resources at the end of this chapter.)

For Conflict Resolution, Address Harmony

When the Great Pyramid Society originally formed, it was ruled by a triumvirate of which one member was a woman. While her name and its spelling has been altered through the eons, she is often referred to by the name Isis. Like none other at the time, she possessed the quality of harmony and endeavored to strike the chord of harmony in everyone.

It was that superhuman effort that led to her appointment on the ruling committee. The word Isis actually meant harmony and was a conscious reference to the Primal Energy, Harmony. The concept of harmonious relations and the Primal Energy Harmony, as well as the other Primal Energies, was passed on from parent to child, from child to grandchild. In time, as the generations began to mix with the original population of Earth, the acceptable way to teach the Primal Energies was to call them gods. Harmony was considered the god that ruled the world. When one is in agreement with Harmony, then things work. Isis, then, was the one to pray to and ask for help in getting along with others.

The concept point of the Blessed Virgin Mary is also that of Harmony, and the ability to harmonize all things together. Appearances or channelings of the Blessed Virgin Mary in recent years are the physical manifestations of a ten-dimensional reality, one primarily of Harmony. (See Note 7.) That ten-dimensional reality is an Akashic Record of all that ever lived in harmony. It is at once a great library, a giant corporation, and a collection of millions of intellects pooling knowledge to give the best answer to the question: how does one live in harmony under prevailing conditions? In our predominantly Christian society, the popular name for the vibration of Harmony would be the Blessed Virgin Mary. In even more ancient times, this energy was know by other names.

Conclusion

At the expense of achieving a focus into the three-dimensional reality, many dimensions are left behind and forgotten. This three-dimensional realm is, in a sense, a dimension of not-knowing. Each person has a perception that what is seen is all there is to the universe, because it is the only thing that can be changed. Because of this, modern humans have tended to manifest with their hands and not with their minds. It is perceived that this is the most reliable method.

The fixation with doing has led to the widespread use of technology and the abandonment of prayer. Especially in Western civilization, medical procedures have become "high tech" and totally scientific, but in some remote locations there does exist "low tech" medicine that works well enough. Increasingly, the wisdom of using both is being seen as the best path. Add meditation and responsible maintenance by proper diet and exercise, and the body will be strengthened to survive the turbulence of the Transition. In all things, avoid the polarities, strive for the balance point.

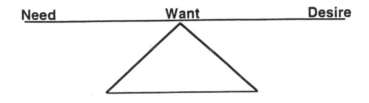

Figure 13.15 Strive for the middle ground.

NOTES

1. Unlike the format used in this book, sacred geometry, the silent language or language of light, was used in those days to teach metaphysics. Primal Consciousness enclosed itself within a tetrahedron (straight lines = male aspect) which spins on three axes forming a sphere (curved lines = female aspect). The sphere is represented in classes as a circle. The first movement of creation was along the axes of spin, from the center of the sphere to the surface. This is depicted as two overlapping circles. The center of the second circle is on the circumference of the first circle as shown here in Figure 13.16.

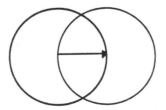

Figure 13.16 The first movement forms the lens-shaped Vesica Pisces.

The overlapping region, the "Vesica Pisces," forms slowly. As it evolves, there is initially one point of awareness, then more, eventually an infinite number, within that single Vesica Pisces. Also, the lens-shaped Vesica Pisces can be outlined by a rectangle to demonstrate an amazing mathematical property. The interesting rectangle has been called the Golden Mean Rectangle.

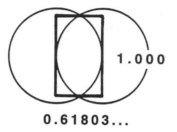

Figure 13.17 The Golden Mean Rectangle fits precisely around the Vesica Pisces.

The ratio of the width/length for the Vesica Pisces and the Golden Mean Rectangle is always Phi = 0.61803..., the magic number introduced in earlier chapters. Each place of self-awareness, a complete life and existence in itself, is represented by the turns in the endless spiral within the Golden Mean Rectangle.

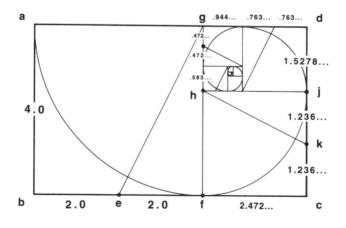

Figure 13.18 An **endless** Logarithmic Spiral fits within the Golden Mean Rectangle.

Consider the Golden Mean Rectangle shown in Figure 13.18. See square abfg. Start at point b and travel along line bf to point e. Notice that line be is the midpoint or one-half of the side of the square abfg. From point e move diagonally to point g. Swing the diagonal eg down using e as the pivot point and g will rest exactly on point c, the corner of the Golden Mean Rectangle.

Any size square, for example cjhf, can be the basis for yet another Golden Mean Rectangle. Using the same method, start at the corner point c, and travel along line cj to point k, the midpoint. Notice that line ck is one-half of the side of the square cjhf. Take the diagonal kh, and swing it using point k as the pivot and h will rest exactly on point d. Notice that the process can be continued to form smaller and smaller Golden Mean Rectangles.

A "Logarithmic Spiral" is formed by drawing a series of radial arcs. Start at point a and draw a quarter circle with point g as the center, and end the curve at point f. Repeat the process once again using point h as the center of a smaller quarter circle from point f to point j. This can be done over and over and forms an **endless**, logarithmic spiral, as is shown in Figure 13.18. The value 0.618..., phi, also is representative of the Fibernachi Series, found in sea shells, plants, and in all living things, if one looks closely enough. Some plants, for example, grow one leaf, then one more, then two, then three, then five, etc. The series is: 1, 1, 2, 3, 5, 8, 13, 21, 34, etc. Notice that the next number in the series always equals the sum of the previous two: $3 + 5 = 8$, $5 + 8 = 13$, etc. If you divide any two sequential numbers you get a value very close to the magic 0.618. The larger the numbers, the more accurate this becomes: $2/3 = .666$, but $21/34 = 0.6177$.

The secret to understanding why all of this apparent magic is found interrelated in everything, is knowing that the Primal Energies are related by the value 0.618. The length of W, plus the length of K, equals the length of H or some harmonic thereof. The length of K, plus the length of H, equals the length of L. This continues all the way to AL. It is in the solid form of everything, as well as the energy flow of everything.

At the two sharp ends of the Vesica Pisces, Creation asks again: "What am I" and these locations become the center of two more circles. The process continues until there are seven circles, the "Seed of Life," as shown in Figure 13.19. Each circle represents one of the Primal Energies. Chaos is the paper that the geometry is drawn on.

2. The teaching of combinational creations, ever-expanding, unending, harmonious, and self-cleansing, was taught in sacred geometry by adding to the above Seed of Life. Each intersection of circles not yet used as the center of a circle was so used, developing another "rotation" — now there are a total of thirteen circles as shown in 13.20.

The idea can be continued and more rotations of circles are added. Each stage of development has a particular name, like the Fruit of Life, the Flower of Life, and so on. Each stage of development is used to give a teaching. Notice that the rotations could continue forever, much like the creations of the Is-Ness. The Flower of Life is found on temple walls in all corners of the world and is shown as 13.21.

Another symbol found throughout the world is designed from the Flower of Life. It is called the Tree of Life, Figure 13.22, and is made up of straight lines that are either the width or length of the Vesica Pisces. The starting or ending point for each line is the center of one of the circles of the Flower of Life.

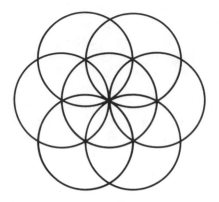

Figure 13.19 The Seed of Life. Each circle is one of the Primal Energies. The paper they are drawn on is the eighth, Chaos.

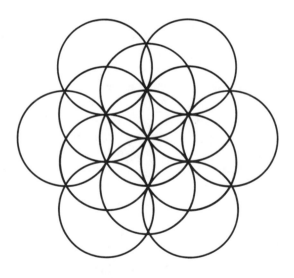

Figure 13.20 Thirteen circles are formed after the next "rotation." Isn't it remarkable that there are thirteen chakra Energy Centers to the physical form — seven major, five minor, and one unifier.

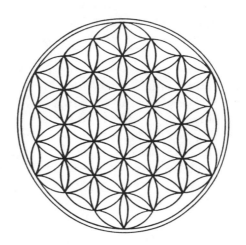

Figure 13.21 The Flower of Life.

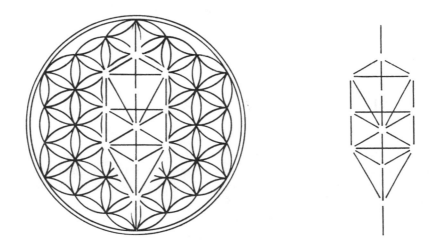

Figure 13.22 Tree of Life, and the Tree of Life superimposed over the Flower of Life.

3. The true base of the Great Pyramid is a contested matter. Some researchers consider it to be the base of the sockets or the base of the pavement blocks. Still others maintain that it is the top of the pavement. (See Reference 31 and Reference 5.) The truth is that the true base of the Great Pyramid is the top of the pavement.

4. Another variation of the symbol is to enlarge and give definition to the crossover point, thus it becomes a circle. This gives proper representation to the energy of Love which stands at the juncture of the Is-Ness and the Is-Not-Ness and gives definition

to all things. (See Figure 13.23.) To give individual definition to the other Energies on each side of the circle, partitioning lines can be added. Each enclosed space represents one of the Primal Energies and Consciousness with Chaos represented by the medium upon which the drawing is made.

The reasoning behind the symbols, however, was not to endure. In time, by reasons of their own desire, and eventually by the force of cataclysmic circumstances, the children of the Great Pyramid Society began to merge with the original population of Earth, degenerating the teaching.

The offspring of the offspring became less and less able to comprehend the concept of "energy" in general, much less Primal Consciousness and Primal Energy, and so it was explained that the Primal Energies were effectively gods. The compartments formed by the partitioning lines of Figure 13.23 were stylized to be feathers, with each feather representing not a Primal Energy, but a god.

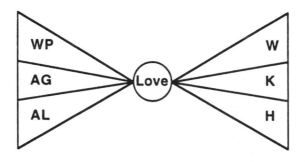

Figure 13.23 All Primal Energies are represented by regions of equal areas

It is easy to see how the binder and separator of all the Energies and all the creations, Love, could be thought to be the organizer, or the principal god, the divine one. It is easy to see how more gods — feathers — could be added to the original symbol.

Col. James Churchward, in his *The Lost Continent of Mu*, Reference 44, gives an excellent list of ancient symbols and his own interpretation of them as well as the interesting story of how he found them. Most of these are the result of retelling the story of the basic infinity symbol. The ancient Egyptian symbol with the divine eye at the center and multiple feathers is a direct re-interpretation of the original infinity symbol. It is not a great leap to see the Egyptian symbol evolving into another symbol which emerged in the middle ages. It has become the popular symbol, decoration, and comforter of today, the cherub: an angelic face, floating on its feathered wings. (See Figure 13.24.)

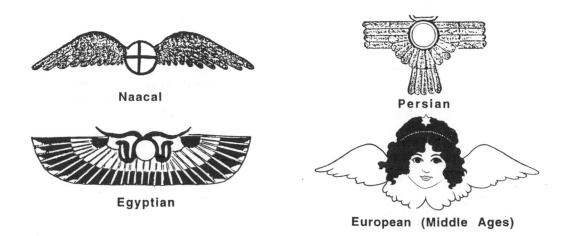

Naacal

Persian

Egyptian

European (Middle Ages)

Figure 13.24 There were many versions of the eye or face of god surrounded by the feathers of the lesser gods (winged circles to some). By the Middle Ages it had become the cherub, a familiar icon even today.

5. The teaching to the children of the children continued for many millennial. However, due to Earth shiftings and the resulting wandering of the vortex, the power of the Great Pyramid dwindled. At present, the experience one feels is very minimal and occurs only during a short period each year. The initiation became one that involved the use of drugs because of the power shift and the fact that as the population began to assimilate the original people of Earth, the character and mental power of the individual mind changed. The drugs were similar to what was used by Imhotep. (See Chapter 12.) The out-of-body experience yielded similar results compared to the electromagnetic shift and the initiated became the priests of the day.

6. Alternate medicine advocates argue about what is dangerous to the human immune system. Books now abound regarding the true horrors of benzene products, parasites, EMF poisoning, and sometimes include isopropyl alcohol. What's the truth?

Protection from Chemicals

Isopropyl alcohol is not the problem. Benzene, found in ordinary gasoline, is the problem. The Ph content of isopropyl alcohol will kill any aerobic or anaerobic bacteria and it is appropriate to use alcohol to sterilize instruments. It can even be used occasionally to kill pathogens that live in the skin. Overusing rubbing alcohol results in skin that is dry and scaling. This psoriasis-like condition is the result of the alcohol dissolving away all of the body's oil that is vital to the health of the skin. Even the fumes from alcohol are not dangerous unless they are breathed for a long time.

Benzene, however, is toxic in liquid and in vapor form. The body does not know how to cope with it. Benzene on its own is the irritant that causes mutation. The body easily absorbs the benzene through the skin or more commonly through the lungs (vapors at the self-serve gas pump) and the cells that try to assimilate the organic benzene (and many other petrochemical molecules made in the distillation process) become stricken with nuclear damage. It is not parasites, but the absorption of toxic benzene that greatly weakens the immune system and causes cancer. If a study were done, it would show a relationship between high incidence of cancer and self-serve gas stations. What is really needed at the gas pump is a service man fitted with a toxic suit that included protective gloves and a charcoal filter respirator. Until then, the individual should at least use plastic gloves and stand upwind of the fumes. Respirators with activated charcoal filters (painters use them — $35.00) are available at hardware stores.

Tiny parasites remain in partially cooked foods, but are easily dealt with by the body. They can be controlled by many common herbs, including parsley, grape juice, and Pau D'Arco tea. The herb formulas used in Hulda Regehr Clark's books, *The Cure for All Cancers* and *The Cure for HIV and AIDS* are not necessarily inappropriate, but used for a long enough time can do damage. The black walnut tincture, if taken daily for an extended time, can be as lethal as taking arsenic. The body has to deal with all of these herbs and get rid of them and that is a burden to the very immune system that is trying to be protected. For this reason, the kidney and gall bladder treatments outlined in the book should not be undertaken by healthy individuals seeking to maintain good health. The extreme formulations should be reserved for the desperate with severe symptoms who are running out of time.

In general, products made from glass or wood are inert to the physical body. Things made from animal products are permeable to the body. Anything that is a combination of the distillation of petroleum into a product that has both organic and inorganic material is capable of being assimilated by the body and is dangerous to it.

Study the composition of products and avoid the toxic ones. A poignant example, "X"..., a petroleun jelly product, is assimilated by the skin, and it contains enough petrochemicals (reads "Petrolatum" on the label) to burden the immune system. Instead, use a natural product like a combination of pure water, vegetable glycerin, and a pinch of ascorbic acid. (Refer to the formulas in Dr. Clark's book for this, it is a treasure. See Reference 42.) The use of "X" and mineral oils containing petrochemicals as a lubricant for sexual enhancement is having a devastating effect on the populace. Small cuts and areas of skin rashes are openings for the petrochemical oils to come in contact with the blood supply. Once these molecules have entered the body in that way, the immune system is burdened with trying to deal with them.

Protection from Electromagnetic Force

A new device is available that encourages the cells to pay attention to a harmonizing frequency and to ignore the 60 cps electromagnetic force (EMF) disturbance. If an individual must work in an environment laced with EMF fields, the use of the device is encouraged. The Clarus Environmental System is available at various suppliers including Balance Productions. (See "Resources" at the end of this chapter.)

Other Resources

When traditional medicine does not resolve a problem and/or if one is concerned with staying in peak performance, then it may be wise to consult with practitioners of alternative medicine. While alternative methods are often referred to as alternative medicine, there is a growing movement to change the terminology to complimentary medicine, implying these compliment rather than replace traditional methods. This expression demonstrates the balance that will enable us to live more harmoniously during the Transition.

Academy for Guided Imagery
P.O. Box 2070
Mill Valley, Calif0rnia 94942

American Academy of Osteopathy
POB 750
Newark, Ohio 43055
614-349-8701

American Association of Acupuncture and Oriental Medicine
1424 16th Street N.W., Suite 501
Washington, D.C., 20036

American Association of Naturopathic Physicians
P.O. Box 2579
Kirkland, Washongton 89083-2579
206-827-6035

American Chiropractic Association
1701 Clarendon Boulevard
Arlington, Virginia 22209

American Holistic Medical Association
4101 Lake Boone Trail, Suite 201
Raleigh, North Carolina 27607
919-787-5146

American Society of Clinical Hypnosis
2250 East Devon Avenue, Suite 336
Des Plaines, Illinois 60018

Ayurvedic Medicine and Health Center
679 George Hill Road
P.O. Box 344
Lancaster, Massachusetts 01523

Biofeedback Certification Institute of America
10200 West 44th Avenue, Suite 304
Wheat Ridge, Colorado 80033

Feldenkrais Guild
14 Corporate Woods
8717 West 110th Street, Suite 140
Overland Park, Kansas 66210

Homeopathic Educational Services
2124 Kittredge Street
Berkeley, California 94704
415-649-0294

Rolfing Institute
P.O. Box 1868
Boulder, Colo. 80306

Trager Institute
10 Old Mill Street
Mill Valley, California 94941

Resources

Earlyne Chaney of Astara channels entities from the ten-dimensional realm of Harmony. Among them are Khutumi, Isis, and the Blessed Virgin Mary. The address for Astara, the Institute for Psychic Learning, is given in Reference 10 at the end of the book.

For a complete source of Yahweh tapes, transcriptions, the Yahweh newsletter, and books, including *The Tool* by Larry Hawes, contact:

Balance Productions
P.O. Box 1681
Vista, California 92085

For products that neutralize the stress and other negative effects of electromagnetic fields (EMF) while improving intuition and creativity, contact:

Clarus Systems Group
1130 Calle Cordiller, Suite 102
San Clemente, California 92673

For professional breath-work therapy, conflict resolution, and alternate life understanding, contact:

Boni Light
Phone: (714) 487-5138

THE FUTURE
Chapter Fourteen
Synopsis

The rediscovery of technology by this society with its emphasis on energy has allowed us to grasp the Primal Energies better than any civilization for thousands of years. The alien visitors have been using Primal Energy directly for millions of years and are watching us wake up to it. During the Transition we will become increasingly aware of the presence of the ET visitors. The benign intent of the Traders is obvious when it is realized that they terra-formed this planet millions of years ago, and repositioned the moon to allow more life forms to thrive on Earth. The Traders visit humans in three ways: four-dimensional visits, three-dimensional visits without movement, and three-dimensional visits with movement. The purpose is to monitor fear, observe DNA changes during the Transition, or gather eggs and sperm. Women who have remembrances of the spaceships and to whom are presented newborns that are more alien than human, are not witnessing crossbreeding. It is an effort to communicate. "Do humans understand that caring for these offspring is a sacred undertaking? What we are doing is making certain that the Earth humans we care for, love, and want to protect, have offspring, and that life goes on. We have visited and have successfully taken genetic material. Here in this dream-state visit, know that the effort has realized fruit and sacred life has been born. This is why we visit and do what we do, to carry on life." The dark thoughts are not in the minds of the aliens, but in the minds of the unaware evolving humans. Cattle mutilations are 85 percent military, the testing of a sonic weapon that boils blood. Some cattle and goats who get viruses and are several days from death are studied by ETs who are cataloging new viruses during the Transition. The purpose of the Traveler ETs is to study and do research, not to help or hinder. In all, there were eighteen pyramids built around the planet. Many are completely buried or hidden by jungle growth. One of them will soon be discovered and unearthed. The hall of records under the Sphinx will soon be found. When humans learn to control their fear, consider themselves equal to the aliens, and learn to cooperate, they too will be allowed to travel among the stars. The first step is to change the hostile intent we have regarding the aliens. The Star Wars space-based defense system, SDI, was aimed at the aliens because we misunderstood their purpose and intent. Let us proceed with cooperation in our heart and use SDI as defense of national borders with the hope that it can soon be dismantled. Nemesis did not go away. It is headed on a trek through the inner planets. It will pass nearest the Earth in the year 2012. The best defense against Nemesis is to live a balanced life with love and cooperation in your heart. Our ten-dimensional nature is actually connected to the sun. If enough of us are united in the balanced way of living life, the output of the sun will change. The sun will alter its output in a way to "air-brake" Nemesis's path into a benign trek through the inner planets.

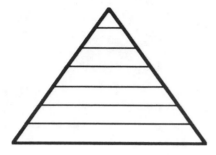

Chapter Fourteen

NEMESIS

The Immediate Future and the Possible End of the World

The Future

The future, at the instant of its realization, becomes part of the past. With only half of the Transition manifested, we have yet to glimpse what the final stages will be like. Earth-shaking events and startling new knowledge will be revealed and become part of the accepted history of the Earth in the next century. The year 2012 will mark the end of the coming major changes.

The Source

Fortunately for humans, a channeled source reveals itself every 200 hundred years or so, capable of disseminating the information and missing perspective to those willing to listen. Not everyone need know about the overview, since most will gain knowledge by direct interaction with life and experience the teaching as it integrates into their cells. In essence, that constantly updates them. Neither form of experience is better than the other, simply different.

The entity behind the channeled source has described itself differently than ever before. It describes itself as one of the eight Primal Energies with a consciousness of its own. The term *energy* was used this time to honor the Earth human's growing understanding of the universe and the laws that govern it.

In the past two hundred years, science has been able to refine the understanding of the laws that govern the three-dimensional reality we exist in. Even without reading these laws in a physics text book, there is now a common understanding that **energy** is needed to get **work** done. That **energy** applied over a period of time is the **power** that gets the job done.

We now understand that at the root of everything is **energy**. **Energy** cannot be created or destroyed, it can only be converted from one form to another. We have every-day practical examples of this important fact. Energy moves into the electric coffee maker and the result is hot coffee. The **energy** in one gallon of gasoline moves a heavy car ten miles, or a light car forty miles. The term **energy** is even used to describe our state of physical fitness. "How's your **energy** level?" — "It's really up. I'll easily get the job done."

This advancement of understanding has allowed the entity behind the channeled source to use more accurate terminology. No longer is it necessary to consider the source as the "One God," or the "many gods," or the "Holy Spirit entering through the chakric system." In the future, huamnity will accept the source for what it is: Primal Consciousness and Primal Energy. All observable and non-observable creations are composed of Primal Energy and Primal Consciousness.

Eventually it will be understood that Transitions are a regular part of the structure of the universe. Traveling ever closer to the speed of light eventually requires infinite energy because, by Einstein's equation, one's ship would become infinitely massive. If one could pass through the speed of light barrier into the dimensional space on the other side, one would enter instantaneously into a different frequency and concept of the universe. The lumbering, massive space ship would appear to transform into a minuscule subatomic particle. Instead of seeming hopelessly compacted, space would appear to be infinitely expansive. The beginning is the end, and the end is the beginning; what is above is below, and what is below is above. Transitions are just like that, and most people reading this will experience a great time shift. Not only will scientists detect time shifts, it will seem more and more difficult to accomplish a task in the allotted time. In the end, by the year 2012, there will be a period of missing time, a full twelve hours will apparently vanish. The midnight darkness will suddenly be the bright noon sunshine. Each person will see life as having limitless possibilities.

In the coming future, the resonate nature of gravity/anti-gravity will be realized, allowing the construction of machines that will provide deep space exploration. It will soon be realized that 30 percent of the bursts of energy, currently a mystery for scientists studying the origin of "gamma ray bursts," are not simply collisions of distant celestial objects, or even the stepping down in energy of high-energy subatomic events. They are instead the result of the great SMS of the Traders shifting from the third- to the fourth-dimension and back again. This excess energy travels either at 90 degrees or 45 degrees from the original direction of its source.

The Traders — Purpose of the Traders

Although it is difficult for earthbound humans to comprehend, the Traders have been trading for at least 500 million years. Their existence is much longer than that, and because of the factor of four error in the current method of scientific dating, events that we consider occurred two billion years ago, such as atmospheric Earth changes, are events that the Traders have had a hand in. Terra, forming and consequent seeding is their major creative effort. They constantly monitor the life forms after cataclysms, help by fine tuning the atmosphere, bringing new seed, and occasionally by genetic manipulation to insure that life forms with a marginal chance of surviving will adapt to the new conditions.

The fear running rampant in some circles on Earth portrays the Traders as cold, heartless, emotionless demons, at best robots controlled by a distant master mind, and possessing no spiritual qualities of any sort. Having observed Earth humans for some time, some people think that the Traders have realized they are missing out, and so, instead of being here to steal our oil, coal, boron, or uranium, they are here to steal that precious little piece of us that is lacking in them. They want to be "whole" again, so they are cutting us up, and doing all sorts of experiments to find that missing piece that will supposedly give them an emotional state of love and spiritual perfection. As humanity becomes more aware of the presence of the Traders, it will become obvious that they intend no harm. Their primary purpose is to insure the continuation of living things, and that is all. Although Earth humans and many of the sentient beings on other planets would disagree about the equality of life, the Traders consider **all life to be equal**.

The Traders do what they do without regard for the populations they interact with, and with respect to Earth they are not here to save humanity as we would understand. Like elsewhere, they are simply preserving life forms of the Is-Ness, all life forms. They do not actively become involved in the affairs of society to "help," other than to observe if the species is able to cope genetically with their environment. They do this throughout the universe and each planet that has been seeded by the Traders is protected against invasion by any other sentient beings that would harm life-forms. It is against the very nature of the Traders to have any malevolent intent on the societies of Earth. The fruits of the Traders proves this.

Terra-Forming

To achieve their goal of preserving all living things of the Is-Ness, the Traders found it necessary to have planets at their disposal with slightly different atmospheres to best match the yet-to-be-placed living organism. An atmosphere primarily of Hydrogen and Helium (similar to Jupiter) can be changed by impacting the planet with large comets and asteroids containing sulfur dioxide. (Since the Traders can harness the power of black holes, directing asteroids is easy for them.) The sulfur dioxide breaks down in the Hydrogen atmosphere and the result is water and some Oxygen. That is just one example of the many processes that they do to prepare the planets. Carbon-based organisms, like ourselves, require an atmosphere with the correct Oxygen ratio — an imbalance could be reactive. In the case of the Earth, sulfur bubbled to the surface naturally, but other fine tuning of the atmosphere has come about by direct Trader manipulation. The most obvious change to help the biosphere support life was changing the orbit of the Moon.

Repositioning the Moon

That the Moon was repositioned can be logically shown. A perfect square is defined as a rectangle with all four sides equal in length and all corner angles equal to 90 degrees. The only possible difference between squares is the length of the sides. All perfect squares have diagonals that have precisely predetermined lengths exactly 1.414213562... times the length of a side. As earlier chapters have shown, the base of the Great Pyramid was designed around the perfect square with each side equal to 750 Great

Pyramid feet. Consequently each diagonal is 750 x 1.414213562, or 1,060.660 Great Pyramid feet. Converting to inches (twelve inches to a foot) yields, 12 x 1,060.660 = 12,727.922 Great Pyramid inches in the diagonal. Thus the sum of the two diagonals is 25,456 Great Pyramid inches. Astronomers and physicists recognize this value immediately as being nearly the precession of the Earth, in terms of years. This fact happens to set one G.P. inch equal to one year of Earth history. (See Note 14.1)

This might at first appear to be an improbable coincidence. If the designers had the intention to define time with the perimeter of the square base representing the rate of angular rotation every two seconds (which is the perimeter of the Great Pyramid laid out at the equator), then the length of the diagonals and any relation to the precession of the Earth would be entirely coincidental. There is only one explanation for the coincidence, the rate of precession of the Earth was made to coincide with this measurement, and that was accomplished by the Traders.

Another overlapping coincidence is the length of a day on the Moon. The Great Pyramid, as already shown in Chapter Five, has many harmonious numbers designed into it. It apparently is written in the key of twelve, along with the harmonic 360. These numbers appear over and over. The Moon of planet Earth apparently faces the Earth all of the time, and astronomers have correctly noted that the Moon is "gravity locked." (During the cooling of the original molten Moon, the magnetic effect of the presence of nearby Earth caused some of the ferrous core to cool, predominately closer to Earth and slightly off center, so the heavier side always faced the Earth.) The scientists, however, never seem to place any significance on the fact that the Moon day and Earth day are different by a factor of 30.

The Moon day is 720 hours long, or 360 x 2, or 12 x 30 x 2, so the orbit and rotation of the Moon is designed in the same "key of twelve, with the harmonic of 360." There is no absolute reason for the Moon to be the distance from the Earth that it is, but the distance determines the orbital period, so change the distance to the Moon and the length of the Moon day changes.

This is not mathematical entertainment. The practical reason, as will be seen, is that the Moon's position is the most favorable for life to flourish here on the mother planet. Secondly, when the rhythm is correct for life forms it is also right for pyramids. The Moon is part of the Great Pyramid power generator. The Moon's orbit causes great gravitational changes on the Earth, this gravitational force causes a bending moment in the outer casing crystals of the Great Pyramid, and this results in a piezoelectric energy flow. Everything about the Great Pyramid was designed to naturally resonate at twelve cycles per second in order to extract the maximum power from the Earth and Moon. The Moon is part of the same machine and scheme, and the system has been fine tuned with the help of the Traders.

The gravitational lock of the Moon provides a convenient Earth monitoring base for the Traders. The far side is always hidden, and there is a portal to a Trader base located there.

Helping to Build the Great Pyramid

The Traders not only helped relocate the second wave to the Nile River region, but also supported them in many ways during the early years. From the Super Mother Ships (SMS), advanced tools were fabricated and delivered, and the power to run the tools was beamed to them until the project was finished and the new society was self-sufficient. Like a doctor monitoring the pulse and pressure of the heart, the Traders routinely map vortex positions on all of the planets. This knowledge provided the ideal location for the Great Pyramid, over the vortex at Cairo.

When a new species is placed on a planet, the first generation is never able to digest food grown there. That adaptation occurs in the second generation. In the case of this planet, the first had to be fed food manufactured on the Mother Ship. The special formula was delivered for the entire lifetime of the 10,000 member second-wave landing party. That nourishment has become known as manna from heaven.

Warning: Electromagnetic Pollution

The goal of the Traders is to wean a new species as soon as possible and to intercede only when extinction is imminent. This means that a species once placed can evolve for thousands of years and never have contact with the Traders at all. Our decision to use electrical energy as we do has caused the Traders to visit, contact the government, and inform humanity that the waves of energy are disturbing in two ways: First because alternating current is used instead of direct current, resulting in a wave form that propagates out and away from the planet in a way that ripples the sails, the sensitive power and detection systems of the Traders. This is not a grave problem, but the Traders and all the Travelers know that we are using electricity, and the curious may someday come to investigate.

Travelers are already here to study our evolving civilization. "Non-Travelers," by definition, still have the tendency to exploit lower animal forms. These Non-Travelers that harm the animals are not allowed to travel with the Traders and so there will be no disturbance from them. If the technology to travel from star to star were ever discovered by these Non-Travelers in the future, they could detect our radio waves and also come to investigate, which might be a problem for us.

Secondly, the alternating current ripples the cells of the human being and all other living things as well. In large doses this can cause certain forms of cancer to develop, as cells fatigue under this constant bombardment. The unit of measuring magnetic induction from alternating current is the gauss. At five gauss the signal is strong enough to be picked up by the Traders and the Travelers, and at this level some sensitive individuals are damaged by the radiating waveform. At 100 gauss, ten percent of the population would develop cancerous tumors after 200 hours of continuous exposure. In contrast there are those who, even at 100 gauss, would not be affected at all.

The Traders have notified the government of this fact, and informed them that a test can be developed to determine if an individual is at risk. As a result, there is a movement on Earth to inform humanity to keep a safe distance from electrical devices because the field weakens dramatically with distance. (At twice the distance there is one fourth the disturbance. At three times the distance there is one ninth the disturbance. At four times the distance there is one sixteenth the disturbance.) Experiments are now being done to pinpoint the effects of periodic exposure and to learn how best to deal with the problem. The Clarus device can be used as a protection. (See Resources Chapter 13.) There are also two books on the subject worth reading by Dr. Robert O. Becker. (See Reference 46.)

Gate Keepers

There exists at present only one method to travel between the stars. To do so, a device is needed to sense the presence of individual gossamer tendrils of Primal Energy and to sense the presence of individual Primal Energy types. Only the ancient Traders have mastered such a device and this is part of their great "Sails." For the foreseeable future, such equipment will remain pure magic to humanity and most other budding Travelers of the universe. Along with the Traders' sensing device, another machine similar to a super computer is needed to remember where everything is. Since everything is constantly moving, it is a task that has only been mastered by the communal mind of the Traders.

Traveling by sentient species other than the Traders, is only allowed once a species has attained a high degree of self-control and can live by the command: **Do not hurt the animals.** Since the gift of individual thought, the mind of the physical body, is essentially a complex formulation of Primal Energy, and since the Traders have devices that measure Primal Energy, all thoughts will ripple their sails. Negative thoughts trigger a sensor and they come to visit to see if it is natural or part of a pattern of primitive behavior. As an example, compare killing a frog to dissect it and learn anatomy and surgery skills to killing simply to inflict pain. The two operations, might look the same from the outside. The Traders, however, immediately know our intention, while we remain unaware of their visit because of its fourth-dimensional nature.

When a high degree of mastery is achieved, one naturally attains a level of vibration that allows the gateway to become visible. It does not resemble a portal to an elevator or an opening to a worm tube as some have suggested, but instead looks like a flying saucer type ship that becomes visible if it is in the area. All that is necessary is to walk on board and, of course, remember your place of origin. More will be given on this, but for now it is only important to realize that the gateway was built and maintained by the Traders, and has existed for hundreds of millions of years.

Genetic Dispersal

If one were a master of cosmic travel and considered all life equal, precious, and even sacred, it might follow that one would constantly guard against damage by natural phenomena, such as galactic collisions, super novas, and planet collisions, and be busy placing valued organisms from places of impending disaster to other places with a promise of longevity. The Traders actually do this all of the time, but the picture of how it is done does not fit the picture most humans would paint. Because it is not done in a method that fits the image and likeness of the human being, it seems beyond the concept of science, and the Traders are misunderstood. In the future, the motives of the Traders, as well as the three kinds of visiting that are done, will be recognized.

Fourth Dimensional Visiting

Here is a working model of creation. Imagine creation to be a large soap bubble. Somewhere within it are vaporous Oversouls capable of migrating around inside the bubble in joyous exploration. Sometimes they experience what is at the very center of the bubble, sometimes they meet others somewhere in the infinite area between that center and the surface of the bubble, and sometimes these souls visit at the surface of the soap bubble. Since the surface is the most dense part of the bubble, it is there a special feature exists. It's called "time." With time, one event follows another, so there is direction and space — height, width, and depth. There is the ability to observe things in a new way with one event following another, which is also what allows for individual creativity to happen. By dipping into that dense, slow moving realm, however, there is an illusion that the film-like surface of the soap bubble is all that exists, and the rest of the soap bubble becomes invisible.

Technically it has already been shown that this happens by quick dips into the Is-Not-Ness and then back into the Is-Ness trillions of times per second, creating the illusion of the Now experience of the three-dimensional reality. The rest of the ten dimensions are only known with a distant intellectual understanding.

During sleep or meditation, there is a release of the subjective mind and its perception that the individual is the only reality. Where one goes at this time is somewhere within the bubble where the soul can have visitations and make friendly agreements. This communication place, or thought communication, is virtually the same way the Traders communicate with each other. Humans can actually have visits there from the Traders, and visit as much as others visit in return. Little of this is remembered. The visitations with the greatest impact are those in the physical realm, and sometimes fourth-dimensional agreements are made to meet the Traders in the physical realm as part of the plan to preserve the living forms of the Is-Ness. These agreement events are sometimes remembered and sometimes not. Sometimes one is left with small anxieties.

Visitations and agreements to meet in the third-dimensional reality can be the grandest experience if one can be there without fear or judgment, but in cooperation with others. It is incredibly fulfilling and worth striving for. Many times the agreement is forgotten, however, and that is why stories of unwilling or incensed abductees originate. In other words, an implantation never takes place by force, they are all made through agreements.

Humans would like the communication to be done in a human image and likeness, but the Traders can only communicate in their way. The Traders can only assume that if the human species is truly sentient, then we will understand. By keeping in mind that the goal of the Traders is preservation of a new, emerging species, the Earth human, some of the things that we might interpret as damage to a human being, are not interpreted that way by the Traders. In truth, the so-called damage is not really damage, because a person only suffers from the loss of the expectation that the Traders would have asked, by phone call or letter at least, if this special service was wanted. The agreement actually was made, fourth-dimensional style, and was simply not remembered.

Three-Dimensional Visiting Without Movement

Another form of contact is an actual three-dimensional reality visit, which occurs when the Traders visit, then leave, while the Earth human remains in one location. The communication is actually a thought communication or silent mind linkage that is intense. There is a lot of information transferred during this mental process, and humans swear much more occurs than actually has happened. In later regression by trained hypnosis experts, the individuals relate stories of absolute realities. They state they were operated on, fertilized eggs were removed, cancer was fixed, and so on, but a medical examination will not reveal any physical proof of the events. Such is the power of the mental pictures that can be transferred by the Traders.

Three Dimensional Visiting with Movement

In another form of three-dimensional reality visit, the Traders actually take human beings to a ship. There are two purposes for these visits. The first purpose is to place monitoring devices, the second is for genetic dispersal. Since this style of visit is the most interesting and is the cause for the most confusion, some detail will be given.

Monitoring the range of emotions of human beings in particular, the version of fear found here on Earth, is of great interest to the Traders. Human fear is of great concern. If our society were to project the fear that we have of each other onto them, in the future humanity would attack the Traders.

They are quite able to defend themselves from any attack from the children of Earth. Since they monitor our intentions all of the time they would simply sidestep any attack. They would simply go fourth-dimensional and return after the missiles had passed. Even if all of our nuclear arsenal could be unleashed against the hull of one SMS, the effect would be far from destructive. Their large ships are designed to withstand the energy density and pressures that exist in the center of suns. They would let the black-hole, antimatter skin of their SMS absorb our missles, beam weapons or whatever we could throw at them. The Traders would simply incorporate that energy and would be that much longer before they needed to gather fuel.

If that were to occur, however, it would have a negative effect on the direction of our evolution. Compared to the Traders, our lack of impact would be perceived as impotence and we would suffer great psychological damage. What we need now is a celebration of our own existence in the universe as a unique design.

Humans are individual physical forms with individual minds, and each one is uniquely different. The group mind of the Traders would be judged to be something superior, instead of simply something different; something unconquerable, instead of something equal. Part of the population would start a new religion that would worship the ones in the Great Ships, the Trader species, and this negative effect could last for thousands of years.

To help monitor the development of that fear, nearly everyone in society has received a small, crystal transmitting device that is located deep within the brain. When the recipient is in fear, this transmitter signals the Traders to come and observe and note whether the source is of natural or human-made origin.

In our present physical form, inherent judgments are made by the visual organ, the eye, and it is important for humans to see things that are familiar. Sightings of unfamiliar creatures normally results in a reactive judgment that yields a fear, and the adrenaline flows. The blunt Earth dictum states: "If it don't look right, shoot it." The thought form does not exist in the mind of the Traders, fortunately, and they have come to accept this odd feature about the evolving Earth human. (See Chapter 12.) As a result, the Traders could not openly expose themselves, because they understand that they would appear to be too frightening. Instead, they discretely appear to a very few. In fact, the general public can easily be convinced that there is no such thing as Traders.

Only within the thought processes of humans does this reactive problem exist, and the Traders have evolved a technique to deal with it. If during a three-dimensional encounter, a person reacts with any judgments, doubts, or fears in the face of the Traders, the standard remedy is to use the aid of a particular friendly Traveler, and this species is far more gruesome than any humanoid-looking Trader. This one, as explained earlier, looks like a huge praying mantis and is larger than a human.

The mantis has the remarkable ability to use the Primal Energy, Wisdom, to reflect back to a prey its own fear. When a human gets a remote glimpse of the creature and reacts with any amount of fear, the fear is intensified 1000 times and mirrored back, and thus the person becomes unable to move. In this condition the person cannot hurt himself, the Traders, or anyone else. Quite often people report waking up in a frozen, panicked state, unable to move. The sensation gradually dissolves and dissipates.

In addition to the fears and doubts generated by the visual reaction to the aliens, a person's own expectations can also yield similar results. If one holds a needful expectation to communicate directly, it will result in paralysis. Dealing with honest human love is no problem for the Traders. Humans who have developed the habit of looking into someone's eye to search for love and understanding will find their experience with the Traders to be quite fulfilling. If a person projects unconditional, total love and understanding, that will be amplified and reflected back. There are many who have the experience of opening their eyes in bed only to exchange an understanding gaze of love with a Trader. They prefer to call themselves experiencers — not abductees.

Humans can project unconditional love, but can also make the mistake of projecting a picture of how that love should be reflected back. An example would be saying, "Here kitty, kitty," to a wild mountain lion. The sight of the cat just poised there looking back might be misinterpreted by the human as, "I love you too, so please come a little closer." But if the cat holds its position and the human approaches thinking perhaps it could pet the cat and convince him of his good intentions, the territorial instinct of the cat might be triggered and lead to an attack. The consciousness of each species is unique, and only humans think like humans, only cats think like cats, and only Traders think like Traders.

The Traders are humanoid in form, have a reverence for life, understand mathematics, chemistry, and the physical laws of the universe. Beyond that, communication with them is very difficult, and the best we can hope for is to share information regarding machines and the mechanics of the universe.

One reason for this is that they share a common mind, not an individual mind. Other reasons are because they are unisex until it is time to reproduce. They never experience juvenile fighting, back-seat romance, or anything considered normal by the standards of our modern day society. They can't conceive of the coping that is part of survival on this planet, nor could humans conceive of what it would be like to gaze on the Andromeda Nebula first hand, or gaze on the Pleiades from a nearby planet on their version of a romantic night episode — whatever it might look like.

It is this very different consciousness that is monitoring the fear of our consciousness. The monitoring devices inserted inside our brains use the body's electrochemical energies for power, no battery is needed. Interconnected hippocampus energies power the device, and the transmitter cannot transmit if the body's emotional energies are continuously in fear or survival mode. Many who are implanted do not know that for certain they are, but do suspect something because in their dream states there is an altered level of conscious awareness. That heightened level, recognized as dream states having to do with flying saucers, emotional encounters in strange places with strange beings, and the like, represents echoes of an actual contact. It is a reporting in. More than 80 percent of humanity has been implanted. Almost all of those in the United States have been implanted. The implantation occurs between the fifth and seventh birthdays. The typical orifices used are the nasal passages or the tear ducts.

In the future, as the benign motivations of the Traders are accepted, the implanting process will be considered a gift. It makes no sense to be insulted at being given a tiny bead-like device that changes and improves the structure and ability to think. In the future, people will be grateful to have been examined by the Traders, realizing they are part of the great experiment to preserve the species of humans and finally eliminate vestiges of the judgments and fear that have prevailed on Earth.

The implants do have an effect on the reality humans experience. The way the tagging devices work is that they find the differences between human beings and enhance those differences. The result is that every tagged individual feels isolated even when they try to find comfort in a group identity. It doesn't last. They eventually notice the differences between themselves and the group, and feel the uncomfortable sense of separation. This, however, has the benefit of making it impossible to be totally lost in a group, and guarantees that every individual will march to his own drummer. Unfortunately, it also leaves each tagged person with an extra stark sense of personal isolation. This might feel like being ignored while standing just outside a group that refused to extend a welcome mat, or like not being invited to the large party that friends were hosting next door.

Tagged individuals can draw extra strength from the understanding that what actually keeps them apart is the belief that this separation is an accurate interpretation of reality and is inevitable. In fact, there is another part, a much large reality. If they could better understand the connection between the third- and fourth-dimensional realities and firmly believe in the cycles of the Oversoul into different physical forms, they would better realize that a unifying-universal consciousness more accurately reflects the way things really are. As a group, Earth humans just haven't experienced that — yet!

Another purpose for visiting the ships is because that is where the process of genetic dispersal takes place. There is a growing understanding among researchers that only a small percent of the population is involved with this. This small group consistently reports that they are visited not once, but repeatedly. They remember having had genetic experiments of some kind done with them, specifically involving the sexual organs.

Some women say they have seen small, child-size aliens or have even been shown a child who is apparently half-alien and half-human. These women feel that a fertilized egg was conceived, altered and taken by the aliens, and they experience a loss.

Because part of the experience is fourth-dimensional, the truth of these events is distorted. Sorting it out requires an understanding of the Traders' consciousness and motivation, which are unlike a human's. The Traders do take genetic material and place it on other planets so that any and all life forms have a greater probability of surviving. The Traders do not consider any particular life form special, even when some demonstrate considerable sentience compared to others. Because they do not practice judgment in this matter, no greater care is given to any one particular species'. The Traders' view of it is that a species body and the genetic material of that animal form, is being revered when they move it to where it will flourish.

Coupling that concept with the way the Traders communicate, by force of mind, and the fact that they share a common consciousness, it is hard for them to conceive of any other state of consciousness. It is equally as hard for the Earth human to conceive of a group consciousness such as the Traders'.

One person dying in their community is like a human losing a hair or a fingernail. It's taken that lightly because the consciousness is never lost. It folds into those who remain alive. The consciousness always was. It is. It always will be. The Traders' consciousness only has an intellectual understanding of what it is like for us, the Earth humans, and so many other species with individual consciousness, to have the inconvenience of having all of our education, hopes, and dreams encapsulated within one finite brain. We dream of immortality — they take it for granted. We struggle to have at least one child, we look in his eyes, and that is our only taste of immortality. The Traders live an effective immortality. Their sandbox is the universe and they have millions of years to see their projects unfold. Our space to experiment is essentially one planet and we must be satisfied with what can be created in one life time — a blink compared to them.

Since they would not be outraged if one person died in their community, they do not have any concept that a human would be outraged if his apparent offspring were to be taken. They do not get that. It is not part of their concept of reality. If they could understand it as the human understands it, they would certainly explain: **"Please excuse the disturbance to your sleep. Surely you must understand that this is a positive accomplishment. You should be excited to know that a genetic dispersal program exists and that you have been selected to be a part of it."**

The last part of the understanding missing to humans is extremely important. A fertilized egg is never taken! The only genetic material taken from any species is the sperm and the unfertilized eggs.

A greater understanding of the Traders' actions can be realized by knowing how the eggs and sperm are treated. If a suitable place for genetic material were not quickly available, humans would launch an extensive scientific effort to preserve the eggs and sperm, perhaps freezing them or attempting some other mechanical technique. These techniques would be unthinkably barbaric acts to the Traders. One avenue they would take to preserve the genetic material for a long time would be to store the eggs as their own genetic offspring.

The Traders have the ability to combine an egg with some of their own genetic material. One effect of this is that the resulting offspring is completely accepted by the society. The offspring carries life with it, then after the planet has been prepared and is ready to receive the new life form, the process is actually reversed. What comes out is a viable egg with the Earth mother's original genetic coding. Because of the nature of their science, this method makes extremely good sense.

Sometimes women who have been on ships, later submit to hypnotic regression to fully remember the event. Sometimes, even without regression, an intense dream state follows and many of the things experienced seem too real to be dismissed. Many women report that they had an experience in which they are shown one of the blended offspring who looks somewhat like a Trader and somewhat like a human. Unfortunately, this dream-state remembrance gets misinterpreted in many ways. One is that the Traders are desperately trying to genetically design a version of themselves that includes human emotional qualities or other qualities that we admire in ourselves. Unfortunately, this attempt to make rational sense of the event sometimes turns it into a nightmare. If the Traders could speak clearly to humans, their explanation for the viewing of the blended offspring would sound like this:

"This is an effort to communicate. This is an effort to ask if you know that caring for these offspring is a sacred undertaking. What we are doing is making certain that the Earth humans we care for, love, and want to protect, have offspring, and life goes on. We have visited and have successfully taken genetic material. Here in this visit, know that the effort has realized, fruit and sacred life has been born. This is why we visit and do what we do, to carry on life."

The reason only a small percentage of the population is visited is because those visited have all of the races in their genetic codes. The blending of the races is a new phenomenon. In a sense, Earth is a melting pot. The blend of the races is being seeded elsewhere.

Once this overall plan is understood, it can lead to an interesting moral dilemma. If blendings are desirable, is there an obligation to do so? The answer is that there is no obligation at all. No one is forced to be a part of it. In fact, since diversity is what allowed the survival of the races to begin with, it is diversity that insures their greatest survivability. The importance of diversity can be seen when it is understood that if the planet were completely blended, a threat to one would be a threat to all. For example, if the blend had the genetic structure that combined African traits with the melanin, then the whole population would be susceptible to sickle cell anemia. What will be required to insure that the population survives is that diversity exists somewhere else and those planets will continue to be protected.

If the Traders are capable of genetic manipulation as stated, and if they are capable of using the timeless aspect of fourth-dimensional travel to move forward and backward in time, it is interesting to speculate if it is possible for them to reverse the outcome of an experiment gone bad by traveling back to the origin of the experiment and simply erasing it? The answer is that although it is very possible, the Traders have adopted an ethic that states: **Once created always created.** Their work demonstrates their commitment to it. The human species can rest assured that it will not be erased.

Origin of the Dark Force

A number of people, including some researchers interested in the UFO phenomena, have examined certain events that are unusual and cannot be explained away easily, and have blamed the Traders. This is especially true if the events are harmful in nature. "When you see the Grays, you know there is going to be trouble." This is far from true. In the future, the truth will be seen for what it is. The problem rests with humans, and humans alone. Consider the issue of missing persons, cattle mutilations, and secret military-research installations.

Missing Persons

The epidemic number of missing people each year, 600,000 cases, has resulted in the Bureau of Missing Persons no longer maintaining records. One prevalent theory as to why so many are missing is that the aliens are using these people in diabolical experiments. Actually, they are being used by other humans. There are hundreds of thousands of people in the United States who take joy in showing their power over others by abduction, stalking, physical mutilation, mayhem, and murder. There are even organizations in society that procure slaves for others or abduct healthy people to use for body parts in medical transplant procedures.

In contrast, none of those who have come in contact with the Travelers or Traders have disappeared, although occasionally some have elected not to return to their native habitat. In some cases those contacted by the Traders have decided to stay on the SMS or other planets where they live out their lives in a state of wonder and exploring. The momentary sense of regret they experience when thinking of what was left behind, is offset by a state of absolute awe for their new surroundings. For various reasons others who desire to return to Earth have a memory mask placed on them that essentially prevents them from remembering the experience. This is done because it would greatly jeopardize their ability to relate to Earth humans in the future if they didn't. No one is ever taken against their will or for any Machiavellian purpose.

Underground Bases and Tunnels

The United States has tunnel boring machines developed by Bechtel Corporation that are capable of cutting 60-foot diameter tunnels. The machines have various applications and have been used to connect military bases by underground tunnels. The longest horizontal tunnel is about seven miles long. Some long tunnels are used to connect test ranges. The deepest tunnel is a hole bored vertically to a depth of fifteen miles. It is a dumping pit for radioactive debris. It was hoped that at that depth the mantle would re-absorb and transmute the radioactivity.

There is a vast tunnel system under a mesa at Dulce, New Mexico which has caused a lot of controversy. Some think it was originally a dumping ground for radioactive waste that was converted into an Air Force/alien cooperative research effort for developing the perfect human. There is no agreement between any alien species and the government to do research or develop a super race. Only on this planet could such erroneous speculation occur. This thought process accuses the aliens of having the same psychological profile as humans, and that projection is inappropriate for aliens.

Some humans have the desire to make friends with the Travelers and Traders, but there is no form of true communication. The reality of true communication depends on some common background, and other than agreement on mathematical and physical principles of the three dimensional realm, that does not exist. Nor is there the desire by any alien species to live enclosed anywhere on Earth. There are some Travelers who share similar DNA with the humans who can and do live side by side with humans. They could not be recognized easily and their purpose is not to be easily recognized. The aliens among us are not here to help nor hinder, but to research for their own purposes. There is really no advantage for the Alien species to having any form of contact at all with the Earth human species.

Those who claim to be living proof and product of DNA research within the caverns of Dulce are actually enjoying the notoriety. The stories of dissected bodies and other biological experiments are simply stories. It is quite easy for anyone in the area of Dulce to hike around and find the entry doors to the underground facility and make fanfare of it later.

This is not to say that the government is not involved in genetic research. There are places on Earth where children are born in experimental laboratories without a mother's womb, and other places where people are being experimented on. In locations where aliens do encounter humans and analyze them and tag them, it is never to the detriment of the person. If there are any painful, violent, or mutilating events, including vivisection, it is not at the hand of the aliens. Harm to human beings comes from other human beings and is not carried on anywhere else, and that is also why we are planet-bound and only allowed to explore this solar system.

Cattle Mutilations

Over the past decades and especially in the 1980's, many ranchers have found some of their livestock missing in different regions of the United States. The animals turn up in odd locations, dead, with organs missing. Since no vehicle entry and egress marks are present, nor hoof prints of any sort, it has been assumed the animals are dropped to the ground after mutilation. The organs are cut out with such precision that even the cells are dissected, quite amazing since no scalpel could achieve what is often observed. Over time, suspicions have developed that aliens are doing the mutilation, but this is not the case. The heart of the cattle mutilation was and is a government research project.

After two world wars, military planners realized that large quantities of advanced weapons used against an unprepared enemy would almost assure victory. An era of secrecy was born in the military, especially in areas concerned with weapon development. Research went on as a safeguard, because it was always assumed that all Cold War enemies were doing the same.

Around 1948, many experiments were done with air pressure weapons. Two methods were tested. One type functioned and killed by imploding, and the other type by exploding. They were tested on living and even non-living structures. One experiment attempted to explode a large ship by quickly reducing the pressure around it. The theory was that if the pressure of the water against the hull could be quickly eliminated, the ship would theoretically explode.

By 1950 another variation evolved which sonically compressed the air to increase the pressure density in a specific, isolated locality to such a force that it could do damage. This came about when it was discovered that the shock wave from jets breaking the sound barrier were causing damage to animals. The effort was made to create sonic shock waves and direct them into a small area. Moving anything in the correct direction and at speed of sound will emit shock waves that can do damage. The velocity determines how much energy is available to kill. This was refined into a short-term, short-distance weapon and, although quite noisy, it was installed onto helicopters for testing.

Eventually the weapon was refined to yet another level. If it were made to be silent, an attack could be made and no one would suspect until the kill was discovered. Instead of a single, powerful and loud shock wave, the idea developed to shake the molecules at their resonant frequency until they broke apart. A human with broken bones is not much of a threat. This was tried first, but eventually it was realized that it was much easier to concentrate on soft tissue damage. An easily produced frequency above the range of hearing was discovered. It was easily focused into a beam, somewhat like a laser although entirely lower in frequency. In principle sonic pulses would have the desired damaging results on mucous tissues.

Early test results were very promising and elite military and special forces thought it would be ideal against mob uprisings or hidden enemies using guerrilla-warfare strategies. Areas camouflaging suspected enemies could be sprayed with the sonic energy leaving the vegetation intact and the bodies, with no apparent wounds, would mysteriously be found dead.

There were many variables that needed refinement and actual testing. The range of the sonic beam in live battle conditions was unknown. It was uncertain how much energy should be expended in different atmospheric conditions and how to correct for differences in air pressure, but no authorization for the tests could be obtained.

Ultimately, a group within the elite military, highly intrigued by the device, decided to test it and obtain the needed data in an experiment of their own design. A clandestine operation was conceived where range animals were killed from a helicopter in remote areas. Unmarked helicopters made forays into isolated canyons under the cover of darkness, making sheep and cattle their victims. What happened was that the sonic energy boiled the blood so quickly that the fluid in the veins, the capillaries, and the arteries vaporized. The animals became extremely hot and quickly died.

The reason tongues and anal tissue from the dead animals were removed is because the cellular effect of atmospheric change is first encountered in the soft tissues, and this was the information needed for calibrating the weapon.

An additional fact is that Earth scientists have laser cutting devices (a classified military secret dating from the late 1930s) that can make fine cellular cuts. The cattle mutilations (in general) were not caused by aliens. Since there was no authorization for the kills, the tissue samples were taken and the animals were dropped. The military didn't want to be caught with the dead carcasses. The weapon has since been withdrawn from general usage. It is no longer installed on helicopters, but the elite military holds the silent mutilator in reserve and is still testing it from time to time.

Chupacabras

The Chupacabra is a mythical creation to stimulate tourism in Puerto Rico and other parts of the world. There is no Chupacabra. During the coming Transition, however, there will be many deaths from new viruses. Animals inflicted by these and other pathogens are often studied and catalogued by certain Travelers. The particular animals chosen are so infected with these viruses that they have only a week or two to live. These animals are given a painless death and the organs taken for study. The bodies are left behind to decay in a natural way — food for microorganisms. These instances are blamed on the Chupacabra. The intent of the Travelers is not to scare the humans of Earth.

UFO and Anti-Gravity Research Areas

The government has the military working on its own version of a flying disc. The design evolved from a study of several alien spacecraft, one of which was recovered almost intact because the Travelers in the craft were susceptible to the microbes in the air, and died. In that case, the bodies were retrieved and taken away by other Travelers. The craft, however, was left because the Travelers feared infection themselves. Only the interior portion of that craft was damaged. Another recovered craft was damaged on the exterior, (Roswell incident) and technicians recognized that the two craft had similar origins. Yet another craft was flown to area 51 by the zetas, who helped engineers for many years try to understand the technology! Engineering knowledge gained from these craft has yielded less than the desired results.

There have been more than two dozen attempts to replicate the craft, but in general, the metal used for the exterior skin prohibits flight into space. In fact, they are useful in only the first 3000 feet of atmosphere, because the actual anti-gravity force has never been understood. The only thing that works is the ionic distortion force. Essentially the surface of the ship is ionized so intensely that the surrounding air also becomes ionized enough so that the repulsion force of like charges floats the craft. Beyond a certain atmospheric density this drive does not work. There is simply not enough air density to float against, and so very little weight can be carried by the devices as they currently exist.

The military is said to have a working craft called the Aurora that can quickly reach a base on the far side of the Moon. The only base on the far side of the Moon now is the one built and operated by the Traders. Humans have gone there, but they do not get there on their own. They are taken there by the Traders, and there are few who will come back from that place and actually remember it. As stated earlier in this chapter, to remove the memory of the visit, the Traders place a mask into the human consciousness, and no human can overcome the effects of the mask.

What Is Big, Black, Dark ,and Ugly?

The Traders, and even the scientists from other planets who come with them, recognize that Earth humans exist in a backward state of development, very unresponsive and very reactive to their own fears, judgments, projections, and expectations. In certain mind control experiments, researchers have been visited by the Traders in the accompaniment of the praying mantis-like Traveler. In those encounters the fears, judgments, projections, and expectations were reflected back onto the researchers involved, causing them to be paralyzed instantly by their own negative projections. The origin of "big, black, dark, and ugly" is in amplifying the dark consciousness of certain human beings.

The Traders appear mysterious and powerful. Their ability to wink in and out of three-dimensional reality is truly awesome. In the mind of Earth humans these are very powerful beings, so powerful as to be unconquerable in any way. Because they work, thrive, and are prolific with a singular mind, there is an absoluteness to them, and because they delve into the very essence of existence, they are to be feared.

Humans can try to blame the aliens for human and animal disappearances and everything that is black, but the Travelers and Traders are entirely innocent. They are here to study and to help life forms survive. Unfortunately, that only leaves us to blame. Some of **us** are the mutilators, the vivisectionists, the conquerors, and the controllers. It's hard to accept, but the dark consciousness is not of alien origin.

The Travelers

There are many different types of Travelers. Since their genetics were brought to this planet thousands of years ago, some have nearly the same physical form as the Earth human. They can and do mingle in the streets almost unnoticed. Some Travelers are humanoid in form, but would be recognized as alien because of the shape of their hands, heads, eyes, and so on.

One form of Traders remains planet bound and has become Travelers. They exist in a gravity field and unlike the Traders, who have weak legs and normally float, they are strong limbed and can walk in the gravity field of Earth. They are from a planet near the star that we call Zeta-Reticulum and are called Zetas. They were already described in

Chapter 10. Because the Zetas have a single mind like the Traders, they cooperate and communicate with the Traders at a deeper level than any other Traveler species.

Other aliens of Traveler status have evolved from the forms that were originally birds, cats, and dogs. They only remotely resemble these creatures now, however. Strangest of all for the Earth human, whose thinking process is directly connected to his eyes, are forms that have evolved from the insect world, the aforementioned praying mantis and even giant 200 pound spiders. (See Note 14.5.) The spider Traveler lays almost 420 eggs per year and, to prevent overpopulation, eats most of them. The spider does not travel much.

The Purpose of the Travelers

In general, the Travelers are doing scientific research and observing to gain knowledge. It will be realized eventually that they are here neither to hinder, nor to help. After all, the reason they are here in the first place is because they have demonstrated to the Traders that they will adhere to the code, **do not harm the animals.** This is an absolute rule that the Travelers and the Traders adhere to. The Traders utilize their sails to communicate, as well as to move between time and space. Because every thought that a Traveler or human has ripples the Energies and is detected by the sails, the Traders will always recognize the mind that intends to do harm. Once detected they visit it. The Traders thus enforce the Travelers, and if any one of the Traveling species were to exercise malevolence of any sort, there would be quick retribution. Their entire race would be planet bound and forbidden to travel between the stars, until a determination of the harm they have caused is made and rectified.

The Pleiadian Purpose

Of particular interest are the Travelers who occasionally mingle unnoticed. Already mentioned is Semjase and her team from the Pleiades cluster. (See Note 14.4.) This tall Nordic-looking blonde has been engaged in contacting Earth humans for a long time although not always with success.

"Several times we have tried to establish contact with terrestrial humans who might want to assist us in our task. We opened contact, but the men selected gave evidence of not being sufficiently willing or loyal. Others were afraid of their own kind (fellow men) and permitted our contacts to go unreported. They explained that their own kind would consider them liars or mad, or would destroy their existence with intrigues." (Pleiadian Traveler, Semjase, 1975, See Reference 25.)

One firm contact was established by the intrepid Eduard "Billy" Meier, who, despite having only one arm, has survived great ridicule and several attempts on his life. He has succeeded in producing valuable photographs and contact notes from Semjase and her team. The notes contain information such as:

"We, too, are still far removed from perfection and have to evolve constantly, just like yourselves. We are neither superior nor super-human, nor are we missionaries . . . we feel duty bound to the citizens of Earth, because our forebears were their forebears . . . " (Pleiadian cosmonaut, Semjase, 1975, See Reference 25.)

The Travelers are quick to point out that they are not super-humans and reaffirm the fact they share genetics with Earth humans. The Pleiadians would like us to know that humanity is not alone.

". . . we have taken on certain tasks such as, for example, the super-vision of developing life in space, particularly human, and to ensure a certain measure of order. In the course of these duties we do, here and there, approach the denizens of various worlds, select some individuals and instruct them. This we do only when a race is in a stage of higher evolution. Then we explain (and prove) to them that they are not the only thinking beings in the universe." (Pleiadian Traveler, Semjase, 1975 See Reference 25.)

The Travelers are also quick to point out that they are not super-missionaries on a mission from God to help bring about peace on Earth.

". . . and neither is it consistent with the truth that our brothers and sisters come from other parts of space on behalf of a God to bring to the world the long awaited peace. In no case do we come on behalf of anybody, since creation, by itself, confers no obligation (on us). It is a law unto itself, and every form of life must conform with it and become a part of it." (Pleiadian Traveler, Semjase, 1975, See Reference 25.)

Semjase and her team teach reverence for creation and all living things, being careful to allow humans to believe what they want and discard the Pleiadian teaching if they desire. Nothing is ever forced. Photos of their ships have been allowed, but photos of those on board have not been allowed as this would compromise their ability to mingle.

Around the world, there are many bases used by the Pleiadians and other Travelers. Some are accessed through underwater portals and others through portals in remote mountainous regions. Tunnels connect the bases. The longest is several thousand miles long. The Pleiadian's purpose is to observe and do scientific research, but not to help the Earth humans through catastrophic times. Observing what happens on Earth is a living history lesson and reminder of what occurred in their past.

Corrections Needed to the Billy Meier Information

The contact notes from Billy Meier were delivered by a form of automatic typing. Meier hears within his brain messages that are a detailed summary of that day's interview with the Pleiadians, beamed down by an advanced technological device on the ships. Then with one hand, he types the text that contains the vital concepts of the meeting. The process is very rapid. The resulting information, consequently, is not the direct speaking of Semjase. In reality, the information has passed through the filter of Meier's thought processes. So the use of words and phraseology represent his best interpretations. In contrast, this work is produced by a similar, although laborious manner, from many cassette tapes recorded of the channeler. Although the purpose of this work is to present the exact phrases as much as possible, it is necessary at times to fill in to complete the flow and rhythm of the teaching. Hopefully this has been done without much distortion.

Several glaring inaccuracies with the Meier information should be addressed. One inaccuracy in his material is a reference to a Giza intelligence, a group that can, by mind linkage, take a potentially gifted healer and turn him into a Hitler. Another inaccuracy is a reference to groups of aliens that will come to Earth with the aspiration to conquer and enslave. Will humanity soon have to deal with extraterrestrials with designs of conquering the planet physically or conquering it by mind control?

The answer is that there is no such threat, and no one can outwit the Traders. Once again, such vibrations will ripple the Traders' sails and they will investigate and make those responsible do retribution. Those that could conquer are already known to the Traders, and they are not allowed to travel, remaining planet bound. Only the Traders have the technique of traveling instantaneously between the stars. Some Travelers could arrive by traveling through time, but it would take a minimum of three generations to arrive and that is too long time to remain angry or desire conquest. Thus, the ones that have the perceptive qualities to come and conquer Earth have no way to get here, any more thanhumans have a way of getting there. (See Note 14.2.)

Moses and the Travelers

One of the stories that has been passed down over thousands of years is that of Moses: the trials of his particular tribe, the parting of the waters to save them, and the swift justice wrought on the Pharaoh's evil army. Is there any truth to the story that Moses was also given tablets containing guidelines for living? Did Moses talk directly to God? Did the Travelers observe any of these exploits? And was the life of Moses important for them to study?

Why the Tablets Were Given to Moses

Moses was the one who came with a plea. He spoke from Love and asked for guidance and the ability to lead his people with discernment and good judgement. In the way he spoke and the way he did what he did, he became resonant to a loftier purpose and became able to call on Primal Energy and Consciousness. (Similar to using "The Tool," see Chapter 13.) In doing the contemplation, his original intention was to discover his place of passion, a place of discernment, and a place of guidance, of cooperation and not control. It was then that the Primal Consciousness and Energy of Love was called forth and heard in his mind.

Yahweh did speak to Moses, and what Moses saw was the Primal Energy and the power of Love. The bush burned later and the rock moved. The flame was modulated to vibrate the air at audio frequencies and this is what Yahweh used to talk to Moses. At another time he came away with the tablets and on them were inscribed the guidance principles. (See Exodus for chronology of events.)

When Moses presented the principles to the people of his tribe, they realized it required a great deal of self-control. Their concept of law included someone always ready to control them, as they had just been released by the Pharaoh. The Pharaoh's rule was firm and if someone did not obey the law, authority quickly controlled that person. Once the tribe was released, they experienced total, unbounded freedom. No structured police force was there to stop mischief. The tribe was used to outside control and rejected the guidelines because they did not feel capable of self-control. Moses received no praise for his efforts, only anger, upset, chaos, and rage.

Moses returned to the mountain, but with a sense of chaos, upset, and a feeling he needed to control his people. Moses once again implored the Source for help and was answered once again by Primal Energy and Consciousness. This time, however, it was not Yahweh, but Chaos. The response from Chaos (in some texts, Jehovah) was that while the people would not see it immediately, in their lifetimes there would be upset. If the people did not follow the guidelines there would be conflict. They would greatly disturb the energy flow around and in their life and would set themselves up to reap the benefits of what they sowed. Not because it was a punishment. Humans have free choice. But it opens a door that allowes that sort of thing to happen. If they did take that step, they should know not to look for someone else to blame. It was true then, its true for us today.

Moses was not getting help, he was getting advice, and it was not given to him because he was a great leader. It could have been any person who approached and asked with deep contemplation in the manner that he did. Anyone would have gotten the same understandings that he did. Considering the intensity of Moses's participation, Primal Energy and Consciousness could not ignore him. Later, after more teachings were presented, Moses understood there were more forms of life than just Earth humans in the universe. He understood the existence of the Traders, the Travelers, and that everything is composed of the Primal Energy.

This one man also managed to focus his energies into intense prayer and meditation, thus generating continued daily guidance in response to his pleas. This is when a group of Travelers, already following the tribe of Moses, made three-dimensional contact, and gave him an electrical device that linked him with the ones aboard the ship. This device has historically been called the Arc of the Covenant. In reality, it was not the capstone of the Great Pyramid, nor anything from the interior of the Grand Gallery, but simply a radio (of alien technology) with a frequency that linked him with the ship.

Once in daily contact with the Travelers, it was easy for Moses to maneuver out of the particularly ominous situation near the Red Sea. The Pharaoh at that time ruled by force, and perceived that conquering was the only method to achieve what he wanted. Although the Pharaoh had let Moses and his people go, his greed and desire to control overcame him. He ordered his military to crush the tribe.

As Moses and his people approached the northern end of the Red Sea, they came on an impassable mountain range to the left, and the wide sea on the right. The valley ahead was getting narrower and the only escape was through the water. They were without boats, and behind them the clouds of dust were rising, signaling the approaching army of the Pharaoh. The situation was desperate. Moses called the Travelers who quickly devised a means of escape. A large mother ship moved in slowly then rapidly accelerated straight up creating a large enough low pressure area so that the atmosphere rushing in resulted in a sudden and violent rainstorm. The wind pressure pushed the water at the north end of the bay, which was only twelve feet deep, to shift to the south for several hours, creating an extremely low tide and allowing the tribe to cross. When the winds subsided, the water, influenced by natural gravity, flowed back north. Unfortunately for the Pharaoh, many of his army were crossing the water basin when it began to refill and they were drowned.

The Morality of the Travelers Helping Moses

It might appear that the code, **do not harm the animals**, was violated since many of the Pharaoh's men died. Why the Travelers were not punished for their part in the event is that their experiment focused on the whole tribe, not only on Moses or punishing the Pharaoh. They had been watching the tribe for some time, and it wasn't really the exploits of Moses that interested them. It was as if a human were interested in a herd of reindeer, for instance, and the experiment, after going on for many years, was about to be cut short due to the extinction of all the reindeer. The event was investigated by the Traders, but because the intention of the Travelers was to allow an escape route only, and not to kill and punish the warriors of the Pharaoh, there was no retribution. The purpose and intention of sentient beings is the important issue, not accidents.

Do the Traders or Travelers Ever Help Individuals?

It might be concluded that Moses was helped by the Travelers, and there are some today who feel that they have been helped by Travelers and even Traders. One case involves a young woman, one B.D., who was severely injured in an automobile accident. With a broken neck, and no vital signs, B.D. was thought to be dead by those at the scene. This was perhaps a valid conclusion since she did experience the complete near-death phenomenon. (See References 11 and 12.) During the experience she revisited old friends, and concluded that alien beings helped mend the part of her neck that was beyond the technology of human doctors. Once mended to that point, she received help to reenter her body, was rescued, and then treated in the hospital. Surgeons and everyone familiar with the case were amazed that B.D. actually recovered. She believes she made Traveler and Trader friends and that this all happened during the period she was considered dead. What is the truth of the encounter?

The Travelers do get involved in some cases, and they do it to see what happens, but entirely for their own purposes, not to help as humans might think of it. The Traders, however, never get involved in such cases. In this particular case, B.D. was not helped in a direct sense. The accident resulted in her having the capacity to see what was going on all of the time. Entities can be in the same space, but not in the same time. The way to become aware of them is to experience them with two or more senses at the same time. In the dream state, which is actually a quickened state of reality, once one's sense of fear is eliminated, the pineal gland and the hippocampic region can be opened. This allows the instantaneous release of endorphins to flow, allowing one to become extremely sensitive to the immediate environment, almost to the point where one can feel a molecule of air moving.

Once in that sensitive state, one can sense and feel other things that are in existence in the same space, but not the same time. The person becomes super sensitive to the ten dimensions, with the capacity to sense that some creations are about to manifest into three-dimensional existence. As long as that state remains, the person can stand close to whatever it is he thinks is going to come into existence before it manifests, and this has the capacity to create some very magical things. So manipulation in the other dimensions creates events that appear to be magical to those standing and observing from the perspective of the three-dimensional reality.

B.D. stood outside of her normal perceptive awareness and became privy to the concept that there are other beings there all of the time. Once she experienced that, she also realized how to deal with the problems of the damaged vertebrae and torn tissue. Through the force of her own will, the changes came into being. Thus the conscious mind of the three-dimensional physical body brings back small portions of the events of the out-of-body experience, but not the reality of the entire event. What is then allowed by her consciousness to shift into the three-dimensional understanding is a construct that returned her to sanity. For her, it was that some Travelers and Traders were concerned with her and made the changes possible.

The Physical Angels

The Traders consider that all life has a right to its own opinion of life. All that they will do is insure the continuation of that opinion and that genetic structure. The Physical Angels, however, have the perception that sentient beings would be better off if they believed in the same form of government and had the same consciousness as they do, and these xenophobic ideas are difficult for them to abandon.

Millions of years ago when the Angels were allowed to return to Earth, they made the final genetic adjustments to the Earth human. The Traders would not have done that. The differing philosophies of the two species rekindled the old disturbance. The Traders elected to restrict the Physical Angels' traveling, not as a punishment, but to quell the disturbance aboard the SMS caused by them and their xenophobic ways. Once again, they were returned to their home planet. Now they are only allowed to make occasional visits to Earth in very small, scientific teams, and the last visit was in 1930.

While on Earth the Physical Angels wear hooded clothing. The hood hides the long head and the bony wing-like protrusion on their backs. In the near future, near the end of the Transition, the tall, hooded Physical Angels may once again make an appearance to see how their experiment, the human beings, fared during the great shift.

Artifacts of Ancient Travelers

The Physical Angels lived for many millennia in this solar system and evidence of their stay is more than just genetic. Their outpost has been detected on the near side of the Moon. Details of the giant dome appear fuzzy on the few research photographs of that area, but the structure is real. It was abandoned millions of years ago. (See Reference 49.) Other moons and planets will reveal similar artifacts in the years ahead, but the effort will be difficult as the surface of some planets and moons rolls, moves, and turns under.

Other species have lived in this solar system, but that was in even more remote times. On this planet their artifacts have had time to travel to the core and return to the surface as component pieces of the original devices. These components were originally designed to withstand temperatures near the Sun, and some of the diamonds and other hard gems made essentially from Carbon, and even some of the radioactivity present on the planet now, are from these ancient devices. Descendants of the original inhabitants of planet Earth are no longer here because there have been cycles of extinction and regeneration, extinction and regeneration.

The concept of this book, that advanced humans were brought here 52,000 years ago, built the Great Pyramid, and had flying discs, does not mean that was the first time humans were brought here. Intelligent human beings evolved quickly elsewhere and were brought back to Earth and lived in small regions of China and Africa long before the Great Pyramid Society existed. These ancient civilizations had craft with wings and moved about much like present-day civilizations.

Those societies, however, could not maintain the civilization. There were cataclysms and a great decline. During the turmoil, which was similar to when the Great

Pyramid Society crumbled, there was a racial blending with the primitive precursors to *Homo erectus*, and that contact actually improved the species. It also was the origin of the many stories that have been handed down through the years of giants, fairies, dragons, and gnomes. Traces of the beasts and also the ancient civilizations will be difficult to unearth, but anthropologists with open minds could piece it together if data retrieved from deep strata that doesn't fit the standard theory is not thrown away. (See Note 14.3.)

Future Discoveries Within the Sphinx — The Hall of Records

The original Sphinx was constructed of a very dense, high quality stone made by pouring an agglomeration slurry into a giant form. The agglomeration, of course, was similar to, but of a much higher quality, than the Portland cement used in the buildings and roads of today. If one keeps in mind that the head was recarved approximately nine times it can be appreciated why the head appears disproportionately small compared to the rest of the Sphinx, which is especially obvious in aerial photographs.

That original body, the three chambers within and beneath the Sphinx, and the connecting corridors, remain to be unearthed. Understanding the relative density is the key to unearthing the original features. Comparing the hard density of the original to the recently deposited soft sandstone features will reveal to researchers what belongs to the original and what came later.

Because of the varying densities, the best analytical tool for searching for the hidden features of the Sphinx is testing with sonar. This method has already uncovered the entry to the subterranean chambers. Future excavation along the side of the Sphinx will reveal original bedrock formations distinct from the sandstone sediment of 50,000 years. Pressure techniques will reveal the true age of the Sphinx and the Great Pyramid to be 52,000 years.

The original head of the Sphinx was almost identical to a monument on Mars, and built by essentially the same people. They look like Akhenaten. (See Reference 5, page 336.) They were on Mars and the fifth planet, now the asteroid belt. Although they visited Earth 330,000 years ago, Earth then had an atmosphere that was too dense and too humid for them. Without wearing apparatus, it was like drowning. They were also allergic to several plants. One of the reasons the Nile River region has turned into a desert is because when they finally needed to settled here 52,000 years ago, they began to get rid of a lot of plant species.

One of the chambers that will be discovered is the legendary Hall of Records. This room is not booby trapped as were many tombs designed by the Egyptians. The ancient Pyramid Society had no understanding of thieves, but did hope to leave an archive. The records are written in a precursor to Egyptian hieroglyphs, a language that the Travelers use, with each other and with the Traders. They recorded how they ended up there, what they did, where they came from, and what they knew about celestial mechanics.

It was left there, along with the Sphinx, as a marker for those who would come after. The intention was the same as someone might have if they were lost in the woods — a little monument with the hope that if someone found it they could find you.

To decipher the time capsule one needs to have a strong dose of the DNA of those from the star Sirius, so that the brain resonates to the original hieroglyphic letter forms. Some humans have that. It is like seeing the infinity symbol differently after reading this book. It is something that one feels and senses. While you cannot justify it to someone else if they challenge it, you will know inherently what those records are all about. It has your "name" on it.

The Great Pyramid — One of Eighteen

How was it possible to travel around the planet with ships that used radiated energy from the Great Pyramid, when distance and the obstruction of the Earth's curvature should have combined to weaken the radiated power? Originally there were eighteen power pyramids located over eighteen of Earth's major vortexes. (See the map of the vortexes in Chapter 9.) Ships could obtain power from many different power pyramids on their journey around the planet. There were, of course, enclaves of the Great Pyramid Society in the vicinity of each of these power pyramids, each was a crystal society with the technology required to maintain the ships. Despite the technology and knowledge of this advanced society, catastrophic Earth changes overwhelmed them. Now only one pyramid is accessible, the Great Pyramid.

What happened to the other seventeen Pyramids? One of the sister pyramids was built on a large island located in what is now known as the Caribbean. The Earth's mantle was thin in that region, so when Earth's molten core reacted to the passing Nemesis, the magma welled upward, splitting the crust, folding a great portion of the Atlantian society underneath itself, and finally sinking far enough to be covered by the sea. Consequently, traces of the Caribbean pyramid and artifacts of that legendary society remain the most difficult, if not altogether impossible, to find.

Another power pyramid survived the Earth catastrophe, but didn't survive the hostilities between the races of humanity. That was the pyramid in China which met its doom when the people there decided that the best way to insure their survival was to build a great defensive wall. The Great Wall of China was built, and part of the stonework came from disassembling the non-functioning China pyramid.

In Mexico near the border of Guatemala, an original Pyramid still exists, but the problem is that it is very difficult to observe. It is partly the jungle that hides it and partly the work of humans. After the catastrophic surface changes, that power pyramid became partly buried in silt and the great quakes of the time caused the peak to fall away. When humans recovered enough to rediscover it, they found a blunt peak protruding from the Earth. The 65-foot high projection was far short of its original 477 feet, because the major portion of the pyramid remains buried in silt. The smooth-sided artifact was, of course, a great mystery to the people who discovered it. They attributed it to be the work of the gods.

To honor this wonder, they built a pyramid around it with a flat top built over it to match the decapitated top of the original. A gap existed between the original pyramid and its new cover. To seekers of that time, a view of the original Mexico pyramid could only be accomplished by finishing an intense initiation. The culmination of the ceremony was to pass through secret passages to the gap to see the original mystery, the ancient power pyramid.

Similar to efforts in Egypt, many pyramids in Mexico were built to mimic the mysterious one that was found. Many such pyramids were built, and they were really double pyramids, composed of one exterior pyramid surrounding and covering an inner pyramid. These recent works are distinguished by the grandiosely decorated inner pyramid.

Locating the remaining fourteen Pyramids will be a rewarding project for future researchers. One will be found within the United States. How to find this buried mono-lith, which can be up to twelve degrees from the regular vortex pattern represented in Chapter 9, and how to properly use a gravimeter to do it, is the subject of a future report.

Future Discoveries of the Great Pyramid

Even the Great Pyramid is partially hidden by silt, and a greater understanding of the monument cannot be acquired until the silt is removed. Again, relative density is the clue, and sonar will be the tool. Simply removing the silt that has filled the subter-ranean passages and re-examining what is already in full view will give a much better understand.

Dating the Great Pyramid

Determining the true age of the Pyramid will be accomplished by a technique other than Carbon 14 testing. The problem with using the Carbon 14 technique in and around the Great Pyramid is that it has produced power for almost 40,000 years. The process of producing power by converting the Earth's vortex energy, Primal Energy, and the gravitational energy involved in resonating the nucleus of atoms, both result in new atoms continually being born, which would alter the test results. Even if researchers could find a piece of wood behind a wall, from that period when the pyramid was constructed, it would only test to be 10,000 years old.

The correct date will be discovered using techniques developed and commonly used in the oil exploration industry where holes are drilled through dense rock structures to great depths. Great pressure develops due to the overburden of rock and soil. Petrologists therefore, understand that there is a relationship between time and pressure and the resulting densification of silt into hard rock and crystals. In other words, by studying the density and crystalline structure of rock, something accurate can be said about how much time has elapsed.

Experts will recognize that the extra compaction of a rock sample taken from beneath the weight of the Great Pyramid will be different compared to rock samples taken from the same strata, but adjacent to the Great Pyramid. A sample taken from the Grotto passage at the same depth as the base of the Great Pyramid, which being nearly under the apex, has experienced a pressure of about 500 pounds per square inch since the Great Pyramid was assembled. When that is compared to a sample at the same level, but adjacent to the Great Pyramid, testing will reveal the true age of the Great Pyramid to be many times older than what has been determined by Carbon 14 testing.

How old is it? The clue to who and when is recorded in the angles of the air shafts. These shafts were actually used for more than air vents. As pointed out in earlier chapters, they were maintenance access shafts, control shafts, and microwave tuning shafts to keep the inner chambers operating at the correct frequency. As such, any angle could have been selected, but particular angles were selected. Although all the angles with respect to the base are different, the angle between the two shafts on the north side as well as the angle between the two shafts on the south side are about 7.5°. It was shown before that the sum of the diagonals are equal to the precession of the Earth, if one G.P. inch equals one orbit of the Earth around the Sun. It was also shown that Sirius, the brightest visible star, has the largest proper motion of any visible star. The amount of travel of this close star is 7.5° in one precession of the Earth. There are two precessions indicated, one on the north side and another on the south side. The builders originated from Sirius and they came here two Earth precessions ago, approximately 52,000 years ago!

The Macros Circuit and the Passage to the Sphinx

The macro circuit hypogeum would appear to be an extensive interconnection of subterranean passages with flaps, valves, and strange doors, some in the floors and some in the ceilings. For the most part these passages were filled with silt and sand and became compacted sandstone. Excavating these passages will be tedious work but, as mentioned, with the use of sonar the complete system will be excavated and one of the corridors will lead to the Sphinx and the complex of rooms located there. Since the builders that came in later times were in awe of the Great Pyramid, its features were copied in one way or another. Because of this there remain to be found many more hypogea under the pyramid of Maidum and most of the other pyramids in Egypt.

The Base Lens

The focusing lens at the base of the Great Pyramid was designed with a radius curvature equal to the base of the Great Pyramid, namely 3,000 G.P. ft, representing *two* seconds of angular measurement at the equator of the planet. (See Figure 14.1.)

Although it is correctly thought to be another method to define the two second time interval at the equator, it also served the double function of honoring the Moon. Part of the energy source was the Moon since its great gravitational effect on the Earth torqued the faces of the Great Pyramid enough to induce large quantities of piezoelectricity. The profile view of the Great Pyramid is similar to tangent lines drawn from the Earth to the center of the Moon. The ratio of the distance to the Moon to the diameter of the Earth is 30, the orbital period of the Moon is about 30 days, and the radius of the lens curvature is a multiple of 30. This design feature not only honors the Moon, but points to the other sources of energy: the Sun, the galaxy, the universe, and even the Primal Energies, which all contributed to producing power. It also honors diversity, since the great power device was built by uniquely different humans!

The exact shape of the base lens, the stepped curvature, will be verified by multiple coring from incremental elevations of the grotto passage and carefully noting the height of the core sample and the distance traveled to the limestone core blocks.

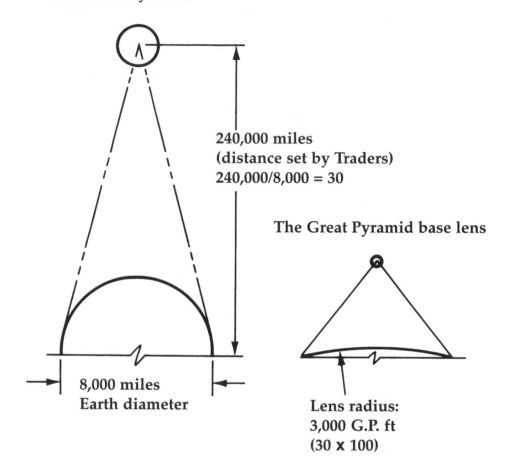

Figure 14.1 The radius of curvature of the base lens is equal to the perimeter of the base, 3,000 G.P. ft, which is a multiple of the ratio of the distance to the Moon divided by the diameter of the Earth, or 30. The period of the Moon is also about 30 days, so clearly the base lens was designed with the Moon in mind.

The Position of the Moon and the Cycles of the Universe

The position of the Moon and even the precession of the Earth are related in subtle harmonic resonant ways. If you have wondered if the gigantic efforts that slowed the Moon and changed its distance from the Earth, could have been mathematical entertainment, the answer is no. There is resonance within the universe, beyond the comprehension of the Earth scientist at this time, that is necessary for the promotion of Carbon-based species. The moon's location serves the purpose of insuring the continued existence of the maximum number of life forms on planet Earth. If the Moon were closer to the surface of the Earth (faster orbital period), the planet would begin to quake with every passing of the Moon and nothing could inhabit the planet. There would also be fewer Oxygen producing life forms and more Methane producing life forms, which would change the atmospheric balance.

If the Moon were moved farther away (longer orbital period), the Oxygen producing life-forms would increase to such an extent that the current life-forms would not be able to live in the resulting caustic atmosphere. Shifting the Moon even farther would cause the tides to decrease in strength, affecting the food chain so much that many of the lower forms, such as spiders, would perish. The Moon is located where it is to allow the participation of all Carbon-based life-forms, such as mankind. Part of the reason it synergistically fits together is because all of it was placed after the Moon was repositioned. The repositioning and the placement has been the work of the Traders. Although species once placed do evolve, scientists must understand that the species that have been cataloged must be constantly recataloged, because the introduction is a continuing process. Eventually this will be recognized, but right now, scientists are discovering new species and dismissing part of the significance by saying it must have existed all along, they simply overlooked it until now.

The Crack in the Ceiling Rock of the King's Chamber

After the great earthquake that destroyed a large part of Cairo, casing blocks from the Great Pyramid were taken to rebuild other temples. A large amount of core material from the top of the Great Pyramid was taken as well, and the removal was not symmetrical. With one side of the structure heavily burdened, the unequal pressure caused stress lines within the Great Pyramid. Evidence of this are cracks in several rock beams in the ceiling of the King's Chamber.

The Assurbanipal Library

There is a great ancient library in the Sumerian city of Assurbanipal where a numeric value is reverently recorded and equals 195,955,200,000,000. The speculation had been that it represented time, seconds to be specific, which when translated into years equaled 6.21 million years. Did some great event happen over six million years ago that is of great interest to humanity?

This speculation is not accurate, although it does have something to do with time. The actual period it refers to is only one second long. In other words, something is happening 195,955,200,000,000 times per second. What that has to do with is the Primal Energies. The clue is the Great Pyramid, which manifests its ability throughout the 52 millennia and stands as a monument to the three-dimensional realm of diversity. The extreme diversity is the result of the bonding of only eight Primal Energies.

The basic Primal Energy that combines with Chaos is Allowance, the Energy that allows all things to flow together and form anything of the three-dimensional world of creations in linear time. Without Allowance there would be no desire, and without desire there would be no creations. That number, 195,955,200,000,000, is the number of pulses per second, the number of reversals from the Is-Ness to the Is-Not-Ness of the Primal Energy and Consciousness, Allowance.

Imagining the universe as a great Christmas tree with the lights all representing where each bit of Allowance is located, the tree winks on and off 195,955,200,000,000 times each second. The logic of recording that fact was confirmed when the value of the second was defined by the perimeter of the base of the Great Pyramid. The Sumerians knew because their ancestors designed and built the Great Pyramid, and knew how this basic unit of time was defined.

Will Humanity Ever Travel?

What could be more interesting than to travel among the stars, to visit the genetic ancestors of humans, to visit species other than humanity, to see such specters as the Magellanic cloud first hand, and to be in wonderment at what will come next in the never-ending exploration of the universe. It would be grand, of course, but it might be some time before the Traders extend the invitation.

Humans by their early nature are voracious hunters without a sense of empathy, community, or much of anything, making them the fiercest predator on Earth. At the same time, humans are physically the most fragile. Around the campfire humans learned a sense of community and began to discover how to exist peacefully in small groups, small communities, and eventually in great societies. Despite civilization's clothing, modern humans are still fearful, reactive, judgmental, and projects fears, always accusing others of the same fear as their own. This, as stated before, is because of the endrocine system, the fight or flight mechanism that allowed us to survive as individuals in the first place. In our civilized setting it puts us at odds with ourselves and makes it difficult to understand aliens.

Holy manuscripts have tried to improve on our condition by teaching virtues and morals. In this country, the Bible is the most well known, and certain passages teach that it is wrong to steal, kill out of jealous rage, and in general conveys a sense of morals. Although the real demon lurks within each one of us, writers have created a mythical demon out there. The devil can infect us. We are admonished in various ways to avoid the demons and their demonic ways.

A poignant example of how this teaching can be confusing is given in a Bible selection from the book of Job. A friend of Job relates a devilish encounter that is still misunderstood by Bible scholars of today. Part of it reads:

"A deep dread came on my bones, and my bones shook. A spirit passed by my face, my hair bristled up, it stood still, I could not discern its appearance, it appeared to be formless before me, silence, then a voice: 'Can mankind be just before God? Can a man be pure before his maker?'"

This was not describing a demon, come to instill fear. It was a visit from a Trader. What the encounter was meant to question was whether humanity could participate with a sense of equality. Can the Earth human stand without a sense of fear? If he can stand without fear, he can also release the fear point. Release the fear point and humans can travel.

Why does man shake with fear before the aliens? The technology used by the Traders and Travelers seems immense and awe inspiring, but it is not immense to the ones who use it. They understand themselves to be equal and that is all. They are here to insure the continuation of all life forms, simply that.

Proof of this is so elemental and simple it escapes some scholars. If the Aliens had the purpose and intent to harm Earth humans, it would already have happened, and very strongly. If humanity is powerless and up against an oppressor, the oppressor would most likely oppress powerfully. If the oppressor is not powerfully oppressing, it might mean their intent is misunderstood. As stated, their intent has to do with preservation of life, but if the DNA they would like to obtain is in a person who is reactive to their presence, the fear is amplified, the person gets frozen, and the aliens get bad press.

This is another example of citizens in the United States of America reacting to the unknown with a resulting sense of powerlessness. Taking an event or an issue and exaggerating it into a newsworthy event is quite common in this country. It is subsequently conquered, and everyone can feel good.

The problem with the alien presence is that aspects of it are so unknown. Inflate that by realizing there isn't much that can be done about it, place that into various conquering scenarios, and suddenly it's as if the military cannot handle an impending, ominous threat. Place that in relationship to the Christian concept (some sects) that consider humans to be the only living, intelligent, sentient, self-aware, tool-creating, society-creating, massive army-destroying creature in existence of all of the planets, among billions of stars and billions of galaxies, and then suddenly realize the truth — that humans are not alone — it leaves us stunned in disbelief.

How can we appropriately play with our brothers and sisters out there with different backgrounds, with different moral interpretations, with different fight or flight mechanisms and consequently, different experiences with fear, when we can't even get along with ourselves? What do we do with aliens who can't communicate in any meaningful way when society teaches that all is lost unless one can communicate? How can we not be afraid when from birth we are taught that religion is the answer, and that religion says that God created humans — no mention of the aliens. So is everything from out there God?

If aliens are equal to humans and tainted with original sin, then how does Jesus get to all of those countless stars and planets and die to remove their sins? Something does not add up. Suffice it to say that religion in its current form, something to join or be persecuted by in one way or another, is a recent development, a poor attempt to control those who will not control themselves. In the past, religion was a concept of how to properly participate in life, a social structure, something to rally around voluntarily.

Blessed Are Those Who Control Their Fear and Walk with Love

Understanding is needed more now than ever before. Some contactees do not call themselves "abductees," but use the positive form "experiencers" instead. They stare at the aliens with love in their hearts, and they never get frozen. They receive caring thought

331

forms: "Easy does it, this won't take long, there you go now, care to look at the power source?"

Another poignant example that shows humans can control their reactive ways is the series of incidents over a ten-year period with the US aircraft carrier, *Franklin D. Roosevelt (FDR)*. The *FDR* was the first carrier to deploy aircraft capable of delivering nuclear weapons. The aliens decided to test the reactive nature of the men in charge of the ship by observing it with scout ships, making close passes. Then the aliens created a massive aerial decoy to see if the humans could be baited into making an attack, especially with the nuclear weapons.

The men aboard the carrier observed a tremendous atmospheric spectacle which was actually a shadow effect of a large Mother Ship. The effect appeared to be a large space ship which created an energy field transforming itself to another location — as awesome to observe as a nuclear detonation. It was the obvious work of the aliens — yet the officers simply observed the phenomena and no jets were scrambled.

Although they were representatives of the incredibly paranoid people of the United States, these officers did not use their most awesome weapons against this possible aggressor. This told the Aliens that those particular humans had the capacity for good sense. The nuclear weapons of World War II were used because of conditions of dire threat, but in this incident those in charge could interpret what dire threat was. So possibly this was a species that could cooperate in the future.

Consider that humans are rapidly changing during this Transition. Man was predominately in a place of conquering, controlling, and exaggerating differences. Now a shift is moving humans towards discernment and individualness, a place that attracts a person to an event because of the desire to participate, as opposed to forcing an individual to participate. This is, however, a time of extremes, and great polarities continue to cause upheavals within societies. Even nature itself is restless and storms are larger than normal.

Future Passing of Nemesis

About four billion years ago, Nemesis became part of this solar system when, as a wandering planet core from an ancient supernova event, it ventured close enough to be captured by the gravity of the Sun, and it orbits in a highly elliptical orbit like a comet. The old ferrous comet has made some of its regular passes directly through the plane of the ecliptic and in some of its eight million penetrations it has interacted with all of the planets, physically, gravitationally, and electromagnetically.

An unusual passing of Nemesis destroyed the fifth planet that was once between Mars and Jupiter. When Nemesis neared the outer planets they were lined up in such a way that the combined gravitational tugging sent Nemesis on a rare figure eight orbit around the Sun. It was actually in retrograde motion as it passed by the inner planets. This unfortunate close pass by the dense ferrous comet sent a shock wave and induced EMF pulse that caused the fifth planet to explode. (See Figure 14.2B.)

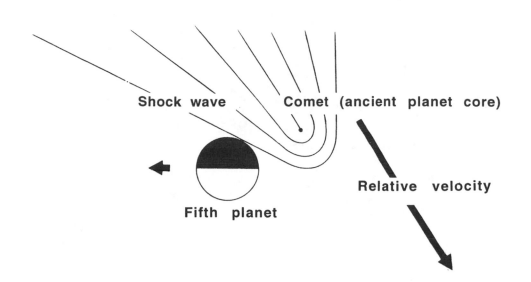

Shock wave **Comet (ancient planet core)**

Relative velocity

Fifth planet

14.2A The dense comet made a close approach at many times the orbital velocity of the fifth planet.

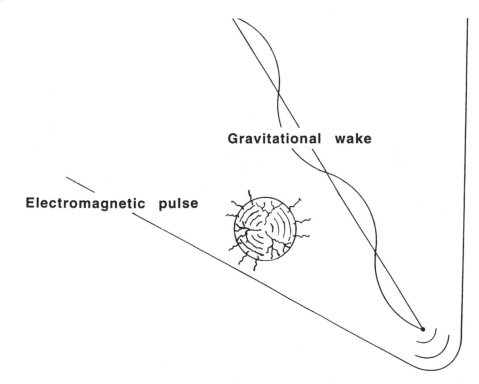

Gravitational wake

Electromagnetic pulse

14.2B The EMF pulse heated and unstabilized the core. The gravitational wake alternately compressing and decompressing the planet, weakened the fifth planet.

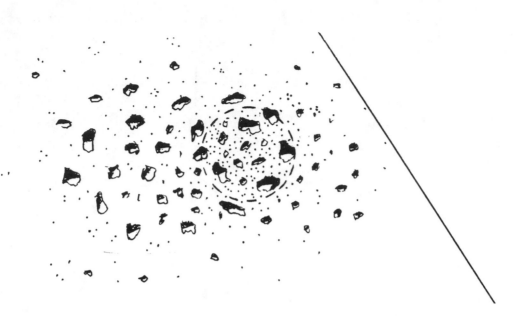

14.2C The fifth planet exploded into fragments.

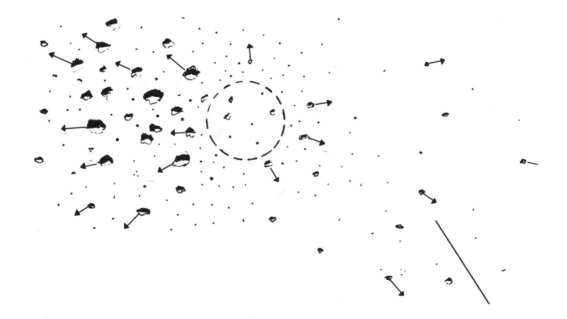

14.2D A small percentage of the fragments went into retrograde motion. Although most spiralled into the Sun, some achieved stable orbits around the planets. This explains moons with retrograde orbits, like Dios and Phobos of Mars.

A percentage of the pieces gained positive acceleration and found looping orbits that carried them beyond the orbit of Jupiter. A percentage were not greatly accelerated at all, continuing to orbit in near-circular orbits around the Sun, forming the main body of the Asteroid Belt. A small part of the material was sucked into the extremely intense wake of the comet, and an even smaller percentage of those pieces still trail behind the comet. The deceleration caused some to spiral into the Sun while still others orbit clockwise (as viewed from the North star) around the Sun, forming the unusual asteroids with retrograde orbit. A few pieces have even been captured by planets, which explains the observed retrograde motion of a small percentage of the moons in this Solar system.

The orbital period of Nemesis, about 500 years, has allowed the comet to make literally eight million passes through the solar system in slightly over four billion years, affecting the planets in many different ways. On one pass the gravitational wake removed most of the atmosphere from Mars. Some of this gas still follows the comet, and part of it has dispersed into the solar system. Mars no longer has a dense atmosphere, so the river basins seen on that planet are now frozen in time. No longer are there seasonal rains to reshape the surface.

Nemesis, the Good

In addition to the destruction of the fifth planet, the effect of other close passes of Nemesis is easy to observe. Each planet has had several encounters with the intruder, and all have altered their spin axis and orbits. They no longer spin on an axis that is perpendicular to the orbital plane, and the orbital planes of all the planets are all different and slightly out of the ecliptic.

It might be quickly concluded that getting rid of Nemesis after its next pass would be a beneficial thing for the living creatures of this solar system. After it rounds the Sun and begins to head out, we could mount a device that speeds it up, pushing it into the distant reaches of the galaxy.

There are two problems with doing that. The first is that it might eventually find a collision course with some other civilization. They would see it coming, investigate, discover the artificial source, and decide to throw a rock at us.

The second is that, all things considered, Nemesis actually benefits this solar system. The worst thing for evolving life forms is to run out of time and be on a planet with a degrading orbit that is doomed to spiral catastrophically close to its sun.

Nemesis actually is part of the mechanism that keeps the planets in stable orbits, countering orbit degradation. Without Nemesis, Earth would be where molten Mercury is, Jupiter would be where Earth is now, and so on. This is because the planets are normally tugged beneficially by Nemesis as it passes by. It is like a juggler keeping a spinning plate on a stick from slowing down. A little tangential tug at the right time does wonders.

It is also during these rare retrograde passes, however, that a lot of damage can be done. Planets can lose their atmospheres, be destroyed, or have their precession so exaggerated that they flip over. This has happened several times to the Earth, and these north/south pole flips are recorded in ocean floor sediments.

Where Is Nemesis Now?

What ever happened to Nemesis? Did it vaporize when it interacted with the 5th planet? Did its small pieces get absorbed by the Sun? Are they harmlessly orbiting in the Asteroid Belt? The answer is fundamental and is of great importance to us now, because it still orbits the Sun like a comet.

The effect of its passing varies in degree from good to bad. A direct hit, and even a pass within several thousand miles, would destroy a planet like Earth by induced explosive energy. Even a close pass within several hundred thousand miles would carry off the Earth's atmosphere. The mechanics of this would look similar to a fast-speeding ship passing an anchored one. The anchored vessel would rock as it absorbed energy from the ever expanding wake of the moving ship. Similarly, the Earth would experience a gravitational wake, a gravitational flux tunnel, of the passing asteroid. Assuming a close pass, the atmospheric gases could float away. Other effects are possible that are almost unimaginable to grasp.

As it passes through the inner planets, it heats up because of its interaction with the solar flux density and the gravitational field of the Sun. The outer layers liquefy, roll off, and leave a lot of small droplets at various distances from the mother. Some pieces may fall into planets, others may fall into the Sun, while the rest tag along a distance behind Nemesis. After eight million passes its orbital path is littered with little pieces. Some are even ahead of the Nemesis, so there is the possibility that a small bit of Nemesis could hit at any time, even before the main body arrives.

What a tiny piece can do is telling. One extremely dense, high-speed piece struck our planet in modern times, hitting Siberia in 1908. The vaporization of the piece released so much energy that 775 square miles of trees were toppled, which is an area of over 31 miles in diameter. (The Tunguska event is discussed in the December 1993 issue of *Astronomy* magazine.) Many speculated that it was an atomic device of alien origin, or a glancing blow from a huge asteroid. What was the actual size of the piece? It was equivalent in volume to an orange, which demonstrates what a combination of speed and density can do — beware of close passes of mother Nemesis.

Direct observation of the Solar System tells us that the probability of a close encounter with Nemesis is extremely remote. Far more likely would be a less severe episode in which the Earth might experience an electromagnetic pulse, minor gravitational disturbances, earthquakes, volcanic ventings, and associated changes to the atmosphere including great storms. Volcanic ash could block the sun to such a degree that the growing of crops would be impossible for months or even years. It is interesting to note what one volcano can do. The volcanic eruption in the Philippines, Mount Pinatubo, in 1989, distributed ash in the atmosphere to such a degree that it blocked fifteen percent of the rays from the Sun. (Source: *Solar Today*, July/August 1993 issue) It took four years for the ash to settle. An even more sobering account of an historical event is given in Chapter 3 of Vice-President Al Gore's book, *Earth in the Balance*, where the story of starvation in China in the year 209 B.C. is accounted:

"Sometime around 209 B.C. there was a huge eruption, believed to be from a volcano in Iceland, which left its evidence deep in the annual layers of snow and ice covering Greenland and the frost-damaged rings of Irish oaks. Two years later, according to the Chinese historian Stu-ma Ch'ien, "the harvest had failed" for reasons no one understood. And two years after that, the Chinese his-

torian Pan Ku wrote in the Han Shu, "a great famine" killed more that half the population, "people ate each other." The emperor, he wrote, lifted the legal prohibitions against the sale of children. It was during this period, according to the Chinese Table of Dynastic Records, in 208 B.C., that "stars were not seen for three months." (See Reference 34.)

Is Nemesis anywhere near, and could its passing trigger calamitous events to Earth any time soon? To answer that consider that every 26,000 years a special type of Transition happens, when the mantle shifts one way or another. There have been many of these cycles. Another transitional cycles occurs every 69,000 years, when the planet experiences electromagnetic upheavals of large magnitude. The reality of this normal 2,000 year Transition is that it also includes the conjunction of a 26,000 year cycle and a 69,000 year cycle. It was during a similar synchronistic resonance when Pangea broke in two! So, will it happen in the lifetime of the reader? The answer is that if one is alive in the year 2011 or 2012, that is when the closest approach of Nemesis will be experienced. This is the eventful time of the Transition; the end of the period will be marked by the passing of Nemesis. The purpose of telling this is not to strike terror, but to sow sober concern. Many outcomes are possible, and concerned Earth humans living in balance can make a difference.

How to Prepare for Nemesis

Astronomers using orbiting high-energy detectors that are sensitive to the X-ray band (more energetic than visible light) will soon detect Nemesis. What can be done about approaching Nemesis requires an understanding of its unusual orbit.

The Sun is actually part of a binary system with a non-luminous shadow sun about 500 Astronomical Units (AU) distant. (one AU is the distance between the Earth and the Sun, approximately 96 million miles. Jupiter is five AU from the Sun.) This large and dense body has never acquired enough mass to begin to shine. Nemesis orbits the binary body and the Sun. The dark body, the Shadow Sun, and the Sun revolve around a point that is about one third the distance from the Sun, the center of mass of the binary system.

When Earth or any other planet is lined up with the two suns, but farthest from the Shadow Sun, the planet gets a beneficial centrifugal boost that tends to fling it outward and away from the system. When the same planets are between the two suns, the centrifugal force is much reduced because it is much nearer the center of mass of the binary system. The differential between the two places in the orbits causes the beneficial force that helps prevent the planet from spiraling into the sun because of the drag caused by impacts with meteors, comets, or anything with mass.

This would suggest that there is no planet with an exactly circular orbit, and in fact, such is the case. A corollary of this mechanical truth of binary systems is that no stable planets suitable for the evolution of life could form except within a binary system.

As Nemesis orbits around both the Sun and the Shadow Sun it has something other than an elliptical orbit. It leaves the immediate vicinity of the Solar system and reaches its slowest speed about one third the distance between the suns. There, the gravitational attraction of the Shadow Sun has a turning effect on the ferrous comet. Unlike comets that only orbit the Sun, it begins to accelerate. Eventually it passes close to the Shadow Sun, speeding at close approach to once again attain escape velocity and is thus "sling shotted" around it and back towards the Sun.

Once again at approximately one third of the distance, it reaches the slowest part of its orbit, but then the gravitational attraction of the Sun starts it racing towards the Solar System, and it enters the solar wind at twice the velocity of an ordinary comet. Ordinary comets orbit only the Sun and have predictable Keplerian orbits. The complete orbit is on the order of 500 to 550 Earth years (depending on the alignment of the planets), and this sling shot-type orbit is not the normal Keplerian ellipse of ordinary comets. It is more like a tetrahedron with rounded corners. (See Figure 14.3.) A closer view of this orbit is shown in Figure 14.4, which shows the Sun, the inner planets, and the path of Nemesis, as well as the relationship to the orbit of the Earth.

The question is, where would Earth be in the orbit to experience the least harmful effects from Nemesis, and where would Earth be to have the most detrimental effects? The answer is that the least detrimental effects will occur if there is a distance buffer, and that is in position A or D, not B nor C. (See Figure 14.4.)

Since the planet might be in position B or C, some would consider it a proper survival strategy to alter the course of Nemesis, thus avoiding the whole problem, now and into the future. A probe launched now, or a series of probes launched within the next few years could encounter the comet when it is six AU from the Sun.

If the effort could be made and enough atomic weapons were thrown at Nemesis, and if they penetrated the shock wave, the object could be deflected away from the Sun forever. It might, however, also break into pieces that could hit the Earth directly and be worse than a near miss. Deflected in the wrong direction, it could hit the Sun. Hitting the Sun at the wrong angle would split the Sun into pieces and that in itself would end the Solar System.

The best time to fire at Nemesis is after it passes, when it is at its turning point and moving at its slowest. That will be about 100 years from now, and also a foolish undertaking, for reasons already given. Our grandchildren and all other evolving life forms actually need Nemesis.

Every day that passes, it accelerates towards the inner planets, requiring more energy to deflect it. The simple reality is that there is no point to launching anything at the Nemesis — not now, nor in the foreseeable future.

Word of the approaching Nemesis should be spread, especially to the planners of all countries. Preparation for food shortages and the like can be made, and knowledge of some of the electromagnetic effects can prevent certain forms of international catastrophes. There will always be people, even ones in positions of power, who believe there is nothing out there that could ever have an influence on us. They believe that all of the large meteors and comets that could damage the Earth did so in the early formation of the Solar System. By being completely ignorant of the sudden catastrophic effects of this passing iron comet, the measurable residual electromagnetic effects could be incorrectly interpreted as a neutron bomb attack. The last thing anyone will need at such a time is a retaliatory nuclear strike!

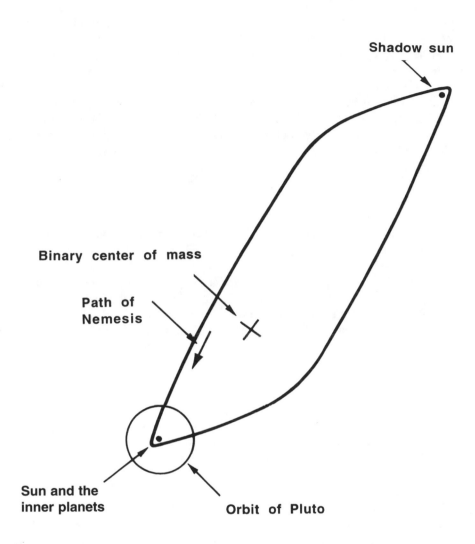

Figure 14.3 The orbit of Nemesis

Referring to Figure 14.3, the interesting effect of the sling shot orbit is that when the comet enters the outer reaches of the Sun, which includes the solar wind and magnetic sphere of the Sun, the incoming body is traveling faster than a comparable comet of identical eccentricity. The solar wind actually modifies the acceleration, and this is an important point. The output of the Sun varies, and consequently, so does the solar wind, which is comprised of highly energetic and charged Electrons, Protons and other cosmic particles. Thus the solar wind has a certain amount of mass and velocity and actually cushions the incoming comet. Its relative density affects the acceleration of the comet. If humans could invent a mechanism to control the solar wind output of the Sun, he could actually affect how close Nemesis would pass.

The Truth of the Revelations

Writings in the Bible called the Revelations and writings within the Koran similar to the Revelations speak of these times. How literal are these descriptions? Knowing about them, how does one prepare?

For one thing, it is important to realize that the visions described are spot reviews of one locality, and were expanded erroneously in the mind of the visionaries to include the entire globe. The entire planet is transitioning, but each individual's experience will be different. Not all will be painful. Some will be quite joyful. Here are some examples from Revelations and an interpretation through the eyes of the present time:

1. Trumpets

Different forms of warnings will enter the reality of each individual. They may be real people, movies, videos, books, newspapers, the media, or other forms. Take note and take steps of action. Without active steps, events will act on the individual and the experience will be one of victimization instead of joyous encounter.

2. Behemoth and Goliath

These are the overwhelming events that are seemingly too large to deal with. Behemoth refers to Earth changes and shifts that will occur, such as volcanic eruptions, earthquakes, great storms, movements of the cosmic bodies, the close passing of meteors, asteroids, and the eventual arrival of the ferrous comet, Nemesis. Behemoths are things that are so large they do not stop to consider how it affects humanity. Goliaths are the intentional acts that affect large segments of humanity, like an invading army.

3. The Seven Candlesticks

The seven candlesticks are also known as the seven daughters, the seven sons, or the seven seals and refer to the seven Primal Energies and Consciousness that combine with Chaos to form everything within the three-dimensional realm, including humans themselves. The teaching has been offered many times and is referred to and recorded in many texts. The seven point to the eight and also to the thirteen. There are eight fundamental Primal Energies and there are five senses of humans. Each of the senses is a combination, as the eyes are a combination of Harmony and Knowledge, for example. This understanding has been taken into other configurations, including the Houses of the Zodiac. All of these teachings and the core teaching for humanity are always the same, how to achieve balanced participation.

4. The 666

This number refers to the splits and the fact that the beginning and the end are essentially the same after 666 splits of the Is-Ness. The inside of the outside is identical to the outside of the inside at that point. Once humans achieve the ability to manipulate the Is-Ness out to the 666th split, to make creations that modify that region, humanity will have the ability to unwittingly move the matter that makes existence happen. Once humans have the ability to manipulate subatomic particles at will, there is a very good chance of unwittingly eliminating the three-dimensional reality. That lifting of the illusion that this dimension is real is a very scary thought, and thus the association of the devil with the value 666. In reality it is a reminder of how powerful humans are. Do not disregard that the part that each individual human is, is a vital part of what God is. Also at this point, humanity will have achieved the ability to travel into fourth-dimensional reality, and accomplish time warps. With true understanding, there is no need to fear.

5. The 144,000 Saved

In the possible event of the complete annihilation of humanity, before that would occur, the Traders would remove a large segment of each of the races of humans. The holding bay onboard each mother ship will support 144,000 people. While there are thousands of ships, there is no promise that the entire population would be taken.

6. The Antichrist

Beware of false prophets and do not follow the Antichrist. The Antichrist are those forms that become dogmas of control, hard-and-fast thou-shalts, and thou-shalt-nots. The original teaching of Christ was how to participate in a joyous balanced way. Beware of religions that do not follow the precepts of Christ, that do not have allowance for another person providing that other person has allowance for himself. Those who don't and who attempt to over-control will find themselves in the midst of their own form of Armageddon.

7. The Single Horseman

Do not think that it is individuals that we referred to in the writings, but instead think about groups. A single horseman will never bring the pestilence, it is the entire realm of men who are trying to carry on with the old ways of control.

8. The Water Turns to Blood

In reality this refers to water turning red because of dying plankton that indicates that air-producing plankton is being reduced. Caused by humanity's pollution of the oceans, when the plankton die on a global basis the percentage of Oxygen will decrease. If a five percent reduction occurs, then no air-breathing animals can live.

9. Disease and Pestilence

The scientific community has "progressed" to the point where genetic structural changes are being done to small viruses without any thought to the magic they are invoking. Pleased with the thought that they can do it, they have now created things in the environment that are not desirable. Nothing can stop these viruses. They are prolific, and some of the new disease conditions are a result of work in that direction. In an effort to fix and heal people, certain vaccines and certain other genetic manipulations have been made that will ultimately prove to be substances that could lead to humanity's destruction.

10. The Weapons of Destruction

Push-button missiles delivering destruction hundreds and thousands of miles away have allowed missile operators to be isolated from the death of other human beings and the general horror of acts of war. Because it does not bother the ones in possession of the devices, it is now less likely that there will be compromise solutions. It is more likely that the weapons will be used to settle conflict.

11. Mass Starvation

The population of the planet has expanded to the point where it is non-sustainable, in fact, over half the population is malnourished and a large percentage is starving. The starving will continue to increase.

12. The Seven Seals

Each seal must be opened and moved through. The seals refer to the Energy centers of the individual. In the old teaching, the Chakra Centers were the focal point of the Primal Energy and Consciousness. Each seal is opened by doing the contemplation, which brings the individual into balance. Once that balance point is achieved the individual will have the capacity, without concentrated effort, to participate in events in such a way that one's active and reactive natures will be in keeping with or consistent with, the wholeness of each one of those Energies. Thus, each day will be conducted in a way that is both gentle and productive for the individual as well as everyone around.

Days with conflict will occur, but those days will be filled with appropriate confrontation. Confronting the issue, not the event, in many cases means simply not agreeing with the projections of others. Those confrontations give one an effect on the world that in turn affects the individual, and results in joyful interchanges. The apparent life struggle is over. When the struggle is over, the transition to Love has been made and that is the "end time" for that person. Societies will transition as well, with the result being that the need for government will be minimal. Members of society will have the natural sense to govern themselves.

Those who do not adapt will at the least experience the worst effects of the changes, or they may well perish. Trying to use the same set of rules they have always used to conduct their lives, they will find they must force things to stay the same as they were. By using force they will be going counter to the nature of how things are now, and they will experience a painful Transition, seeing the worst of the visions of the Revelations.

Here is an example of applying the teaching and achieving that balanced point. If one does ecological changes to save the world (selfless) then one is unwittingly helping to destroy the world — totally selfless action is unbalanced. If one is doing ecological changes to be seen as a good person (selfish), that also insures his non-existence — again, there is no balance. If one is doing ecological changes because of the understanding that ecology is part of everyone and the efforts do not hurt the individual or those around him, then that is appropriate.

One of the great problems humans face in the process of coming into balance, is what to do with their superior attitude. Human beings have still not accepted that physical existence is a physical Earth biosphere phenomena, so they have not accepted that they are actually no greater a part of the food chain than any other living creature. Humans, as far as the Earth is concerned, are identical to the ant, but humans will consider themselves to be superior because their myopic thought is that no creature manipulates the environment quite as well as they do.

How many people are aware of and can name the seven sentient species, besides humans, that exist on Earth? There are other creatures as conscious and appreciative of nature who possess the ability to experience as much pain and pleasure as do humans! Most humans still do not consider that, and this superior thinking is brought into every aspect of life. There is even the comparison to every other human being — is that one above or below, or how can he be truly sentient if he has a different skin color? Has each human learned to tolerate other nations, the opinions of others and the different lifestyles, or do they feel attacked simply because someone else has a different opinion? When will the use of reason and the conscious mind be considered a tool, rather than considered the absolute of reality?

Equal in the Eyes of God

While looking for that superior or inferior level, the reality is that everyone is equal. The difficulty is to see it. Each person is equal in being different, equal in their capacity to participate, but not equal in life experiences. Humans are equal in their capacity to experience, but not equal in their capacity to interpret those experiences, because each one interprets them from a position that says: "I am the center of the universe and everything exists to support me." Holding that thought process almost assuredly guarantees the extinction of humans as they presently exists.

Practicing the art of equality is far better. Start with the simple process of greeting each other by looking into the other's eyes and noticing that, while each person is different, the intrinsically equal part is the same. That is, feeling love equally, feeling anger equally, feeling starvation equally, and so on. The capacities are equal, the abilities may not be. Judgment based on abilities will mean the spiral back into conquering and enslavement. By contrast, participating from the place that sees all individuals as equal, is the most that humanity can do and nothing else matters. When it feels like fun, it is being done appropriately.

Achieving Balance

Hopefully the end of this process will be joyfully experienced by each individual as well as society itself. What it will look like gives a hint at what goals there are to achieve. Here are a few:

For societies and nations, it may be that strong central governments will finally change into minimal governments, because individuals will naturally cooperate. Competition in every realm, will be changing into a world of minimal competition and increasing cooperation.

Trade and exchanges made using currency will be changing to a world in which part of the trade is accomplished without currency. There will be some equal exchanges of goods and, when labor is involved, remuneration will be part goods and part currency.

Giant corporations that are above the law, will be moving into a world where the law affects everyone including the corporations. Corporations and individuals owning vast resources of land and/or mineral wealth, will be changing to a world where humanity is paying only for the service of the delivery of the mineral wealth. Food from good food-growing regions distributed to people in need, will change to a world where people in need are distributed to good food-growing areas.

The media, used to controlling humans and reinforcing thier limitations, will change to a media that teaches responsibility to humans.

Industry using polluting fossil fuels, will change to a world where industry is switching to Solar, Hydrogen, and other alternate, non-polluting technologies.

Industry continuing to do DNA research, will be changing to a world where industry is abandoning DNA research and concentrating on techniques to keep humans in a constant state of health.

The health industry professionals, seen as superior beings to worship, will be changing to a world where the health professionals are seen as equal.

For the individual transitioning into Love, the changes also will be dramatic. Maintaining a superior attitude towards the animal kingdom and nature in general, will be changing to a world where people master the art of being equal with all beings and nature in general.

Working under conditions of drudgery for personal profit, will be changing to a world where people work for the community and for the pleasure of it.

Living to the age of 75 years, and considering that old, will be changing to a world where living to the age of 125, and eventually 225 years, is commonplace.

Forcing one's ideas on others, will change to a world where seeing and relishing the differences between the people of Earth will be celebrated as a great advantage.

Using money to get things, will change to a world where the general well-being is served by exchanging labor to get things.

Being susceptible to old and new viruses, will change to a world where the general condition of all people will have an immune system capable of dealing with virtually all viruses that exist.

Getting caught in the shifts of the Earth, will change to a world where individuals will feel and become sensitive to electromagnetic waves and intuitively move to a safer spot.

General ignorance and disregard for the ecology, will change to a world where each individual will have a growing reverence for the biosphere and everything within it, and treat all things as equal.

Being awe-struck and fearful of the aliens, will change to a world where all people will welcome the appearance of the ships as natural. Although noticeably different in form and nature, the aliens will not be considered as superior nor as inferior, but simply equal.

What the end of the Transition will mean for Earth itself is very dramatic. That Earth would move into an unsafe region and lose part of its atmosphere, will exchange for a planet that moves into the safe region, near position A or D of Figure 14.4 with no great cataclysmic effects.

Living in Balance with Nemesis

The celestial spheres are recognized as having very precise and regular orbital periods due to the incomprehensible mass and speed of the orbs. Humans, by comparison, even nuclear equipped humans, are puny. Orbits are beyond the power of humans to alter. If the position, direction, and velocity of Nemesis were put into a computer the distance it would pass by Earth could be calculated with great precision. Nothing can change that fact, but can we affect it? How can the Earth get from an unsafe to a safe position?

Considering that the solar wind is variable, if controlled properly, it could "airbrake" the entry of Nemesis, dramatically changing doom to victory. Remember also, that every human is a free-willed being existing within the three-dimensional realm, but at the same time existing in all of the other dimensions through a soul linkage. The key is recognizing the powerful effect of the piece that exists in all the other ten dimensions.

Decisions made here mesh with the ten-dimensional realm. If the overwhelming consciousness on Earth is to achieve balance, the Primal Energies will cooperate. There does exist a Primal, celestial, ten-dimensional mechanism that can help us. By doing the contemplation, the individual and then society achieve the balance point, activating the region beyond the three-dimensional realm of the logical and rational, and a great change in the "magical" realm, that of the entire ten-dimensional spectrum. The answer will come in the form of a change in the Solar output. The output of the Sun will appropriately increase or decrease as needed and coax Nemesis into a safe passage.

This is the greatest interactive game of the Solar system, and if enough individuals come into balance, the positive change will occur. The reality is there is no stopping Nemesis, it is just a question of how close it will pass.

Approximate tragectory parameters
1. **Eccentricity = 0.9988**
2. **Major axis = 500 AU**
3. **Perihelion = 0.3 AU**
4. **This portion is elliptical**

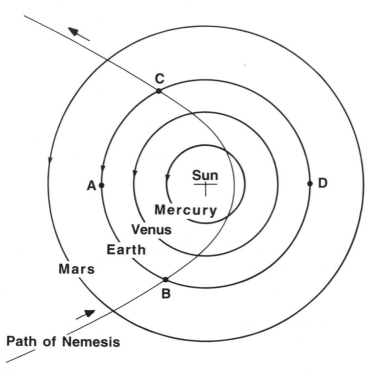

Figure 14.4 The orbit of Nemesis through the inner planets

The Clock Is Ticking

Humanity is in the middle of making a great decision, and the effort that will be necessary, if done without reactive fear, will collectively form a new civilization. This collective action must not be based on feared reprisal from the aliens. If we come together armed, mindlessly conquering, and vanquishing any alien species that does not think like us, we will be contained and restrained to travel within this solar system until that warring survival strategy is recognized to be a dead end. (According to Col. Philip J. Corso (Ret.) in his book, *The Day After Roswell*, the Strategic Defense Initiative (SDI) is not a defense against, any missle attack, but the hostile aliens! See Reference 52.) If we come together based on inner change, however, the aliens will finally trust the Earth human. If

346

we unite together for the purpose of overcoming our own natural fears of not being equal, or overcoming the need to justify that we are worthy, then we will be welcomed as a favored child is welcomed.

As it is now, if the aliens contact humanity openly on a grand scale, humans will go through distinct stages: panic at the thought of their awesome power, depression because it didn't happen in a way that we pictured it, sad because we are not allowed to ride with them, anger because the lid has been placed on the sandbox and we are not allowed to star hop, and finally we will try to buy them and convince them of our value. Alas, that human manipulative trait will not work either, there is nothing we have that they can't find elsewhere.

Balanced Isolation

Our state of existing as a single physical form with a single mind is designed to give us the greatest range of creation and emotional experiences. Often, however, it leads to a state we describe as loneliness. The confusion that sometimes results when we miscommunicate with words means that part of our existence will be in isolation. Some even seek isolation in order to achieve heights of creativity. Seeking the solitary state is not in itself to be admonished as some in society currently teach. The solitary state is in itself a precious state of creation, because each human being has the ability to be a galaxy, a complete universe unto themselves. We cannot use mind force, as the Physical Angels do, to come into union with others. Instead we use words and pictures, but these are sufficient.

Only a few species in the universe have the ability to exist in the three-dimensional as well as the fourth-dimensional reality. Few have what humans have — the ability to dream.

Accepting fully what we are, will help achieve the balance point. Every Earth human can dream of a balanced outcome and a safe passing of Nemesis. Many future realities are forming, one for each one of us. As the song from the musical "South Pacific" says:

> *"You got to have a dream,*
> *If you don't have a dream,*
> *How you gonna have a dream come true?"*

Achieving the pinnacle of a balanced society begins with each individual. Step one is always taking a deep breath and the acceptance of the knowledge, and step two is beginning the process of action, doing the contemplation. Get involved, come into balance and learn how to participate and enjoy every moment of life. If you're having fun, then you're doing it right.

If your goal and hard efforts are aimed at achieving a glimpse of the ships, then that puts a need to it and it will not happen. Change your focus to simply being in balance with yourself and others. When even a single individual reaches that point, the Traders recognize it. As others join in, the vibration intensifies, and eventually the whole planet will shine and we will be of a different vibration. When that is achieved anyone in the vicinity of them will be able to see the ships.

Once they are visible, it is as simple to walk aboard a Trader ship as it is to take an elevator. That is how it will happen, and one day when we can congratulate ourselves that we are equal, we'll realize that the key was always within our mind. As each new Earth Traveler succumbs to the curiosity and walks aboard a ship, his distant remembrance will begin to resonate strongly and, like a loudspeaker, will shout this clear understanding:

"Welcome to our ship. Please joyously join the nest. Feel at home. Have what you like. Get off when you want. Get back on when you want to. Be sure to go wherever you would like to go. Go home whenever you like. Take what you like. Whatever is ours is ours, but you are welcome to it. We have been waiting for you for a long time. What took you so long?"

NOTES

1. The Earth is a large gyroscope since it has mass and is spinning on its axis. The axis of every gyroscope "precesses," which is a slow re-orientation of the axis. Precession is the "wobble" that is observed when the toy gyroscope slows down. A close inspection of this wobble reveals that the axis of the gyroscope is defining a cone-shaped orbit about a vertical axis. The Earth is tipped approximately 23 1/2°, the axis of the wobble or precession, and according to astronomers one rotation equals approximately 25,600 years. It is this precession that causes the stars in each hemisphere to change slowly. Astrology has cataloged the ever-changing observable stars into twelve categories or "ages." The astrological "signs" have names, such as Aries, Taurus, Gemini, and so forth. Each age is 25,600/12 = 2133 years long. (Note that this system is another based on the key of twelve.)

2. The Traders have the technology to monitor all thought on every planet. They are quite aware of what planets have barbaric races. Such groups are kept planet bound where they can evolve without harm to the other species who are part of societies that live in peace. With this in mind, it can be seen that the words written on page 37 of *Message from the Pleiades,* cannot be taken literally. (See Reference 25.)

The literal translation is that "rather nasty contemporaries" may soon be on us (Earth humans), that we must "be on guard before these," and that it was "one of our missions to warn you of these." This is an error in communication. In reality, those who "live in certain barbarism" are not allowed to be Travelers.

The only way to get to this planet from another star (this is also true for the Pleiadians themselves) is by invitation on board the Super Mother Ships of the Traders. This is how the warring types of societies are kept planet bound. Like us, they are not invited. At most they can only travel one light year from their own sun, which keeps them quite bound to that solar system.

It must be remembered that Billy Meier typed his notes via a transmission that he heard in his mind. Everything he wrote is an interpretation on his part, and in this case he unfortunately left the wrong impression. If anything, we are the ones who will be visiting those barbaric races soon, and when we do we had better remember to keep our force shields activated. (Page 29, Reference 25, "Message from the Pleiades," gives an adequate description of a force field/shield in operation.) The Traders, remember, have the capability to float and protect their fragile bodies by living in a bubble-like force field/shield that protects them against any aggressive acts of life forms with hostile inclination.

3. There are some technological devices that have survived the demise of the Pyramid Society which were used for thousands of years around the Pyramid enclaves, and to a lesser extent, even into the time period we have defined as ancient Egypt. These devices were secrets known to the priesthood and handed down through the millennia.

Their technology provided such things as heating and cooling, light, and even superior metallurgy, which was used in such things as swords and knives. Demonstration models are now being constructed and it is the intent of the author to publish another book outlining the success of the devices, the key to how they are constructed, and how they could be integrated into today's society.

One device is a battery that operates on a principle quite different than lead acid or similar batteries. Once the energy density is calculated it might be a better alternative to the batteries now proposed to power the electric vehicles that our society sorely needs to relieve the smoggy cities. The book has been tentatively titled, "Devices of the Ancient Pyramid Society."

4. George Adamski's book *Inside the Saucers* is an encounter with a Nordic looking group, and one of the attractive females he described, although he assigned a different name for reasons he outlines in his book, is none other than the famous "Semjase" of the Billy Meier case, about 20 years later. (See Reference 22.)

These space ambassadors affirmed Adamski's notion that Venus and Mars were inhabited by humans. They led him to believe that they were from Venus. Others were not only from Mars, but Saturn and other planets of our solar system. This seems to conflict with what we are told about these planets — too hot, too cold, and with unfriendly atmospheres. Could it be that these planets are, in fact, more habitable than we've been led to believe? (See Daniel Ross, *UFO's and the Complete Evidence from Space.*)

It could, as I was told, mean that the aliens use "Venus" as a code to mean second planet from their sun, "Mars" to mean fourth planet from their sun and that their sun is in some other solar system. The future may prove both realities to be true!

5. Not all the Travelers who visit Earth are blue-eyed, blonde female beauties with gentle manners. There are also beings quite unlike Earth humans, and they are almost incomprehensible to us. One small example is a being that humans have the capacity to incarnate into because it is of the same type of soul that empowers us. The animal form is approximately six feet tall and as mentioned earlier, looks much like a praying mantis.

On the planet of its origin it lived and attacked its food, and it ate living things. The way it trapped its food was that it had a small resonance similar to a human's ability, via the chakric system, to sense another human being. Its ability to sense fear in another triggers an instinctual neurological reaction, amplifying the exact pattern that it feels back to its prey. That larger fear in the prey gets amplified again, until there is a sensory overload that freezes the prey. At that point, the praying mantis, could easily reach out and take its lunch, but the mantis-Travelers gave up eating food acquired that way 500 million years ago. They cherish the frozen animal and send it Love, even fondle it, and hope that it understands that by being frozen it cannot hurt itself or any other nearby species.

This ability of the praying mantis and the ability of the Traders to travel instantly around the universe has combined into a interesting relationship. If during a visit some animal species, including humans, appears to be so afraid that it could hurt itself or another, it is automatically frozen. The process is similar to what humans would do with tranquilizers for animals at the zoo, or animals being tagged in the wild. In short, the mantis is the anesthesiologist for the Traders. Many humans have the experience of waking up in a frozen panic state. The eyelids do not move, nothing moves, and there is an electricity in the air. Something unusual is happening. Gradually the sensation fades and the normal reality returns. That experience was merely the end of the visit, the conscious mind remembers only that small three-dimensional part.

Some are able to overcome their fear and experience a deeper interaction when around the mantis. The mantises have almond eyes similar to, but larger than the Traders'. If an experiencer is convinced the being has three fingers then that is the true form of the mantis. The Traders and Zetas have four digits. Unlike the hands of the Traders and Zetas, the hand of the mantis does not hang down close to the hip. Instead, in the relaxed state, the mantis hand is at shoulder level with the three digits pointed forward.

Yahweh Speaks

"If a rock speaks and it gives you something of value then take what it gives you. Leave the rock so it does speak of value to some other. If you happen to find a little joy, a little enjoyment, a little pleasure, a little sense of wholeness, then listen to it, but place it in relevance to your own life, because yours is the value point, not what is given to you, but what you take from it.

"There are no Travelers nor Traders that know more about you than you. There is not a hierarchy of power, whereby some celestial being knows the secrets of the universe more than the secrets you know yourself. There is not a race of beings out there that knows the answers and if you could just get to them you would get an answer and save yourselves. That is not what it is about. Although there are some races that have conceivably been out there an infinite variety of times, they have learned to accept themselves to a wholeness that they never actually even think they should be different. They do not look on it in that way. They do not actually discover in quite that way, they do it much differently than you. Just because you cannot understand them does not make them either superior or inferior. Consider any difference that you might encounter as a celebration of the uniqueness of you.

"There is no third dimension. There are three dimensions, there are four dimensions. there are five dimensions, there are six, seven, but when you see from a single dimension, you are seeing one-dimensionally. You can not see one-dimensionally. The most narrow you can observe is a three-dimensional spectrum of existence. That is where your sanity arrives, the conjunctive place of three dimensions. Each person sees through three dimensions, always. Your body exists in that space. Your spirit exists in a space, also of three dimensions. For your limited thought processes, it is supposed to.
"You are capable of at least realizing things out to as much as five dimensions. You can imagine time: future, past. When your sense of awareness of all of those things moves synergistically together, you can actually intuit a wholeness, and that becomes your five-dimensional senses. But, essentially with your five senses you are able to sample the three-dimensional reality and you are intended not to be able to sample the other seven dimensions. Therefore, you have the viewpoint of three-dimensions.

"The question is, which three dimensions? Your anchoring dimension is your essence. Then around that, you choose two other dimensions that overlap, and that becomes your emotional three dimensions. Your physical three dimensions are bounded somewhat with the Earth's energies in terms of which three dimensions you will use. Typically, you humans do not alter those three dimensions very much with your emotions, but you can. This is an overlay of dimensionalities.

"Your world is constructed, essentially, physiologically, molecularly, in such a way that you are bonded to a three-dimensional reality spectrum that is essentially Allowance (AL), Allegiance (AG), and Will and Power (WP). That has been your history, but it shifts. Your Earth energies shift a little bit. The world that it is going into is losing WP and thus everything is breaking down. What is replacing it is Love (L). Eventually you will be AL, AG, and L. The next shift will be in 2,000 years. At that point you will be losing AL, more WP again. Notice you always have three dimensions. It will be this three (Body = AL, AG, and WP), this three (Body = AL, AG, and L), or whatever. It is a shifting thing that occurs. This is the physical.

"Now the spiritual or the emotional. It comes from you as an anchoring point, and it is an overlay of dimensions. While the body has these three (Body = _AL_, AG, and WP), the spirit might have these three (Soul = Knowledge (K), L, and _AL_). The anchoring point being, in this example, _AL_. You must share one of the dimensions or you can't be a human being in this three-dimensional spectrum of existence.

"If the one you happen to share at this time is _WP_ (Example: Soul = K, Harmong (H), and _WP_, with the Body = _WP_, AG, and AL), you are going to be in deep trouble as a human being. Unless you share another one to go along with _WP_, you are going to not exist. That means that for many it is necessary to develop an ability to share L, or to share a more appropriate version of _WP_. It is an overlapping thing. In no case will you be able to really perceive life with four dimensions, except as a subtlety. In effect, this does make you be something, but it is only your existence. Your existence is a background for you to live with it. What you do with that existence is up to you."

Hint: In all future creations, monitor your intent. Your daily mantra should include: "for the common good and benefit of all."

About the Cover

In honor of the first split, there are two crystal obelisks, representing all Energy and Consciousness divided into two realms, the Is-Ness and the Is-Not-Ness. The obelisk forms the portal through which God might discover all that He is.

In honor of the second split, the title is composed of four words representing all Energy divided into four distinct groups of Energy and Consciousness.

In honor of the third split, the subtitle is composed of eight words representing all Energy divided into eight distinct groups, Primal Energy and Consciousness.

In honor of the 34th to 36th splits, where we exist and create, and all of the precursor creations that have made it possible, the drawing depicts a complexity of forms, composite in nature, representing that the three-dimensional reality exists because of combinations of all eight Primal Energies.

The Sphinx is shown in its final representation, the human head and the recumbent feline body representing God-Human, Human-Animal, and in general all creations, especially those with a soul connection. Behind the Sphinx is the Great Pyramid, identified by its slope angle of 52 degrees, and the top third is bright representing the original gold cap. The Pyramid gives free power to the society and reminds them by the geometry and other secrets encoded within it of the basic secret. It resonates to Allowance, the Primal Energy that is most abundant in three-dimensional creations on this planet, and it points to the other seven.

The greatest meditation is to imagine your astral body, sitting lotus style, merging with the Great Pyramid so that your Chakric System will be energized with Primal Energy! Allowance is represented by the toroid at the bottom. Allegiance is represented by the toroid above that, and Will and Power is represented by the next toroid. Love is represented by the lavendar toroid around the sphinx head. Love lines up with the face of the Sphinx because the Sphinx grandly represents Love, which straddles the Is-Ness and the Is-Not-Ness and bonds all things, such as the lion body and the human head, together. Love gives definition to any new creation.

Harmony, Knowledge, and Wisdom are represented by the toroids around the Madonna. The Madonna represents the soul that empowers the physical body, and it lines up with the apex of the Great Pyramid. The facets of the Great Pyramid emanate energy for the society living in the three-dimensional plane of existence, and the apex emanates energy to communicate to distant worlds. The latter beam of energy and opening in the head of the Madonna represent the future creations, which are endless, and spirit awaits spellbound, in anticipation of what we will create.

Humans of planet Earth should rest assured that in all of the universe there is no dark force or dark light. There is only light, white light, seeking limitless creation.

The three chambers within and beneath the Sphinx represent not only the real chambers that exist, but also the ascension principle. Each one of us will eventually make that journey, when we are ready and chose to do so. A small ascension that awaits us in the not-too-distant future is joining with the rest of the human beings who, having successfully mastered the contemplation, are already exploring the universe.

REFERENCE LIST

1. John Baines and Jaromir Malek, 1986, *Atlas of Ancient Egypt*, Phaidon Press, Littlegate House, St Ebbe's Street, Oxford, England OX1 1SQ.

2. Francis Crick, 1982, *Life Itself . . . Its Origin and Nature*, Simon and Schuster, NY.

3. I.E.S. Edwards, 1972, *The Pyramids of Egypt,* Viking, NY.

4. Lawrence Fawcett and Barry J. Greenwood, 1984, *Clear Intent*, Prentice Hall, Englewood-Cliffs, NJ 7632.

5. Peter Tompkins, 1978, *Secrets of the Great Pyramid*, Harper/Row, NY.

6. Wendelle C. Stevens, 1981, *UFO . . . Contact from Reticulum*, Genesis III Publishing, Inc. P.O. Box 25962, Munds Park, AZ 86017.

7. Joseph Davidovits and Margie Morris, 1989, *The Pyramids: An Enigma Solved*, Hippocene Books, NY.

8. George C. Andrews, 1987, *Extraterrestrials Among Us*, Llewellyn Pub., St. Paul, MN 55164-0383.

9. Charles Berlitz and William L Moore, 1988, *The Roswell Incident*, Berkely Pub. NY.

10. E. Chaney, 1989, Astara, School of the Ancient Mysteries, Institure of Psychic Research, 800 W. Arrow Hwy., P.O. Box 5003 Upland, CA 91785.

11. Shirley Maclaine, 1986, *Dancing in the Light*, Bantam Books, NY.

12. Kenneth Ring, 1986, *Heading Toward Omega and Life at Death*, Quill, 105 Madison Ave, NY.

13. H. Janson, 1965, *History of Art*, Prentice-Hall, Englewood Cliffs, NJ.

14. Timothy Green Beckley and Arthur Crockett, 1984, The *Great Pyramid Speaks*, Inner Light Publications.

15. Max Thoth and Greg Nielseen, *Pyramid Power*, Destiny Books, Rochester, VT.

16. Henry Semat, *Introduction to Atomic and Nuclear Physics*, Fourth Edition, Holt, Rinehart, and Winston, NY.

17. David Hatcher Childress, *Anti-Gravity and the World Grid*. Adventures Unlimited Press.

18. Hardy and Killick, *Pyramid Energy: The Philosophy of God, The Science of Man*, Cadake Industries & Copple House, P.O. Box 1866, Clayton GA.

19. *Mysteries of the Unknown . . . Mystic Places*. Time-Life Books, Alexandria, VA.

20. Rev. Clarence Larkin, *Dispensational Truths*, P.O. Box 334, Glenside, PA 19038.

21. Larry Hawse, Balance Productions, P.O. Box 1681, Vista, CA 92085, (760) 630-9247, or (760) 940-8910.

22. George Adamski, *Inside the Spaceships*, The George Adamski Foundation, P.O. Box1722, Vista, CA 92083.

23. John G. Fuller, *The Interrupted Journey* (Betty and Barney Hill Abduction Case), Dell Publishing Co., Inc., NY.

24. Raymond E. Fowler, *The Watchers*, Bantam Books, 666 Fifth Ave, NY.

25. Wendelle C Stevens, 1988, *Message from the Pleiades*, The Contact Notes of Edward Billy Meier, Genesis III Publishing, Inc., P.O. Box 25962, Munds Park, AZ 86017.

26. Sean Morton, UFO Excursions, 2207 Hermosa Ave. Hermosa Beach, CA 90254, (310) 217-7579.

27. Shakti Gawainm, *Creative Visualization*, Whatever Publishing, P. O. Box 137, Mill Valley, CA 94941.

28. Jeff Hecht and Howard W. Sams & Company, *Understanding Lasers*, 4300 West 62nd Street, Indianapolis, IN 46268.

29. John E Pfeiffer, *The Emergence of Man*, Harper and Row, NY.

30. Gabriel Ward Lasher, *Physical Anthropology*, Holt Rinehart, and Winston Inc., NY.

31. Wm. R. Fix, *Pyramid Odyssey*, Mercury Media, Inc., Urbanna, VA.

32. George C. Andrews, *Extraterrestrials Among Us*, The Llewellyn New Times, P.O. Box 64383-010, St. Paul, MN 55164-0383.

33. Eugene A. Avallone and Theodore Baumeister III, *Mark's Standard Handbook For Mechanical Engineers*, Ninth Edition, McGraw-Hill Book Co., NY.

34. Al Gore, *Earth in the Balance*, Penguin Books USA, 375 Hudson Street, NY.

35. Robert Burnham Jr., *Burnhams's Celestial Handbook*, Dover Publications, Inc., NY.

36. Meir H.Degani, *Astronomy Made Simple*, New Revised Edition 1976, Bantam Doubleday Dell Publishing Group, Inc., 666 Fifth Ave., NY.

37. Marlo Morgan, *Mutant Message From Downunder*, MM Co., P.O. Box 100, Lees Sunnit, MO 64063.

38. Chet Raymo, *365 Starry Nights*, Simon and Schuster, NY.

39. G. & C. Merriam Co., *Webster's Seventh New Collegiate Dictionary*, H.O. Houghton and Company, The Riverside Press, Cambridge, MA.

40. Kenneth R Lang, Astrophysical Data: *Planets and Stars*, Springer Verlag, NY.

41. Udo Erasmus, *Fats and Oils*, Alive Books, P.O. Box 67333, Vancover, British Columbia, Canada, V5W 3T1.

42. Hulda Regher Clark, Ph.D., N.D., *The Cure For All Cancers, The Cure Fore HIV and AIDS*, Promotion Publishing, San Diego, CA.

43. Andrew Weil, M.D., *Natural Health, Natural Medicine,* Houghton Mifflin Co,, Boston, MA.

44. Col. James Churchward, *The Lost Continent of Mu*, Be Books, Albuquerque, NM.

45. Deepak Chopra, *Ageless Body, Timeless Mind*, Harmony Books, NY.

46. Robert O. Becker, M.D. and Gary Selden, *Cross Currents, The Body Electric*, Quill, William Morrow, NY.

47. Nancy Appleton, *Lick the Sugar Habit*, Avery Publication Group, Inc. or Dr. Murphy, (619) 450-5959.

48. Burton Boldberg Group, *Alternate Medicine*, The Future Medicine Publishing, Inc., Puyallup, WA.

49. Richard Hoagland, *The Moon/Mars Connection*, P.O. Box 2284, South Burlington, VT 05407.

50. Hancock and Bauval, *The Message of the Sphinx*, Crown Publishers, Inc., NY.

51. Raymond E. Fowler, *The Watchers, The Secret Design Behind UFO Abduction*, Bantam Doubleday Dell Publishing Group, Inc.

52. Col. Philip J. Corso, (Ret.) with William J. Birnes, *The Day After Roswell*, Simon and Schuster Inc., NY.

Update Before Going to Press

1. The Zetas, with the understanding of the Traders, have given advanced technology since the late 1950's to the researchers in Area 51. The intent was two fold. One, to let us know that we are not alone. Two, to let us get used to actually exploring our solar system with scout craft. In fact, this flying-disc technology will take us beyond this solar system to as far as a few very close stars.

2. Flyovers, similar to the March 1997 flight over Phoenix and other cities of the world over a two-week period, will continue to increase. Soon, nearly everyone will witness them, and know that we are not alone.

3. In time, the next level of technology — attaching to the SMS and traveling with the Traders to explore the far reaches of this and other galaxies — will be given.

Appropriate Behavior for the Earth Human

In light of this astonishing disclosure, what is expected of us? The author suggests that there is much for us to do to become responsible citzens of the inter galactic community. First we should welcome any extraterrestrial that visits our solar system. The obvious way to do this is first to stop chasing scout craft and second, to change the intent of the Strategic Defense Initiative (SDI). This spaced-based weapons system, popularly called Star Wars, should be changed from an active defense against the extraterrestrials to a technology for simply enforcing the borders between nations. Eventually it must be abandoned.

To show that we will be responsible citizens of the galaxy we must prove that we can achieve a sustainable planet. The population should be reduced and maintained at less than two billion people. In the process we must rediscover the steady-state economy of the Great Pyramid Society. That means we must abandon the throw-away fossil fuel and nuclear economy and focus on building things that last. It means we must convert to a Hydrogen economy as soon as possible.

In the process we will clean up the environment that has been so badly neglected. The planet we design and nurture will determine whether the door way to the inter galactic community will open and it is entirely up to us. Meanwhile, they patiently wait and watch — from a distance.

"Cross-breeding" is really transferring DNA technology. It best ensures human DNA gets to planets where humans will flourish."

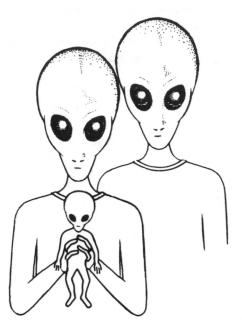

"This is an effort to communicate. This is an effort to ask if you know that caring for these offspring is a sacred undertaking? What we are doing is making certain that the Earth humans who we care for, love, and want to protect, have offspring, and life goes on. We have visited and have successfully taken genetic material. Here in this visit, know that the effort has realized fruit and sacred life has been born. This is why we visit and do what we do, to carry on life."

About the Author

Reg T. Miller was born in 1942 with an ancestral background that includes French, British and German. A conservative upbringing taught hard work and lots of study. This was easy for Reg whose fascination with machines led him to dismantle old clocks, motors, radios and televisions to understand how they worked. As a teen, a correspondence course taught him the fundamentals of electronics and by sixteen he had a First Class Radio Telephone license. One of his old televisions was soon transformed into a working radio transmitter and, suddenly, a small rural town in Michigan had another AM station with "top fourty" music and no commercials! Soon after, he won first prize at a science fair in Bay County.

In college he majored in physics and minored in mathematics. During college he did fit-and-function studies for a company that did huge dome tents for the military. He went on to work for the Department of Defense collecting radio active samples from A-bomb testing in the atmosphere and later, worked as an engineer for Rohr — a mojor sub-contractor for Boeing.

Because of health reasons which could not be explained or treated by conventional medical science, Reg took an early retirement and became interested in traveling to the ancient power spots in Egypt. He had heard that many physical healings were taking place with a group called Astara. He had, as he calls it, a fourth-dimensional experience within the Great Pyramid and soon became frustrated trying to explain to his science minded friends that he had been visited by an ancient pharaoh, had lived many life-times in Egypt and believed in the existence of UFO's!

The experience of Egypt and the pyramids sparked an intense quest for metaphysical knowledge. While immersed in this search, Reg met Chuck Little, an engineer and channeler of Yahweh. Yahweh appears every thousand years or so and teaches at the level that can be understood at the time. Now that we have some understanding of energy, Yahweh has explained the Primal Energy connection between the occult and what has been discovered by science.

Reg has spent many years devoted to this project because he believes that it is important for us to grasp the technology of the extraterrestrials and realize their basic peaceful intent. We must also have the knowledge and tools for peaceful coexistence with ourselves and with the extraterrestrials.